# Dynamic Psychiatry in Theory and Practice

# Dynamic Psychiatry
# in Theory and Practice

—•—

## EDWIN R. WALLACE, IV, M.D.
Director of Psychotherapy Education
and Associate Professor
Psychiatry Department, Medical College of Georgia
Augusta, Georgia

*Formerly*, Chief of Individual Psychotherapy
Connecticut Mental Health Center
Assistant Professor, Department of Psychiatry
Yale University School of Medicine
New Haven, Connecticut

Lea & Febiger • 1983 • Philadelphia

Lea & Febiger
600 South Washington Square
Philadelphia, PA 19106
U.S.A.

**Library of Congress Cataloging in Publication Data**

Wallace, Edwin R.
    Dynamic psychiatry in theory and practice.
    Bibliography: p.
    Includes index.
    1. Psychoanalysis. 2. Mental illness—Diagnosis.
3. Psychotherapy. 4. Insight in psychotherapy.
I. Title.
RC504.W27   1983             616.89'14               82-14880
ISBN 0-8121-0856-6

PRINTED IN THE UNITED STATES OF AMERICA

Print Number:    3    2    1

To the two Lauras,
Win,
and Paula

Let a full and careful treatise be constructed . . . so we may have a scientific and accurate dissection of minds and characters, and the secret dispositions of particular men may be revealed; and that from the knowledge thereof better rules may be framed for the treatment of the mind.

Sir Francis Bacon

*The Advancement of Learning*
*Book VII, Chapter III*

# Acknowledgments

I want to begin by acknowledging my great debt of gratitude to two physicians, now deceased: Edwin R. Wallace, III, M.D., my father, and Cyrus R. Friedman, M.D., my analyst. Next my thanks go out to a master clinician and pedagogue, George E. Gross, M.D., of the New York Psychoanalytic Institute and the Mt. Sinai Medical Center. Dr. Gross will recognize his own voice in much that I say. I value Professor Philip Rieff, of the University of Pennsylvania, and Stanley W. Jackson, M.D., of Yale University, for upholding standards of excellence and thoroughness to which we should all aspire and for providing mentoring at some crucial points in my career.

I wish to acknowledge the beneficent impact upon my professional education and career in general of: Joe E. Freed, M.D. and Lucius C. Pressley, M.D., both of the William S. Hall Psychiatric Institute and the University of South Carolina School of Medicine; Ilhan Ermutlu, M.D., of the Georgia Mental Health Commission; Oscar Sachs, M.D., of the New York Psychoanalytic Institute and Society; Gordon Crandall, M.D., of Charlotte, North Carolina; Gloria B. Green, M.D., of Norman, Oklahoma; and Stephen Fleck, M.D., of the Western New England Psychoanalytic Institute and Yale University.

I want to thank the following supervisees for asking the impertinent questions that led to this book and for allowing me to borrow from their own clinical work: my third-year clinical clerks in psychiatry at the University of South Carolina School of Medicine; psychiatry residents whom I supervised at the William S. Hall Psychiatric Institute in Columbia, South Carolina; those Connecticut Valley Hospital residents who spent their outpatient year with me at the Connecticut Mental Health Center: Inn Seok Oh, M.D., Wayne Andrus, M.D., Eloina Wieland, M.D., Alnoor Ramji, M.D., Idel Beer, M.D., Leela Panoor, M.D., Nanita Simon, M.D., Erlinda Paseos, M.D., Romeo Villar, M.D., Jay Shetty, M.D., and Nam Sik Chang, M.D.; and my psychotherapy supervisees and participants in my psychotherapy seminar at the Connecticut Mental Health Center, especially Ms. Mary Doyle, Ms. Margaret Russell, Ms. Michele DeVoe, Ms. Laura Hansen, and Ms. Kathy Paul, and two of the Yale residents whom I had the good fortune to supervise: Michael Sherer, M.D. and Frank Gawin, M.D. My patients, who have taught me so much about themselves, myself, and humanity in general, must of course remain nameless.

I want to thank George E. Gross, M.D., and Professor Philip Rieff, again, and Charles Gardner, M.D., of the Western New England Psychoanalytic Institute and of the Yale Psychiatric Institute, for kindly reading and commenting upon the manuscript of this textbook. I value Mrs. Edith Wolkovitz, of the Connecticut Mental Health Center, for her expert typing and patient decipherment of my handwriting. I am grateful to Ms. Lenora Hume, of Lea & Febiger, for her skillful editing of this manuscript.

Last, but hardly least, I want to acknowledge the forbearance of my family, who appear in the dedication, during the difficult gestation, labor, and delivery of this volume.

E.R.W.

# Contents

# Introduction

Good intentions, while indispensable, do not a psychotherapist make.
Ideally, all the therapist's interventions, whether in supportive or insight-oriented treatment, should flow from his theoretical understanding of the case. This does not mean that there is no place for "common sense" reactions or the rapid and intuitive response, but that some overall conception of the patient's lifelong development and action-reaction patterns should govern the therapy.

Facts, in psychiatry or elsewhere, do not simply arrange themselves but must be met halfway by mind—a mind with a theory. Without a theory, one is confronted by a morass of meaningless data. Solely by refraction through the selecting and ordering lens of theory do data become comprehensible and usable information, or facts. The scientist does not first passively collect the data and only later theorize about them; theorizing and data-collecting are in an active and mutually conditioning interrelationship from the start. Even a bad theory is better than none at all since at least it enables the investigator to *organize* his observations and *test* its claims against the behavior of reality. Only through the disconfirmation or radical reconstruction of unsatisfactory theories has science moved closer to that elusive entity known as "truth" which, as Bacon said, is more likely to emerge out of error than out of chaos. A good theory has explanatory power, leads one to ask questions and to see data one would not otherwise, enables one to make predictions and "retrodictions," is amenable to testing against subsequent data, is capable of modification and development, leads to maneuvers that improve one's effectiveness in the internal and external worlds, and last, but hardly least, serves the practitioner-investigator as a beacon and a mooring in reality's sometime stormy sea.

There are, of course, many theories of psychopathology and psychotherapy, each of which values some sorts of data more than others, asks some questions, and neglects others. Each of the established theories

1

grasps a certain plane of multifaceted reality and any of them serves the therapist better than none at all. In this book I shall confine myself to that hypothesis which I feel is the most holistic and operational in psychiatry: the dynamic model.[1] Like all scientific models, it is not a system of revealed truth or concrete entities, but merely a set of abstractions or *theoretical constructs* designed to help us understand and, by understanding, to influence *interpersonal relations,* which are the only *real* things in psychiatry. It will stand or fall upon its ability to do so. It is essential that you do not view the dynamic model as a static and fully formed affair. It has undergone continuous development and modification since its inception at the hands of Freud, and it will continue to do so.

Dynamic psychiatry consists of a theory of normal and abnormal psychology and a therapeutic-investigative philosophy and technique. It is *an historical and interpretive method for the study and therapeutic transformation of interpersonal relations.* It is not, as is too commonly supposed, antagonistic to the data of biological psychiatry, social psychiatry and sociology, systems approaches, and behavioral psychology. Rather, it is interested in, and incorporates, data from them all. It takes exception only when the adherents of any one of these orientations claim to have the whole truth. For example, it recognizes both the biological and the social factors that function as motivators in human behavior, conceptualizing the id as the predominant locus of the former, the ego as the common ground between the two, and the superego as the headquarters of the latter. It acknowledges that the forces with which the family and social systems theorists are concerned are also those which are active within the psyche and that there is a subtle and inextricable interaction between the persons within our heads and those without them. It does not deny the applicability of learning theory to the cognitive functions of ego and superego nor that conditioning and modeling play a role in human behavior.[2]

Indeed, I maintain that the dynamic model is the *final common pathway* through which the information from these other approaches must be filtered if it is to be meaningful within the context of the total human-

----

[1]Throughout this book I shall use the term "dynamic," or "psychodynamic," rather than "psychoanalytic," because I wish to avoid the excessively biologistic or instinctivist connotations of the latter as used by Freud. The dynamic model is what I consider to be the solid and usable core of Freud's teachings, as embellished by the interpersonal psychiatric theorists such as Sullivan and, more recently, by the ego and object relations psychologists from within psychoanalysis itself. From my use of the term "dynamic," it follows that this book is not, strictly speaking, a textbook of classical psychoanalytic theory and technique, of which there are texts aplenty from which you may choose. You will find references to many of these at the close of the chapters.
[2]See page 3.

being-in-a-society. This model appreciates, better than any other, that human behavior is an epiphenomenon of neither culture nor biology, but of the *interaction* between the two. At the same time, since dynamic psychiatry is concerned with the sphere of meaning, purpose, feelings, and symbolic communication, that which most differentiates our behavior from that of the rest of the animal kingdom, it is the most *human*istic theory in psychiatry. It is, in every sense of the words, the "species-specific psychology" of Homo sapiens.

Learning dynamic psychiatry takes place *affectively*, as much as cognitively. It is acquired as much through the observation of *oneself* as of any outside object. What you will read in this volume applies to you as much as to your patients, and the more you appreciate this the better clinician you will be.

I have written this book for three reasons. First of all, I wish to reassert the primacy of psychodynamics in a time of headlong rush into one-sidedly biological and descriptive approaches to the understanding and treatment of behavioral disorders. I shall not be asking you to "believe" in any of the concepts presented herein. I am only asking you to acquire a working knowledge of them and to test their usefulness against your concrete clinical and personal experience. If you explore your patients' lives and your own life in sufficient depth and make a concerted effort to understand them using this model, then I have no doubt that you will emerge from your encounter with dynamic psychiatry as enthusiastic about it as I am.

Second, although there are textbooks that treat the theory, those that present the evaluation interview, and those that expound the therapy, there are virtually none that adequately treat all three. As a student you should be able to read one book of manageable length that gives you an

---

[2]There have been several excellent attempts to demonstrate the complementarity of psychoanalytic theory and behaviorist theory. One of the first was Dollard and Miller's (1950) *Personality and Psychotherapy*. Books and articles continue to appear (see Wachtel's [1979] *Psychoanalysis and Behavior Therapy*). For example, the similarity between the analyst's concept of "transference" and the behaviorist's concept of "stimulus generalization" has been pointed out. Connections have been drawn between the dynamic notion of "identification" and the behaviorist one of "modeling." Much of the dynamic therapist's work has been reinterpreted as systematic desensitization. The concept of conscious and unconscious factors in reinforcement has been introduced into behaviorism, and the punitive role of the superego has been taken into account by many learning theorists. However, the major difference between analytic terms such as "transference" and behaviorist ones such as "stimulus generalization" is that the former take account of the dimension of *meaning* in human behavior. In other words, a rat's observable behavior can be treated simply as what it appears to be, whereas a human's has a historical, often unconscious, dimension related to the feeling-toned contacts with the persons from whom it was learned and to the situations in which it arose.

overview, a gestalt, of dynamic theory and practice. It should present only the *basics*. In my experience teaching psychiatric residents and other mental health trainees, it is usually the most basic and elementary concepts that are the least understood. I have been astonished by students who bandy about the complex jargon of ego, object relations, and self psychology without being able to give simple, operational and, at the same time, theoretically precise definitions of terms such as "symptom," "conflict," "neurosis," and "character." I shall therefore confine myself to a bare-bones presentation of dynamic psychiatry, to which I shall apply the flesh of clinical examples,[3] but which you must clothe with what you glean from supervised clinical work, case conferences, taking and formulating psychiatric history, reading and, last but hardly least, your own "patienthood."

Third, there is much common sense, philosophy, and practical wisdom, which is known to and transmitted by every good clinical supervisor, but which for some reason never makes its way into the textbooks. Perhaps this is because it is considered too simplistic or self-evident. While no book can claim to replace clinical supervision, where dynamic psychiatry is actually learned, a text should strive to approximate it as closely as possible. I have attempted to do so, to convey as much of the "feel" for what it is like to practice this model as possible. Consonant with this aim, I have embedded the exposition of both theory and technique in a clinical matrix.

This book presupposes no prior knowledge or experience in the field, although it assumes that most readers will be studying to be mental health professionals of some sort. If it is successful, it will shorten, but not replace, the painful trial and error process of feeling one's way into dynamic psychiatry. Because this volume is a concentrated dose· of complicated material and an introduction to a mode of thinking quite foreign to that habitually practiced by most of us, I urge the student to read it more than once.

This book is divided into three sections. The first, comprising three chapters, presents the theory. The second, also made up of three chapters, discusses evaluation interviewing and diagnosis. The third, composed of six chapters, is concerned with treatment—both supportive and insight-oriented therapy and the relatively neglected, but important, role of the dynamic model in hospital psychiatry. A list of suggested readings follows most chapters.

*After much deliberating and after writing many clumsy sentences, I decided, in the interest of readability, to use the masculine pronouns "he," "him," "himself," when referring to the generic patient or therapist. Please understand this to be an inclusive reference to both men and women, as shorthand for what would otherwise be phrased "he or she," "him or her," "himself or herself."*

---

[3]The identifying data on all patients cited herein have been omitted or altered sufficiently to protect their anonymity.

# SECTION

# I

# Theory

# 1

# The Unconscious, Mental Forces, and History

Dynamic approaches to the understanding of human behavior have existed since at least the turn of the nineteenth century. In 1824 the German philosopher-psychiatrist Herbart, who coined the term "repression," published a theory of dynamic psychology surprisingly similar to the one we use today. Schopenhauer, Nietzsche, Hartmann, Heinroth, Carus, Fechner, and many other nineteenth-century philosophers, physicians, and scientists anticipated certain psychoanalytic ideas. Lancelot Law Whyte (1960) has enumerated some 70 individuals who possessed a concept of the unconscious before Freud. Henri Ellenberger (1970) has taught us that other aspects of dynamic theory and practice had been grasped by Mesmer and other eighteenth- and nineteenth-century hypnotists.

My intention is not to detract from Freud's genius, but to give the reader a sense of the power and persistence of dynamic modes of thought. By 1900 the pressure of ideas and observations was such that if Freud had not developed psychoanalysis, then someone else probably would have! In any event, Freud deserves our everlasting credit for systematizing, from his reading, clinical experience, and personal creativity, a dynamic psychiatry that was not purely a speculative or academic enterprise but an empirically based therapeutic and investigative tool. Freud began this work in the early 1890s and by 1899, the year of appearance of *The Interpretation of Dreams*, the foundation was laid. By 1926 most of the ideas which I shall impart in this chapter were raised. Freud achieved this synthesis almost single-handedly, although his theory and therapy have undergone considerable development and modification at the hands of his disciples.

Dynamic psychiatry is a theory of *normal* as well as *abnormal* psycholo-

7

gy and applies as much to you as to your patients. Indeed, it teaches you, the therapist, that there is no wide and comfortable berth between yourself and your clients and that many of their preoccupations are also yours. The dynamic model conceives of the mind as a system of *forces in motion*. Observable or self-reportable behaviors (including acts, feelings, and fantasies) are conceptualized as *vectors* between two or more *underlying* (often *unconscious*) *conflicting* or *complementary* forces of *varying magnitude* and with a *history* in the life of each individual. These forces[1] may be biological, social or, more commonly, an inextricable combination between the two. Dynamic psychiatry concerns itself preeminently with the human organism's attempts to effect some sort of *equilibrium* among its internal forces and between these forces and those of the environment. It is preoccupied, in other words, with *adaptation*, a concept which the reader should keep in mind throughout this volume.

Freud's theoretical writings, as opposed to his more purely clinical ones, are called the "metapsychology." We continue to use this word to refer to the theoretical system which organizes and explains the observations of dynamic psychiatry. Metapsychology is subdivided into six complementary orientations: genetic, dynamic, economic, structural, topographic, and adaptive or adaptational. "Genetic" refers to its historical or developmental approach to human psychology and psychopathology. "Dynamic" alludes to the concept of mental forces and "economic" refers to the variations in magnitude of these forces. The "topographic" and "structural" theories are models of the mind, or "psychic apparatus." The former refers to the conceptions of "conscious," "preconscious," and "unconscious" modes of mental functioning, the latter to the 'id," "ego," and "superego." The "adaptational," which was the last of the approaches to be formulated, is concerned with the psychic organism's attempt to come to terms with its environment.

Ideally, the dynamic theory of character and psychopathology should be presented at once with the basic concepts of the dynamic model in place within it. How this might be accomplished is completely unknown to me. Consequently, in this chapter and the next I shall first hew out the blocks with which I shall build the dynamic theory of character and psychopathology in Chapter 3. These blocks will be "the unconscious,"

----

[1]It should be understood that terms like "force" or "magnitude" are used in the metaphorical sense. They are theoretical constructs, or heuristic devices, and not quantifiable realities. Their sole purpose is to convey an operational *understanding* of "mind," another theoretical construct, whose substrate is not merely the brain, but the entire human body and sociocultural and physical environment as well. We shall often speak of "the mind," "the unconscious," and so forth as if they are places. Again, this should be taken only metaphorically, for they are understood as qualities rather than entities.

"mental forces," "history and psychic causality," "the structural theory of the psychic apparatus," and "developmental psychology." Some repetition has been unavoidable in bringing this story to its climax in Chapter 3. Nevertheless, this repetitiveness may not be undesirable since, if the student is to make these ideas part of his blood and bone, he must partake of them frequently and in different, ever richer, contexts.

## THE UNCONSCIOUS

The proposition that unconscious forces determine our behavior quite as much as, or even more than, conscious ones and that, indeed, our conscious motivations are themselves usually *derivatives* of unconscious ones is the cornerstone of dynamic psychiatry. Often called "depth psychology" for precisely this reason, it is the theory which looks *beneath* the act and recognizes that the same observable unit of behavior in ten different individuals may yet be determined from ten different directions and serve ten different purposes. Just as likely, it is present in *each* of these ten persons for ten different reasons and means ten different things. It is aware that Don Juan behavior may cover up an unconscious sense of inadequate masculinity in one man, while impotence may be a reaction against underlying intensely masculine sexual and aggressive strivings in another. Some psychologists believe that dynamic psychiatry's dogged insistence on looking *inside*, as well as *at*, the human actor needlessly complicates matters and makes psychology less scientific. Their reaction would be similar to that of an anatomist who becomes indignant when told by a physiologist that, even though two particular cells look identical under the light microscope, they actually behave quite differently when treated with the same chemical reagent. What "surface psychologies" gain in scientific elegance they lose by inadequately reflecting the complexity of human psychological reality and by excluding from their purview that sloppy, subjective arena in which we play out our day-to-day lives.

The idea of the unconscious is considered outlandish by many and an insult to the notion of free will. Nevertheless, its truthfulness has been grasped for centuries and can be easily demonstrated inside or outside the therapeutic situation. The concept is necessitated by otherwise inexplicable phenomena of, and discontinuities in, human behavior.

Every reader has forgotten someone's name or misplaced an object and later unexpectedly and spontaneously remembered it. Since the information *returned*, it must have been in the mind all along, or it was nowhere. It was, in other words, in a state of *unconsciousness*. Many of us have misplaced objects and, in searching, mentally retraced our steps or followed our associations, or train of thought, until we recovered them. This is an example of the unconscious becoming conscious and it is the basis for psychodynamic psychotherapy. In Chapter 3, in our discussion of the relationship between psychopathology and conflict, I shall dem-onstrate that there are good, albeit unconscious, reasons for simple acts like misplacing one's keys or forgetting a name or appointment—in other words, that forgetting is an *active* and not a passive process and that, like other human behaviors, it *serves a purpose*. To cite only two examples, forgetting the name of a person who unconsciously reminds us of a detested uncle from childhood can be a way of avoiding painful memories associated with him. Misplacing our car keys when we have a meeting with the boss may be a way of dealing with unconscious apprehensions about him, apprehensions perhaps based on still earlier ones toward a parent.

Posthypnotic suggestion is another example of how an idea, feeling, or impulse can be unconscious and yet mightily influence our behavior in consciousness. Here one gives the subject a command, while he is in a hypnotic trance, that he is to carry out upon awakening. At the same time, the hypnotist tells him that he will not *consciously* remember that it was suggested to him. I have witnessed this phenomenon and it is amusing to see the perplexity of the subject when asked why, for example, he walked to the window and raised it in midwinter. His initial confusion is usually followed by a trumped-up explanation, a conscious "rationalization" of what is actually unconsciously determined behav-ior. However, as in the case of the misplaced object or forgotten name, if you can get him to "free-associate," to follow the ideas that arise in his mind wherever they lead, he will often succeed in consciously remem-bering your command.

One of the most dramatic demonstrations of the unconscious that I have seen occurred during hypnotic "age regression," where the person is instructed to go back, mentally, in time. A 21-year-old hysterical woman, baby-talking in hypnosis, disclosed several traumatic memories from her third year, memories that had been inaccessible to her waking consciousness for years. The validity of the events to which they re-ferred was confirmed by conversations between the social worker and the patient's aunt and older sister. Other ways in which the potency of the unconscious manifests itself are *parapraxes* or slips (of the tongue or pen), a sudden loss for words or loss of one's train of thought, dreams (in which material of which we are unaware in waking consciousness emerges) and, of course, psychopathology. In Chapter 3 I shall describe how an unconscious conflict between a man's desire to beat up his wife and the internal prohibition against it brought on an hysterical symptom.

Outside of hypnosis, which rips through our time-honored resis-tances against becoming aware of conflictual unconscious material, we do not view the unconscious directly but rather come to know it through its *derivatives*. For example, repeated conflicts with one's employers could be a *derivative* of unconscious conflicts with a parent. Repeated relationships with older women might be a *derivative* of a man's unconscious incestuous desires for his mother.

The following is an extended clinical example of the power of the unconscious:

> Mrs. A., a 21-year-old woman, presented with depression secondary to marital problems. A few months before, she had impulsively proposed to a man who had "stepped out" on her repeatedly during their long and stormy "steady" relationship, who abused drugs and alcohol, who was a "con artist," and who often went many evenings without seeing her. She could not understand: 1) why she sought out such a man in the first place; 2) why she precipitously asked him to marry her even though she had previously resolved to break off with him; and 3) why she stayed in this marriage despite considerable unhappiness. In the course of a few sessions I found that she proposed to him *only days after learning that her recently divorced father was marrying a 20-year-old woman.* It developed that this father had been alternately seductive and rejecting to the patient in her childhood, that he "ran around" on the patient's mother, abused drugs and alcohol, and was a "confidence man." In a nutshell, she experienced her father's divorce and almost immediate remarriage as yet another case of his teasing and rejecting her. She responded to this frustration by marrying a man, incidentally ten years older than she, who *unconsciously* represented[2] her father, and yet of whom the father disapproved. It emerged in the course of treatment that her unconscious purposes were twofold: 1) to marry a man like her father and reform him, thus gaining the ideal father-husband she never had in childhood, and 2) to "get back" at the father for deserting her by marrying a man he disliked.[3]

In short, this patient's behavior was motivated by powerful, though *unconscious*, fantasies, feelings, and preoccupations. I was able to *infer* these unconscious factors from what I knew about the relationships with her father and husband and from the temporal contiguity between her father's remarriage to a woman about her age and her own decision to marry. It was relatively easy to help her become *affectively* and *cognitively* aware of these factors and, when she did so, her behavior changed markedly. Interestingly, when she told her older sister, who was not a mental health professional, what had gone into her marriage and depression, the latter replied, "I suspected it all along. *I* could have told you that."

Later in this chapter, when we discuss transference, we shall see that among the most important things which can be unconscious are one's assumptions about oneself and one's environment. These amount, in

---

[2] I shall often refer to persons in one's current, external reality as "unconsciously representing" certain figures from one's past. Please take this as a shorthand reference to what would otherwise be more accurately, but clumsily, expressed as "individuals who represent, in one's unconsciousness," certain figures from childhood.

[3] See page 12.

effect, to sets of historically determined *rules* for perceiving and conducting oneself in the world (see Schafer, 1976, 1978), e.g., "all men will
reject me like Daddy," "if you get too close to women they will trap
you," "it's a jungle out there and you must continually be on your
guard," "if you show your emotions, you will be ridiculed," and so
forth. Much of the therapist's business is inferring, from observed and
reported patterns of behavior, the conscious, preconscious and, especially, unconscious assumptions and rules upon which these actions are
based.

Freud believed that unconscious material obeys its own laws, which
are different from those of waking, adult, syntactical logic and in many
ways are closer to the thinking of childhood. Popularly, it is often called
the "logic of the emotions." This *primary process* mode of thought and
handling of feelings and impulses is discussed in the section on the
psychic apparatus. At this point I shall elaborate on only one special
characteristic of unconscious material: its timelessness. Unconscious
strivings persist year after year, relatively impervious to modification by
the influences of reality and by the higher functioning of the intellect.
Indeed, as is evident in the previous case, these strivings are more likely
to affect the sort of reality a patient chooses and lives in than to be
affected by it. Insight-oriented psychotherapy is about the only way of
effecting some change in these perennially striving unconscious wishes.

There is a *continuum* from consciousness to unconsciousness with
points all along the way. There are varying degrees of unconsciousness.
Some ideas, feelings, and actions are not conscious at any given time,
but are quite capable of becoming so. The best examples of these are
automatic acts like starting and driving a car. Unless we are learning to

---

[3]My explanations of clinical case material will often sound rather pat. This is in
the interest of brevity and clarity and is not meant to imply that my formulations
speak to all the dynamics at work or that equally reasonable supplementary (or
even supplanting) hypotheses might not be proffered and tested against the
data and the patient's subsequent responses. Each human being is too complex
to be tied to a *uni*vocal formulation. Indeed, one of the beauties of clinical case
conferences is that the student is forced to weigh the clinical evidence for his
particular formulation and to consider alternative—sometimes complementary,
sometimes contradictory—hypotheses for the same set of data. Although hy-
pothesizing and interpreting in dynamic psychiatry is, as I shall repeatedly
demonstrate, rule-following behavior with explicit evidential criteria (with the
obvious corollary that some formulations will be more data-connected, comprehensive, and useful than others) any fundamentally interpretive enterprise
always has room for another perspective on the phenomena under consideration. To think otherwise is to fall into the trap of intellectual hubris and
authoritarianism with patients. Tolerating the ambiguity inherent in the work
while at the same time respecting and refining one's interpretive approach is the
most difficult dialectic for the dynamic therapist—and indeed, since Heisenberg
and Einstein, for the scientist in general.

drive, we are not consciously aware of the innumerable thoughts, motions, and reactions necessary to operate an automobile. Nevertheless, we can effortlessly direct our attention to this behavior and become conscious of it. Another, slightly more unconscious, example would be the name on the tip of the tongue, which comes to us after only an instant's reflection. Such ideas are what Freud called *preconscious*. Freud believed that virtually all feelings, ideas, and impulses *begin* at the unconscious level and, if they or their representatives (*derivatives*) reach consciousness, it is by way of the preconscious. I shall give a clinical example of an idea and affect moving from unconsciousness through preconsciousness to consciousness.

> A 34-year-old man entered treatment for marital problems. He was involved in an affair and strongly considered leaving his wife and children. It became apparent that he was recapitulating the behavior of his own father, who cheated on the patient's mother and who finally deserted the family when the patient was ten. He had never come to terms with his feelings about the parents' divorce and was completely *unconscious* of the role that event was playing in his own distress. At one point, after a number of sessions, he said, "You know, I think my school problems and nervousness started when I was in the fourth grade." So I asked, "What else was going on then?" and he replied, "My father left home!" After recovering his breath, he stammered, "Gee, Doctor, I feel like I've just been hit by a ton of bricks!"

When I asked my question, I had decided that his long-repressed knowledge of the *connection* between the paternal desertion and his childhood and current problems had moved to the preconscious level of awareness and that, with only the slightest encouragement, he could reach out and grasp it. Incidentally, letting the client arrive at this insight was more therapeutic and better for his self-esteem than simply giving it to him.

The rest of this book will be replete with examples of the potency of the unconscious, both in psychopathology and in our everyday lives.

## MENTAL FORCES

What is the nature of the "forces" operative within the psyche? Freud tended to dichotomize them into the biological on the one hand and the cultural on the other. Equilibrium existed when there was a state of truce between culture and biology, and conflict when there was a state of war.

Most people today, including myself, believe this is a much oversimplified view. In reality, it is not possible to clearly distinguish between *biological* and *societal*. Most of our impulsions, or *dynamics*, are composed of biological and social elements inseparably intertwined. For example, "ambition," as a motivator, is a function of biologically based aggression and societal and familial injunctions. Conflict may exist between two primarily cultural impulsions, as much as between a purely biological and a purely cultural one. An example would be conflicts between social injunctions to intensely competitive strivings and those to charity and altruism (each of which, incidentally, possesses biological elements as well).

Indeed, the ultimate nature of the forces which drive us is, in most respects, a purely academic question. What we, as dynamic psychiatrists, are concerned with is *mental experience* and the fashion in which it is integrated and differentiated (i.e., *mind*). We are not now, and may never be, able to make definitive statements about the nature of its biological substrate. What is important to know operationally is that we are driven by at least four sorts of dynamisms: 1) conscious and unconscious affect-laden *fantasies* ("wishes," in plain English); 2) *defenses* against these fantasies and their associated feelings; 3) *current forces* impinging upon us from the outside world; and 4) the *commands* and *prohibitions* of the outside world as internalized in the form of conscience (both conscious and unconscious). Interactions between these forces can produce new forces, as we shall see in our discussion of conflict and defense. For example, the interaction between an unconscious affect-laden fantasy and a (conscious or unconscious) moral injunction against it leads to *anxiety* which itself motivates the psychic organism to a variety of defensive maneuvers.

The concept of "dynamic," or "mental force," must also be understood as intimately related to that of "psychic tension." The needs, desires, and external and internalized social pressures that function as mental forces are associated with *increments* in psychic tension. They disturb that state of minimal tension or homeostatic constancy that the psychic organism strives to maintain. Since this psychic tension is unpleasurable and since the personality strives to minimize such sensations (e.g., the "pleasure principle," discussed in Chapter 2), the individual responds with behaviors aimed at reducing the tension or, from a different perspective, satisfying the need or requirement. The tensions associated with mental forces elicit need-satisfying or need-attenuating behaviors (ranging from still more fantasies to overt actions or, as we shall see, to maneuvers designed to inhibit awareness of these needs and pressures and/or substitutively gratify them). For all these reasons we conceptualize these mental forces as the "motor" of human behavior.

It is essential to know that these forces do not exist in a vacuum, but within the context of *interpersonal relations*. In other words, the affect-laden fantasies or prohibitions are directed toward, or derived from, people who are *now* or *once were*, in our physical environments. Thus, raw sexual and aggressive drives do not sit about in our unconsciouses, waiting to attach themselves to, or be pulled out by, any object that presents itself. Our unconscious sexual, aggressive, and other impulses are directed, from the outset, to the *internal representations* (the feeling-toned "pictures" within our minds) of particular important persons from our past and present. In the technical sense, we express all this by saying that quantities (metaphorically speaking) of psychic energy or forces *"cathect,"* or attach, themselves to the internal representations of objects[4] from the environment. The original objects of these fantasies were, of course, the central figures from our childhoods, and these fantasies remain bound, at least to some extent, to internal representations of these objects all our lives. These unconscious fantasies are constantly scanning current reality for persons sufficiently resembling these prototypes toward whom to express themselves. (Recall the case of Mrs. A.)

Dynamic psychiatry recognizes that these forces within the mind are in a delicately balanced *equilibrium,* both with one another and with the forces of the environment. This is a *dynamic,* not a static, equilibrium and its maintenance requires a good deal of hard work. Dynamic therapists recognize that one does not alter one force in the patient or his environment without affecting its relationship with many others. For this reason, they respect the equilibrium, however maladaptive, each patient has been able to work out on his own. They do not go in willy nilly supporting one force and attempting to weaken others without first considering the total impact on the balance of forces within the patient and its relationship to the environment.

The constellation and balance of forces can change over time. Old forces can gain or lose in magnitude and new ones can arise. The most dramatic example of the former is the sudden strengthening of sexual fantasies at the time of puberty. The most dramatic example of the latter is the new demands placed on us by society at the moment of early adulthood. These drastic shifts in the strength of biological and social forces can lead to disequilibrium where none was before and account for the fact that many psychiatric disturbances first manifest themselves in adolescence or early adulthood.

When the forces, whether conscious or unconscious, active at any moment are moving toward the same goal, and when that goal meets with the approval, or at least not the condemnation, of society, then we have a mind at harmony within itself and with its environment. We

---

[4]The term "object" is used in a highly specific and technical sense in psychoanalysis to refer to those "persons," or rather internalized *representations of them* (we never relate to reality directly but only to our perceptions and interpretations of it), with whom we interact or have interacted. I shall reserve my discussion of object relations theory for the section on the psychic apparatus and on psychological development.

have, in other words, a mind in a state of optimal *adaptation* and adaptation is what we are all striving for, the psychopathological no less than the healthy. (In the third chapter I shall demonstrate how symptoms can be viewed as miscarried attempts at adaptation.)

On mornings, for example, when our impulsions to earn a wage, reassert our professional identities, socialize with our fellow workers, and satisfy our consciences converge, we are "propelled" effortlessly into our jobs at the clinic. Unconscious motivations may conspire *as well* (e.g., identification with helping and nurturing figures from childhood, attempts to give to others what we ourselves were deprived of, the desire to surpass and triumph over our parents occupationally, needs for the approval of a boss who unconsciously represents a parent)—but as long as they mesh with our conscious ones, there is no problem. This is, of course, the state of affairs in mental health or normality, and it is hoped that we all approach that point at least part of the time.

If, on the other hand, we experience ourselves torn between the aforementioned pressures toward work and the desire to call in sick so we can meet our friends at the beach, then we are in a state of conflict. This may be painful but, since the conflict is quite *conscious*, it is not, by definition, a neurotic one.

If the forces stream toward a common goal which nonetheless runs counter to the best interests of our family, fellows, and society, then we may find ourselves in conflict, not *within* the self, but *with the environment*. This would be the case should we decide, quite placidly, to "rip off" the clinic, our professional peers, and patients in any number of ways. This is still not neurosis, since the conflict is not *intrapsychic*. Furthermore, it is not associated with the anxiety, psychic pain, or *ego dystonia* of the neuroses. It is, instead, a classic example of so-called sociopathic, psychopathic, antisocial, or "character-disordered" behavior, to which we shall return in Chapter 3.

If the forces within the mind are striving in different directions and if any or all of them are unconscious, then we speak of a state of *unconscious intrapsychic conflict*. This is the hallmark of *neurotic*[5] behavior, of which all of us are capable at times. As discussed in the third chapter, unconscious conflict can manifest itself in several ways: indecision; widely contradictory feelings, behavior, and points of view toward the same person, issue, or thing; slips, or *parapraxes,* of the tongue or pen; misperceiving, misremembering, misplacing objects, forgetting names; alternating severe inhibition of certain affects and impulses (e.g., anger

---

[5]Psychosis is also characterized by unconscious intrapsychic conflict, but the barriers against the intrusion of unconscious material are weakened. The psychotic is likely to be consciously aware of conflictual forces that in the neurotic are deeply unconscious—e.g., incestuous or murderous fantasies.

and sexuality) with episodic eruptions of them; and neurotic symptoms and character styles.

To illustrate, if the forces driving us to the aforementioned clinic include unconscious sexual fantasies for a patient who (consciously or unconsciously) reminds us of a parent or sibling, or unconscious aggressive fantasies toward a supervisor who represents a hated childhood authority figure, or an intense, unconscious desire to gain the attention of the authorities (parent representatives) at the expense of our peers (sibling representatives),[6] and if these trends are opposed by a (conscious and unconscious) set of values that says "thou shalt not do, or even think, such things," then we are in a state of *unconscious intrapsychic,* or neurotic, conflict. We may be intensely aware *or* totally unaware of the *anxiety* that accompanies every neurotic conflict. We may be aware that we are anxious and that it is somehow related to ambivalence about work. We may even know some of its *present-day,* as opposed to its *historical,* roots. For example, we may be *aware* that we have been troubled by sexual dreams about a particular patient, but *unaware* that this is because the patient represents our sibling or parent. In any event, for this to qualify as a genuinely neurotic conflict we must be *unconscious* of at least some of the elements that constitute it. You should also know that conflicts in which all the elements are seemingly conscious (e.g., whether to accept a major promotion that involves a long move) can still rest on unconscious pillars (e.g., father conflicts or dependency issues).

Much of Chapter 3 is concerned with painting a clearer picture of the relationship between unconscious conflict and psychopathology.

## HISTORY AND PSYCHIC CAUSALITY

Strictly speaking, dynamic psychiatry should be called "dynamic-historical" psychiatry since it places greater emphasis on the patient's longitudinal development than any other school of psychiatry or psychology. There is a circular relationship between history and *psychic causality,* the idea that human behavior is *caused* by *mental* events. The latter is the rationale for taking a history, and yet the operation of psychic causality is revealed only by taking that history. Consequently, in this section I shall go back and forth between the two.

Dynamic psychiatry recognizes that virtually all psychiatric patients are not born with their difficulties, but acquire them. This does not mean that hereditary and constitutional factors may not play a role. Rather, they almost never play the total, or usually even the most important,

---

[6]The technical word for those figures in adulthood who unconsciously represent important persons from childhood (e.g., parents, siblings) is *imago*. Thus, we would speak of the boss who represents the father as a "father imago," the patient who represents the sister as a "sister imago," and so forth.

part in the so-called "functional" (as opposed to organic) disorders that make up the majority of what the psychiatrist encounters. People are the way they are because of the interaction between their biological endowments and their environments—because, in other words, of their *experience*. None of the important and repetitive experiences in life, however actively or passively we participate in them, leaves us completely unaffected. No one would dispute that to understand the current economic, social, and cultural scene in the South, one must take into account the colonial and antebellum periods, the Civil War, and the Reconstruction. How then could anyone presume to understand why his patient behaves as he does without knowing how his environment has acted on him and he on it from his earliest years?

Before Freud, most psychiatrists cared little about *what* their patients were exposed to, what it *meant* to them, and *how* they attempted to adapt to it. Emil Kraepelin, the exemplar of late nineteenth- early twentieth-century descriptive psychiatry, was interested in what the patient *looked like* at the present point in time. He did not care to know much about what went on *inside* him, and his history-taking was largely limited to that of the present and past overt psychiatric disorders. Nor, unfortunately, do many present-day descriptive and biological psychiatrists take much history other than that of the manifest psychiatric disturbance itself. Furthermore, recent years have witnessed a proliferation of "here-and-now" therapies which give short shrift to history.

History-taking is an arduous and time-consuming task, but it is indispensable for one who really wishes to know his patient. Indeed, the most important reason to take a history is that it is not dead, but rather is alive in the "here and now," both because the patient continues to be driven by, and preoccupied with, historical factors *and* because he usually arranges to find or create current environments that resemble those in the past. (Recall Mrs. A.)

The theory of psychic causality, or psychic determinism, is the primary rationale for taking a history or conducting psychotherapy in general. It asserts that human behavior is the product of mental events and that these mental events themselves have *causative antecedents*. It holds, in other words, that events in the mind, just as in the physical, biological, and world historical spheres, do not occur without reason or purely by chance. Human behavior is *meaningful* and must be explained with reference to the *historically determined* set of meanings of the actor.[7]

In the case of the mind, these *causative antecedents* are the unconscious, affect-laden, goal-directed fantasies (wishes) about which I wrote in the previous section. The wish is the mother to the deed. These fantasies, which are the true motor of human behavior, can emerge in response to *internal* pressures—impulses originating in still deeper layers of the

---

[7]See page 19.

psyche and with the participation of the biological components of drives such as hunger, sex, and aggression. Or, they can arise in response to stimuli from the environment. Or, more often, they emerge in response to a subtle interaction between pressures from the two.

Before continuing, I wish to emphasize that this usage of "causality," or "determinism," is not identical with that in the physical and biological sciences. There are significant differences in the nature of causation between the two. Among the most important of these are that the conscious and unconscious fantasies that precede and lead to *all* human behaviors (except the most grossly neurological and purely physiological) are not simply blind mechanical forces but *strivings* to bring about a longed-for *future* state of affairs. In other words, our fantasizing, or wishing, is *goal-directed* and *purposeful*. Therefore, when we ask what "causes" a particular behavior, we are also asking what *purpose* it serves and what it *means*. In this sense, the theory of psychic causality is also the theory of psychic meaningfulness or psychic purposefulness. When we speak of "cause," we mean something more akin to what the historian, rather than the physicist, means by the word.

Whether one chooses to speak in terms of "causes," "motives," "motivations" or, like Schafer (1976),[8] of "intentionality" and "reasons"

---

[7]All this may seem trite today, but when Freud began work, psychologists and psychiatrists were explaining most normal and abnormal mental phenomena neurologically. For example, dreams were taken to be the meaningless epiphenomena of random neuronal firing in the cerebral cortex. Hysterical symptoms resulted from "hereditary neuropathic degeneration." Schizophrenic speech, or "word salad," as it was called, was a psychologically meaningless product of toxins or brain lesions. By contrast, for the dynamic psychiatrist, trying to explain a paranoid's or depressive psychotic's delusions solely with reference to his catecholamines, without taking account of what he has experienced in his world and what it means to him, is on the same order of fallacy as attempting to explain Plato's philosophy solely by reference to the neurological and muscular apparatus that subserved his manipulation of language and the writing down of his thoughts. For good examples of the role of actual experience in childhood in the formation of adult delusions and hallucinations see Hannah Green's (1964) *I Never Promised You A Rose Garden* and William Niederland's (1974) *Schreber Case*.

As one moves up the scale in terms of organization of matter and energy (from physical to chemical to biological to psychological to social), the higher level is never sufficiently explained by invoking the principles and processes of the level below it. Dynamic psychiatrists do not deny that there is an inextricable, although as yet inexplicable, relationship between "mind" and "body." Nevertheless, they believe that the symbolic is adequately reducible to the biological no more than the latter is adequately reducible to the chemical, or the chemical to the physical.

[8]Schafer's two books, *A New Language for Psychoanalysis* and *Language and Insight*, are high on any list of those which any student of dynamic psychiatry "must come to terms with." Although I disagree with many of his contentions, he has influenced my conceptions of history and causality. For further treatment see "Historiography in History and Psychoanalysis" (Wallace, 1983).

makes little practical difference as long as one accepts that all observable and self-reportable behaviors *result* from *mental antecedents*. This is what I shall mean in this book when I say "psychic causality." These antecedent, causal, fantasies themselves are a function of historically based preoccupations and of the forces of current reality. Insofar as the former is the case, we speak of "historical determinism." By "historical determinism," the handmaiden of psychic causality, I shall mean that the present-day configuration of any personality has arisen out of previously existing ones, and that one cannot explain any individual's current (conscious and unconscious) interpretations of self and world and present desires, fears, inhibitions, and behavior patterns without understanding the history of his actual and fantasied interpersonal relations. Although all of us consciously and unconsciously wish and act to fulfill or inhibit our desires, much of what we both long for and fulfill, and what we refrain from, are themselves functions of our history. In other words, we do not simply freely choose, in an historical vacuum, what we want and abhor. This is not the same as denying our subjective sense of volition and willfulness. It means only that our experience largely determines what we want, where and how we want it, and whether or not we choose to indulge or deny ourselves.[9]

Psychic causality operates on both the microscopic and macroscopic levels. As to the former, it reveals itself in the patient's free associations within the therapeutic hour. Psychic causality assumes that there is some sort of connection between statements that are uttered in temporal contiguity with one another. Every clinician soon learns that the manifold productions of any patient, in any hour, group themselves around particular themes and preoccupations, that they are a *function* of central

---

[9]It is not my intention to enter into the free will-determinism controversy. Let me say merely that in focusing on the historical, unconscious factors that *limit* the range of our *conscious* volition, dynamic psychiatry does not thereby dispute the existence of the latter. If we write briefs for the former, it is because there is no lack of advocacy for the latter. People have always known about conscious volition; Freud taught them about unconscious determinism. Nor is to avow historical determinism at the same time to disavow the self-originating (albeit not always consciously so) character of our actions. We are, after all, one-half of those interactions which have determined us. It is thus correct to say that we are, in a real sense, part of that history which determines us. It is always *we* who will or cause *our* behavior, sometimes more consciously, other times more unconsciously. If by "free will" one means that certain behaviors of the human being escape the causal nexus into which the rest of existence is thrown, I would deny the plausibility of the concept. However, if one means "*conscious* self-determination," then I would endorse it. The point to be differentiated is not whether a given behavior is "determined or free," but whether (or, more accurately, the degree to which) it is consciously or unconsciously determined. The idea of a conscious ego whose powers it is the aim of psychotherapy to augment, and of a "therapeutic alliance" between patient and therapist presupposes a degree of conscious self-determination in the client.

underlying fears and fantasies. The same can be said of the infinitely more variegated data of an entire human life.

I shall illustrate first with reference to the microscopic, then to the macroscopic, with the same patient, Mr. E., a brilliant graduate student in art whose most immediately striking characteristics were his obesity and slovenliness. I shall frequently have occasion to refer to him in this book.

> He began the hour by talking about his piano teacher whom, he said in passing, I physically resemble. He suspected this teacher did not think him very talented, but doled out false praise so he could continue to earn a fee. Mr. E. then began complaining about his graduate adviser who did not seem to listen to, or be interested in, him. Then he railed out about a fellow art student who would twist his statements around to resemble what the latter wanted to hear. From there he moved on to anger at an uncle who he feels is his parents' agent. Next he spoke of conversations with his father in which the latter seemed to be feigning interest. It was only in the last five minutes that he became aware, and communicated, that he had similar concerns about me (who unconsciously represented all these figures). From Mr. E's past history I knew that both parents had very rigid and definite ideas about how this, their first, child was supposed to behave. Because of their own agendas, the patient was never responded to as a separate person in his own right, and such affection and nurturance as he received was "conditional." When it became apparent that the patient had neither the desire nor the ability to meet the parents' expectations, they lost interest in him.

In summary, one can see how the themes of the hour were a manifestation of the themes of an entire life. In other words, there were good historical reasons or underlying "causes" for the train of associations within the session.

In another meeting Mr. E. arrived 30 minutes late. The following interchange occurred:

*Patient:* Sorry, I'm late because I misread my watch. You probably don't believe me.

*Interviewer:* No, I believe you misread your watch. The question is, "What led you to do so? What purpose did it serve?"

*Patient:* It means nothing. There is no reason. I just misread my watch, that's all. I do it all the time.

*Interviewer:* Yes, but the question is, "What went into it this particular time?"

In the course of the remaining minutes he became aware that he was paying me back for being out sick at the time of the previous session. "I felt abandoned, left in the lurch." In other words, an unconscious fantasy something like "I shall be late and give that bastard a dose of his own medicine" was the causative antecedent (or the purpose) of his misreading the time. This particular fantasy itself was determined not merely by my absence, but by a history that left him with strong feelings of insecurity in relationships and with exquisite sensitivities to loss and rejection.

The following are some additional concrete clinical examples to drive home what I mean by "cause" in psychic causality. Mr. D.'s father died on Monday, and two days later he attempted suicide. When we say this external event "caused" his suicide attempt, we do not mean that it "caused" it in the same way that a gamma ray "causes" the transmutation of a molecule. What we actually mean is "a set of *internal processes* set in motion by the father's death led Mr. D. to attempt suicide." What these internal processes were could only be divined by knowing his history.

> Mr. D. had been ignored and intimidated by his well-known and highly successful father throughout childhood. He reacted to this by developing powerful fantasies of murdering and surpassing the father. Because these fantasies aroused the fear of his father's retaliation and the condemnation of his own conscience, they were *repressed* (unconsciously warded out of awareness). However, they continued to thrive in his unconscious and drove him to enter into and rise in his father's profession. When the combination of his own success and his father's death fulfilled his unconscious wishes, the patient reacted, equally unconsciously, with an inordinate sense of guilt. This unconscious sense of guilt led him to punish himself by attempting suicide.

Mr. D.'s case illustrates that what functions as the "causal" or precipitating event in any psychiatric disorder depends upon the system of meanings and motivations of the patient, and that that system, in turn, depends upon his history.[10] In other words, because the early interaction between Mr. D. and his father led him to guilt-ridden murderous fantasies about the latter, he reacted to the father's death as if he were actually responsible for it. Another man, with a different history, would have dealt with his father's death in a quite different way. One can predict that certain types of external events, such as the death of a family member, will have an impact on anybody, but the specific effect depends very much on the *meaning* of the event, and that depends on the *history*.[11]

The case of Mrs. F. concerns the patient's response to the therapist's interventions. It also illustrates the following general principle: reactions that follow immediately upon certain events in the environment, such as

---

[10]This is as true of the precipitating event in those supposedly more biologically based mental disorders as it is of the precipitant in the neuroses. For example, in order to understand what constitutes an environmental stressor sufficient to precipitate an endogenous depression, one must know the *history* of the prior traumata of that individual.

[11]See page 23.

(even apparently unrelated) statements that occur in temporal contiguity with one another, can be assumed to be somehow connected with each other, even if that link is unconscious.

> During the early evaluation and therapeutic sessions with Mrs. F., I noticed that every time I broached anything having to do with sexuality she shifted in her chair, averted her eyes, and coughed nervously. She did this, for example, when I questioned her about menarche, early relations with boys, and her current relationship with her husband. From this I concluded that there was some sort of cause and effect relationship between my questions and her agitation. When I knew her better, it became clear that my questions had impinged upon anxiety-laden unconscious conflicts over sexuality, stemming from her origin in a family which was preoccupied, negatively, with sex. Her mother referred to her own menses as the "curse" and a "sickness" and constantly lectured her on the "nastiness" of sex, at the same time that the parents' marital discord and her father's blatant affairs titillated her with the knowledge of his availability.

Still another example of oblique connection between the therapist's statements and the patient's response is that of the aforementioned Mr. E., who dealt with his strong unconscious yearnings for dependent intimacy with others, and attendant fears of rejection, by generally denying that people held any importance for him. When I informed him of my impending summer vacation, he was silent for a few minutes and then looked toward the air conditioner and said "I hate that damn thing. It's too cold in here. Will you cut it off?" He was utterly unconscious of the connection between my announcement and his reaction, and was totally unaware that he was displacing his anger at me onto an inanimate object. Such events occur all the time in psychotherapy and if you do not believe in psychic causality you will never make sense of them.

In line with the principle of psychic causality, the therapist should know that when he takes the patient's history he is getting not so much a chronology of the actual events in his life as a record of the *meanings* of these events. Meaning occurs within the matrix of *interpersonal relations,* within the context of one's relationships with important persons from past and present, and his feelings about them. The most withdrawn schizophrenic, reclusive scholar, or eremitic monk lives in a world richly populated with persons (and parts of persons). An individual's very withdrawal must be understood in terms of those *from whom* he is

---

[11]The precipitant in the so-called "traumatic neuroses" must often be understood symbolically. For example, one bank clerk's anxiety attacks, following a holdup at gunpoint, were a manifestation, not merely of unresolved feelings about the incident itself, but of conflictual incestuous fantasies stirred up by the symbolic, sexual meaning of a man "sticking her up" with a pistol. In another case, a man's latent homosexual issues were set off by being mugged, in the dark, from behind.

withdrawing. Fantasies are nothing more than, as Sullivan renamed them, "private interpersonal experiences."

None of our daily activities can be understood without reference to this current and historical nexus of relationships with persons both inside and outside our heads. For example, the meaning of my profession to me cannot be understood merely with reference to the intellectual pleasure I derive from its theory and practice, nor even to the prestige and satisfaction derived from playing some role in alleviating the misery of others (the current interpersonal context). It can be understood only by knowing something of the interpersonal context in which my desire to be a physician *arose,* with reference to the "physicianship" of my father, the esteem of physicians by my mother, and the conscious and unconscious complex of my relationships with them. All of our behaviors continue to carry meaning from the interpersonal situations in which they were born.

The dynamic psychiatrist is the historian of the *real* and *fantasied* interpersonal relations of his patient. It is less important to sort out neatly the reality and fantasy elements in a patient's story than to grasp his view of the world from the inside. Indeed, since our experiences with people influence our fantasies and vice versa, there is usually an inextricable and circular relationship between actual and psychical reality.

In short, the patient does not give you a flawless chronicle of the actual events in his life. He gives you something much more important and therapeutically relevant: an historical account of himself and the world *as he sees them.* Of necessity, this story bears some relationship to what has actually transpired, but it also reflects what the patient wanted and feared. It is *in accord* with this view of self and world that he frames his actions. Everything that he does *makes sense within this context.* It is this psychical reality that is the true engine of his psychopathology.

If you take a detailed life history, you find *patterns* of stressors and coping repeating themselves. Often the patient plays an active role in manufacturing these stressors. There are themes in the story of the environment's action upon, and reaction to, the patient, and of his action upon, and reaction to, the environment. From recurrent linkages between certain classes of actions and external events and between external events and reactions, you infer things about what the patient's world means to him. You learn that each person's conflicts, as well as his coping mechanisms, are a function of the history of the early interaction between the driving forces in his psyche and the impulsions, inhibitions, and reactions from the outside world (family, culture, and physical environment).

Most importantly, you discover that each person develops certain *expectations* and *evaluations* of himself and of others based on how he was treated in childhood by, first his family members, and later his peers and outside authority figures. These evaluations and expectations function as a lens through which all one's perceptions of the real world are filtered. Because of historically based distortions in this lens, we selectively inattend to data that run counter to our expectations and evaluations and absorb that which conforms to them. Those who unconsciously remind us of these prototypical actors elicit expectations and reactions similar to those evoked by the originals. Often our reactions actually induce them to behave toward us as we expect—the classic neurotic self-fulfilling prophecy, of which this book contains many examples (see Ms. H.). You see it all the time: the thrice-divorced woman with an uncanny knack for choosing abusive, alcoholic husbands; the bright young job-hopper continually "harassed" and unappreciated by his employers; the "unfortunate" woman whose boyfriends all "just happen to turn out to be homosexual." The list is endless. Each of them, seemingly pursued by a relentless and demonic fate, is unconsciously reenacting and "coming to terms with" conflict-laden infantile experiences. As Jung said, it is psychological law that we are doomed to encounter from without that which we do not confront from within.

Indeed, the farther you go in this field, the more you will be impressed by how adept people are at finding and creating present-day environments that resemble the pathogenic ones of their past. Quite apart from this reflecting a perennial attempt to fulfill cherished childhood fantasies, it seems as if there is some mysterious, fundamental drive in the human being to reduce any dissonance between one's view and expectations of self and world and that self and world themselves, even if it means making one's reality a thorny bed in which to lie. Perhaps it is associated with fear of the unknown. We prefer the familiar, old, painful, predictable reality to the risks and uncertainties of a future in flux.

In part, however, this recreation of past in present stems from an attempt to actively master one's *passively experienced* traumata, to go back and improve the past this time. This is what Mrs. A. was trying to do by marrying a man like her father and attempting to reform him. One of my patients, enacting a more potent variation on this theme, actually moved back in with her father after her parents' divorce and tried, much to the distress of both her father and herself, to exact from him the interest and affection she had never received.

There are also, of course, adaptive ways of coming to terms with one's history, but the psychiatrist is less likely to encounter these than their maladaptive counterparts. For example, some abused and neglected children become child-care or social workers, rather than child abusers, as a way of actively mastering the traumata that they have undergone. Some children of alcoholics become addictions counselors rather than alcoholics. One young woman became a career diplomat, in part as a way of mastering feelings about her family's frequent and difficult moves in her childhood. She still felt like an outsider, but this time *she* was in control of the situation. One boy's interest in atlases and travelogues, a means of mentally escaping from a turbulent home, developed into an adult career in geography.

This unconscious *acting out* of the past in the present is what the analyst calls *transference*. Wishes, fears, expectations, and feelings are *transferred* from the childhood objects toward whom they were originally directed to present-day people who represent, unconsciously, the originals. This "acting out" takes the place of a conscious remembrance of, and verbal communication about, the past. In this sense, it figures as another one of the *resistances* to the emergence and expression of unconscious ideas and affects with which the therapist must contend. At the same time, however, the analysis of this particular resistance (the transference) constitutes, as we shall see, the vehicle of insight-oriented psychotherapy.

The most striking example of transference was told to me by a psychiatric resident I was supervising. When the patient came for his first appointment, he greeted his therapist with, "You don't like me, do you, you son of a bitch!?" This patient was telling his therapist, in eleven words, that he had been exposed to such disappointment in life that he expected the resident, a total stranger about whom he knew nothing and who knew nothing about him, to instantly dislike and reject him. A man on the street, confronted with a similar communication, would probably have responded with, "You're right, I don't, you son of a bitch!" However, the resident, fortunately, was able to contain his feelings enough, and believed in historical determinism enough, that he and the patient were able to spend the next three years working to understand what went into the patient's "Hello."

The next example illustrates not only transference and the power of history, but also the concept of psychopathology as "atavism"—the persistence of formerly adaptive behaviors into the present, where they are no longer necessitated or advantageous.

> As a small child, Ms. H. was rejected by her busy and alcoholic father. Still she loved and longed for him and, when she reached out to him, his rebuffs brought pain, humiliation, and impotent rage. To avoid the pain of future rebuffs and the attendant anger (which was itself conflictual for her since she was enjoined against even feeling, much less expressing, such things), she eventually withdrew from her father and repressed her needs for him. One must admit that, under the circumstances, there was a certain adaptiveness in this. However, such expectations of, and behavior toward, the first important male in her life became so ingrained in her that, when she left home, she *transferred* them to men in general, particularly those who might in some way be significant to her. She would do one of

two things: either withdraw and be coldly aloof from men who unconsciously interested her or else, by identifying with her father, let them briefly into her life and then actively reject them before they could reject her. By so doing, she ensured that men ended up being as cold and indifferent to her as her father was—the famous neurotic self-fulfilling prophecy. Thus, a behavior pattern, appropriate to an admittedly inappropriate situation in childhood, continued into adulthood where it was no longer adaptive. Before long she began treating me similarly. She was late for and cancelled sessions, "tuned me out" during the meetings, accused me on several occasions of being inattentive and uncaring, derogated the value of the treatment, and contemplated dropping out. She was, in other words, *acting out*, rather than consciously remembering and talking about, the complex of feelings and expectations associated with her father's rejection of her. When I translated her *behavior* into *words*, her tardiness and withdrawal ceased and she began working in therapy.

Transference reactions are not limited to psychotherapy; they occur in day-to-day life as well. All of us react toward important people in our present not solely out of who they are, but in part out of who they consciously and, especially, unconsciously represent to us. Transference accounts for the instant like or dislike of a person upon first encounter. We even have transference reactions toward our own patients, based on our histories, and these are termed *countertransference*. Patients can evoke sexual, rageful, competitive, parental, fearful, jealous, or other feelings in us depending upon *their* behavior, *our* psychodynamics, and *who* they represent to us. The most important difference in the transference reactions in the patient and those in the well-analyzed therapist is that they are *conscious* in the latter. There is also a difference between the transference reactions that develop in everyday life or in brief therapy and those that develop in long-term insight-oriented psychotherapy. Those in the latter are more intense and less disturbed by intrusions on the part of the more neutral therapist. We shall return to, and broaden and deepen, our concept of transference again and again.

I shall close the section on history with two clinical vignettes that illustrate many of the principles to which I have referred. The themes will appear obvious to the reader, but they were not to the patients and they had to be picked out from a morass of other data. In order to spot themes in a life, you must combine a passive receptivity to the data with an active restructuring of it.

Ms. D., a 30-year-old divorcée, was referred by her employer for absenteeism secondary to a series of accidents sustained on the job over the previous four months: sprains, jammed fingers, tripping over furniture, and the like. A *history of the present problem* revealed that the accidents started some six weeks after the drowning of her boyfriend on a fishing trip in which she was present. Apart from an initial state of shock and a very few days of crying, the patient thought or felt little about the episode and said she had "worked my grief out."

Upon taking a *past history of the problem,* I found that there were at least two earlier occasions when she had been involved in numerous accidents. The more recent followed her discovery that her husband was having affairs and intensified during the separation and following the divorce. The first episode began at age 12, when her parents were having numerous fights, and continued for several months following their divorce.

Upon taking her *past history in general,* I found that even before age 12 there were many minor illnesses, cuts, and bruises that caused her to miss school often. There were two other pertinent pieces of data as well. The father was alcoholic, had affairs, and was generally absent. The mother was so preoccupied with her own hypochondriacal complaints and *minor injuries* that she had little time for the patient except when the latter was hurt or sick.

Only because I took histories of the present problem, previous similar problems, and her childhood experience did I become aware of the similarities in the relationship between the three external events and three major episodes of accident proneness. To wit, each "run" of accidents followed a loss. The discovery that her even earlier patterns of injuries occurred in a setting of deprivation and rejection clinched my hypothesis that it was a set of unconscious feelings and fantasies elicited by losses that led to her accidents.

During the course of treatment she began to develop strong dependent and affectionate needs for me which were accompanied by the expectations that I would respond to them in the cold and rejecting manner of her parents (transference). These needs and expectations gradually moved into consciousness and she considered leaving treatment ("reject you before you reject me"). The accident proneness, which had subsided in her work environment, began manifesting itself in relation to the therapeutic hours. She would bump her head on the roof of the car when getting in to drive to the session, trip when coming up the steps of the building, and so forth. Then, on June 4, six and a half months after entering treatment, she came in my office with her arm in a cast, explaining that she had slipped while fishing from a rock the day before. She had no idea why and was at first loath to attribute it to psychological factors. Only after a few minutes did she and I realize that June 3 was the anniversary of her boyfriend's drowning! Indeed she had even been fishing in another section of the same river! When I pointed this out to her, a wealth of affect poured out and our work began in earnest.

It seems incredible, but people can be quite unaware of such connections. Magical things can happen with numbers which one discovers only if one looks for them. Anniversary phenomena are the most dramatic demonstration of the time-keeping mechanism in the unconscious and of the power of history in our lives. The case following this one also contains some uncanny examples of this.

In the final weeks of therapy, Ms. D. became aware, first, of a good deal of rage toward her boyfriend for leaving her (dying) and, second, of a wealth of guilt feelings in reaction to this and over her inability to save him. Then she became aware of hurt, rage, and guilt toward her ex-husband, then toward her father for deserting her when she was 12. Eventually she also became cognizant of similar feelings toward her inattentive and self-centered mother. She recognized her accident proneness as, in part, a way of getting attention, acquired by identification with the mother. (Recall my discussion of coping mechanisms, as much as conflicts, being functions of one's history.) Finally, she discovered that accident proneness was a form of unconscious self-destructiveness, a means of discharging aggression toward others by turning it on herself and a way of absolving her guilt feelings through self-punishment. The accidents in relationship to our sessions were in response to her unconscious expectations that I too would treat her as did the others, thereby resurrecting the constellation of rage and guilt which she dealt with through self-destructiveness.

I shall present one final example of the power of the past over the present, exemplified in anniversary reactions in the life of one of my patients and in that of her ex-husband and daughter. As I just described, such phenomena are more prevalent than one would suspect. We do not learn about most of them because we neglect to obtain precise dates for major events and reactions. (Most gaps in the history occur because the therapist either did not listen to the patient or did not ask the right question.)

Mrs. E., a 34-year-old woman with hysterical back pain and depression, presented after a suicide gesture precipitated by a chance meeting with her former husband. After her first suicide attempt at age 16, she was admitted to a psychiatric hospital. This followed an elopement with her boyfriend who soon mistreated, disappointed, and rejected her. A few years later she married a man whose father had deserted his family when he was eight years old, leaving his mother with himself and two brothers. When the patient and her husband had three children, one of them a boy eight years of age, the husband deserted the family, quickly remarried and, like his own father, established a new family and had no further contact with the first one! Lifelong problems between the patient and her daughter intensified after the divorce. When this daughter was 16, she ran away with a boy of whom her mother, my patient, disapproved, took an overdose of the *mother's* medication, and ended up in the hospital where her mother was first admitted, but on a different ward and under the care of a different physician!

Such examples seem supernatural, but they are not at all. I deliberately chose this case for its dramatic quality. Usually the numbers do not work out so well, but the themes are there nevertheless. Rather than demonstrating the operation of a mystical principle, such cases support the dictum that "being done to is the best way of learning to do unto others." This woman raised her daughter in the aloof yet authoritarian way in which her own mother reared her, sought out a man similar to her distant and womanizing father, and nagged and rebuffed him so that he became even more so. The daughter in turn was unconsciously identifying with the mother and learning from her how to "cope" with distress. The ex-husband was merely behaving as his father had taught him a father was supposed to behave. The presence of three children, one of whom was a boy of *eight*, was sufficiently similar to the situation when his own father left him that it functioned as the *stimulus* for what he would probably have done sooner or later anyway.

However, in being history-ridden, our patients do not differ *qualitatively*, only *quantitatively*, from us. Each of us is a product of the history of the mutual interaction of our biological endowments and our environments. On the commonsense level, we can see our friends and ourselves recapitulating, less blatantly perhaps than Mrs. E. and her husband, aspects of our parents' marriage in our own. It may be sad but it is true that none of us lives totally in the present. We perceive others through a filter of our conscious and unconscious historically based preoccupations, wishes, fears, and expectations and react to them on this basis. Our spouse is never solely our spouse, our colleagues never only our colleagues, our boss never just our boss, our physician never only our physician, our patient never merely our patient, and so forth. We live, simultaneously, in two worlds—one unconscious and one conscious, one past and one present. If we seem to manage better than many of our patients, we should not become too self-righteous because it means largely that our history has been more benign, or at least less malignant, than theirs and because we have been taught and have modeled more adaptive coping skills than they.[12]

I do not want to close this chapter before relating seemingly contradictory remarks from two medical students, previously antipathetic toward psychiatry who, as a result of a detailed study of their patients' biographies, became enthusiastic about their psychiatric clerkship. One student, struck by the ubiquity of certain issues in human development, said "This business is so fascinating because all these people keep telling the same story!" The other, quickly disagreeing with him, replied "No, psychiatry is interesting because *no* two people tell the same story." In fact, both were right. Being human and growing up with humans ensures that we shall all face certain universal and enduring tasks. At the same time, human lives, like world myths and great works of literature, are complex and creative *variations* on these themes. The dynamic psychiatrist is continually encountering the universal in the

---

[12]Woody Allen says there are two classes of parents: the miserable and the horrible. Fortunately, the parents of most mental health workers seem to fall in a category which might be termed the "optimally miserable."

particular and the particular in the universal. *This* is what makes this work so interesting.

In the third chapter I shall relate what I have said about history, transference, and psychic causality to conflict, symptom formation, and adaptation. In Chapter 4 I shall elaborate upon the role of the history in dynamic psychiatry.

## SUGGESTED READINGS FOR CHAPTER 1

Brenner, C.: *An Elementary Textbook of Psychoanalysis*, New York, International Universities Press, 1973. The most lucid and complete elementary presentation of classical Freudian theory.

Fenichel, O.: *The Psychoanalytic Theory of Neurosis*. New York, W. W. Norton & Co., Inc., 1945. An advanced textbook and reference manual.

Freud, S. (1916–1917): *Introductory Lectures on Psycho-Analysis*. Standard Edition of the Complete Psychological Works of Sigmund Freud, Volumes XV and XVI. London, Hogarth Press, 1961. A must.

Sullivan, H.: *The Interpersonal Theory of Psychiatry*. New York, W. W. Norton & Co., Inc., 1953. The core of Sullivan's revisionist viewpoint of psychoanalysis. Excellent.

# 2
# The Psychic Apparatus and Personality Development

## THE PSYCHIC APPARATUS

The psychic apparatus is what is called "mind" in common parlance. In 1899 Freud introduced the *topographic* model of that apparatus. This conceptualized the mind as consisting of three systems: the *conscious*, or Cs; the *preconscious*, or *Pcs.*; and the *unconscious*, or *Ucs.* When conflict was present, it was hypothesized to exist between the Cs. and Pcs. systems on the one hand, which represent the defensive requirements of reality, and the Ucs., on the other, which harbors the turbulent forces of the instincts striving for expression. In the course of continued work, Freud found that this model did not do justice to the facts, which suggested that defensive processes and moral commands may be quite as unconscious as that which they oppose.

Consequently, in 1923 Freud formulated a new theory of the psychic apparatus. This *structural theory*, as he called it, has stood the test of time and is the one used today. The terms conscious, preconscious, and unconscious have, of course, been retained, but they are now used descriptively to refer to the degree of consciousness or unconsciousness of the contents of the psychic apparatus. The new subdivisions of mind are termed *id, ego*, and *superego*.

These "structures" do not correspond to discrete anatomical entities within the brain nor are they conceptualized as fixed and static "compartments" within the mind. Like most of the concepts in dynamic psychiatry, structural theory is nothing more than an abstraction, a model which helps us to make sense of the manifold behaviors of human beings, and it should not be reified or concretized. At times I shall refer to id, ego, and superego almost as if each represented a discrete human being with a mind of its own. However, this is only for heuristic or explanatory and practical purposes. It should be understood that we are never confronted merely by an id, ego, or superego but always by the behavior of a total personality. Id, ego, and superego are only abstract ways of comprehending that most complicated of all realities—the human actor in his surroundings.

Each of the "structures" should be understood as a *group of functions.* They may exist in dynamic equilibrium or in conflict with one another. The chapter on psychopathology describes how conflict may exist between id and ego, id and superego, id on the one hand and ego and superego on the other, ego and superego, and between any or all of these agencies and the outside world.

### The Id

The *id* is that portion of mind, unconscious by definition, wherein reside many of our oldest and most powerful impulses. Freud saw these forces as largely biological[1] (sexual and aggressive instinctual drives), but I see them as unenmeshable mélanges of biology and culture. What is important to know, for all practical purposes, is that the id is the locus of powerful unconscious, affect-laden, wish-fulfilling fantasies: dependent, sexual (in both the genital and pregenital sense), murderous, ambitious, competitive, and so forth.

Among the strongest and most important of these fantasies are those in existence since childhood. At this point I wish to reemphasize what I said in the section on "Mental Forces": that these fantasies are directed toward internal representations of objects which are now, or once were, in the real world. In the case of impulses like hunger and thirst, these objects are impersonal, inanimate ones, though even they can include interpersonal elements, e.g., slaking one's thirst on grandmother's homemade apple cider. Most of the fantasies in which dynamic psychiatry interests itself, however, involve *persons.* For example, fantasies of owning a Rolls Royce or becoming president take as their objects not so much the car or the office as the acclaim and admiration of important others that accompany them. In the case of the infantile wishes that

---

[1]Or, rather, Freud did not view the id itself as the repository of these biological impulses but rather of the *mental representations* of them. This was his way of acknowledging that the psychiatrist does not deal with biological phenomena directly but with *mental experience,* which he viewed as their epiphenomena. However, what Freud never explained was how one moves from purely somatic, supposedly instinctual, processes to the mental experience that is our primary datum.

form the nucleus of most of our fantasy life, the original objects were the members of our immediate family.

All such wishes begin unconsciously in the id and, if they have sufficient strength and do not offend our moral sensibilities or the requirements of reality, are permitted entry into the consciousness of the ego. For example, biological drives such as hunger and thirst somehow become psychically represented (depicted) in the id as wish-fulfilling fantasies. Thirst might represent itself as the unconscious *image* of oneself drinking a glass of water. This fantasy, since it obviously offends the requirements of neither reality nor conscience, rises effortlessly into the consciousness of the ego, where it is fulfilled in the real world. Other fantasies, however, are not viewed by society or by our internal police so innocuously, and these are debarred from consciousness altogether. It is, by and large, only in psychotics, psychopaths, small children, and people in exploratory psychotherapy that we find conscious awareness of incestuous, cannibalistic, parricidal, fratricidal, and other antisocial fantasies. However, as mentioned earlier, such fantasies can still reach consciousness, and even be acted on, in the form of *derivatives*, e.g., conscious fantasies of having intercourse with a woman who unconsciously represents a man's mother or of taking the place of a boss who unconsciously represents his father.

The forces of the id operate differently from those of the conscious adult ego. I shall elaborate upon this in the next section but, to oversimplify, the id is the small child who lives on in each of us. It proceeds in accordance with the *primary process* and the *pleasure principle*. "Primary process" refers to both a *method of handling mental forces* and a *mode of cognition*. In regard to the former, the id, like the small child, is incessantly striving to fulfill its desires. In this quest it brooks no delay, takes no account of the requirements of reality, and repays frustration with rage. If the primary object of its fantasies is absent, it will take another. If the spouse toward whom one is angry is out, the children will do as well. When the mate is away and one has sexual and affectionate needs, a "pick-up" will suffice. The idea of postponing gratification and enduring present pain for future gain is totally foreign to it.

This manner of handling one's wishes accords with the *pleasure principle*. Basically, this means that the human organism strives to maximize pleasurable sensations and minimize unpleasurable or painful ones. Internal needs and noxious environmental stimuli are associated with an *increase in psychic tension*. This is unpleasurable, and the mind seeks to reduce the tension by gratifying the need or moving away from the offending external stimulus. The pleasure principle applies to the ego, as well as to the id, but the former functions in symphony with a modification of it known as the *reality principle*, which is discussed subsequently.

The primary process mode of cognition, as opposed to that of handling psychic energy, is characteristic not only of the id, but of unconscious parts of the ego and superego as well. It is, however, more purely represented in the id than elsewhere. The primary process is called, in common parlance, "childish thinking," "wishful thinking," or the "logic of the emotions," and hearkens back to the early years of life. It is characteristic of the conscious lives of children and psychotics, the symptoms of neurotics, and the dreams, daydreams, wit, artistic endeavors, and unconsciouses of all of us.

Primary process thinking is dominated by *affect-laden, wish-fulfilling fantasy*. At the level of the id these fantasies are expressed in pictures, the earliest form of thinking in us all. It is only when these fantasies, or their derivatives, reach the level of the ego that they are translated into words. Intimately related to this pictorialization is *symbolization:* expression by way of similes, metaphors, and allusions. Freud opined that there were certain universal symbols, e.g., snake for penis, or house for body or woman. However, for the most part he believed that a symbol could be understood only within the historical and current context of the particular individual. Neurotic symptoms are symbolic communications. The next chapter describes, for example, a man whose hysterical paraplegia expressed the unconscious idea, "I can't stand up to my wife." *Condensation* and *displacement* are other primary process mechanisms and are closely connected to symbolization. The former is the telescoping of several ideas and feelings into one symbol or communication. For example, an elderly gentleman in a dream might personify, simultaneously, one's father, boss, teacher, the policeman who ticketed one the day before, as well as certain split-off parts of oneself. Displacement is the disassociation of an affective charge from the idea with which it belongs and its transfer to an item with which it is unrelated. An example would be a dream in which the most intense affect was associated with the least significant content, while the important fantasies were accompanied by tranquility or boredom.

In primary process cognition the *sense of time* is absent, or at least distorted. This is best exemplified in dreams where persons from the remotest past and most recent present rub shoulders with one another and where cause and effect relationships and chronological orders are often reversed. Diametrically opposing and logically incompatible ideas may coexist peacefully, as is best illustrated in the apparent absurdity and contradictoriness of many dreams, in the communications of children and psychotics, and in many puns, jokes, and riddles.

The impulsions of the id scan, via the perceptual apparatus of the ego, the environment for suitable objects toward whom to express themselves. Conversely, external cues may stimulate its fantasies from a state of quiescence to one of intense activity, e.g., the sight of a man resembling her father may excite a woman's unconscious incestuous fantasies. Apart from this, the id is relatively uneducable by, and impervious to, the demands of reality. Left to its own, the id would ride roughshod over all the traditional taboos and imperatives of society. In classical political metaphor, the id is the energetic yet raucous mob while the ego is the organizing and governing elite.

Freud viewed the fantasies and preoccupations of the id as timeless. For him, childhood wishes continue to strive for expression, their intensity and content unaltered by the passage of time, like ancient relics safe from decay in their tombs. Actually, these fantasies are not so timeless and static as Freud believed. They continually jostle up against other fantasies, the forces of ego and superego, and perceptions from the real world (as represented to it by the ego), and inevitably undergo some alteration in the process. Nevertheless, it is useful to conceptualize them as *relatively* timeless and *relatively* impervious to the demands of reality. The perennial pressing of these prehistoric fantasies for expression *is* responsible for a good deal of the recurrent themes one encounters in any history. Whole lives can be organized around a few powerful unconscious fantasies. Freud would come to view the persistence of these fantasies and of the primary process into ages and situations where they are inappropriate as the hallmark of psychopathology.

## The Superego

The *superego* is that portion of the psychic apparatus, partly conscious, mostly unconscious, which represents to us the *pre*scriptions and *pro*scriptions of the outside world: the "thou shalts" and "thou shalt nots." The former, the positive goals and aspirations toward which we strive, are often considered a subcompartment of the superego, the *ego ideal*. The superego is roughly equivalent to what is popularly termed "conscience," though this is both more and less than the superego. It is more in the sense that conscience includes ego, as well as superego, elements. It is less in the sense that it does not take in the unconscious aspects of our morality that are so characteristic of the superego.

The superego arises from the child's interaction with the authority figures in his environment. In early life these are, of course, parents and parent surrogates, whereas in later life fresh increments to the superego are absorbed from those who unconsciously represent these primal authorities. The superego is formed by *identification* with the parents. It is as if each of us carries around our parents inside our heads where they subject our fantasies (conscious *and* unconscious) and actions to constant scrutiny. The small child actually sees his parents' pointing fingers and hears their scolding voices in his mind's eye and ear respectively. In the course of time these commands become largely depersonified and abstracted, as they are in the adult. Nevertheless, in the most unconscious layers of our superego they retain their personal characteristics and, in psychotic states of regression, may become personified in consciousness once more—the hallucinated "voice of conscience."

The superego exacts the same things of us as did our parents and in the same manner. If they were benign and understanding in their correction of our conduct, then our superego will be likewise. If they were harsh and punitive, then so will our internal moral watchman be to us. If they treated the slightest flickering of sexuality or aggression as anathema, then our superego will too. If they regularly allowed us to carry our impulses beyond the point of no return and then battered us down for it, then so will our superego. If their discipline was fraught with inconsistency and their ideals with hypocrisy and deceit, then our superego will be likewise. If our morality was inculcated through punishment and negative reinforcement, at the expense of positive reinforcement for desirable behavior, then our inhibitions will be strong but our ego ideal, or positive aspirations weak, and we might end up as morose and saintly incompetents. If they were inappropriately indulgent, then either our superego will be correspondingly weak or, if we felt ourselves and our environment insufficiently protected from our fantasies, it will be excessively strong. If they represented values harshly dissonant from those of the culture at large, then the seeds will be sown for conflict between ourselves and our society. If they were either coldly aloof or malignantly present, then there may be insufficient positive affect to nourish the growth of much superego at all.

In the chapter on psychopathology I discuss how the superego may participate in conflict with the id or the ego. The interaction between id and superego is basically the interaction between parent and child. Since large parts of the superego are unconscious, like the id, it is privy to information about our unconscious fantasies to which our ego is not. The superego may be aware of antisocial fantasies of which the ego is not and an *unconscious sense of guilt* and need for punishment can result.

A good example of this is the man who, following a confrontation with his father in which he triumphantly refused to enter the family business, held up a local gas station and virtually waited around for the police to arrive. The psychiatric evaluation of this college graduate, with no prior criminal record, revealed that his assertiveness vis-à-vis the father was a derivative of unconscious patricidal rage. His superego, rooted in the same unconscious, was cognizant of this and a crushing unconscious sense of guilt and need for punishment resulted. It was only after these factors were revealed to him that he accepted legal counsel and strove to advance his case.

This "criminal out of an unconscious sense of guilt" illustrates one other important facet of the superego: that it operates by the principle of the *omnipotence of thoughts* and the *"talion law."* The former is the idea that "wishing makes it so," that the *wish* is not merely the mother to, but is also the equivalent of, the *deed*. The omnipotence of thoughts is characteristic of childhood and its persistence in the superego is an indelible mark of that agency's origins in our distant past. In the aforementioned patient the superego reacted as if unconscious fantasies of murdering the father were tantamount to ending his life. It responded, in accordance with the primitive talion law ("an eye for an eye and a tooth for a tooth"), by leading the son to commit a crime in reality that would net him the sort of punishment he would have deserved had he actually killed his father.

If Freud's initial depiction of the superego as a rigid and unrealistic instrument was in a rather pessimistic light, he came to believe that it was capable of considerable modification within the analytical treatment itself. This was hypothesized to occur in part because of the incorporation of the therapist as a more benign and realistic agent into the superego and ego ideal.

## The Ego

The *ego* is that segment of the psychic apparatus, often referred to as the executive function, that mediates between the forces of the id, the superego, and the current reality of the outside world. It is the ambassador that represents the claims of each upon the others. It is the organ of *adaptation* and strives to keep the forces of the three in some sort of *equilibrium*. The ego aims to secure the maximum amount of gratification of our affect-laden fantasies that is compatible with the demands of internal morality and the environment.

The ego is the locus of the perceptual, motor, mnemonic, affective, defensive, and secondary process intellectual functions. It has *both* conscious and unconscious portions and the latter are characterized, like those of the id and superego, by the operation of the primary process.

Freud saw the ego as emerging out of the contact of the id with the environment. Current psychoanalytic theory contends that the ego, like the id, differentiates itself from an infantile id-ego matrix. In commonsense terms, I view the ego as that set of functions which arises from the interaction between one's biological endowment and one's experience. The bedrock of the ego is, of course, laid in the interface between our heredity and *early* family environment, but the ego is, to some extent, in a process of continuous growth and development throughout life. Its form and content are the *fruit of one's relationships*. Apart from occasional bursts of personal creativity, insight, and synthesis, the ego operates with what we have been given by, and allowed to take from, others. It is acquired by identification with,[2] and learning from, our parents. It is as if we have a crowd of persons within, each lending us their coping skills, for better or worse.

Freud believed that most of the energy for the formation and operation of the ego was borrowed, or rather enticed, from the aggressive and, especially, sexual "drives" in the id. He thought this was the case because the nucleus of the ego is formed by representations of our parents and the id impulses simply cathect, or direct themselves toward, these representations. In the course of time the ego functions become relatively independent, or *autonomous*, of their power plant in the id. This he called "deinstinctualization," "neutralization," or *sublimation* of drive energy. Nevertheless, in times of conflict this energy might be recalled by rebellious forces in the id or might become bound up in defensive maneuvers of the ego, at the expense of the higher functions of the ego. This he termed *reinstinctualization*, or *deneutralization*, of drive energy. This is why the functions of intellection and judgment can suffer in severe psychopathology. The zone of the ego which is not subject to periodic exaction on the part of the id and the defensive processes is known as the *conflict-free sphere*, and its territory varies from individual to individual. Processes such as locomotion, perception, and logical thinking are relatively autonomous in most of us, though conflicts over aggression or sexuality can lead to hysterical paralyses and sensory deficits, while strong feelings, fantasies, and fears can affect our perception of, and intellectual action upon, reality.

> A good example is the schizophrenic graduate student who was still living, at age 26, with her parents. Her field, reproductive biology, was a thinly veiled sublimation of her preoccupations, present since childhood, about what her parents did in bed. As her repressions began to fail and her incestuous fantasies started surfacing, she became unable to study. What was previously a conflict-free sphere of her ego, her intellectual function, became reinstinctualized.

Conflict is not the only process that can interfere with the functioning of the ego. Fatigue, organic illness, toxic substances, extraordinary ex-

---

[2]Freud believed that there were two ways of relating to objects: by identification and by object cathexis. The former is historically older and can be seen quite clearly in the interactions of small children with the objects in their environment. Normally, it is supplanted by true object cathexis in the adult. Certain adult characters, called by Deutsch (1965) the "as if" personalities, retain this earlier style of relationship with others and change, chameleonlike, with the company they keep. In schizophrenia and other severe psychiatric disturbances, we see a persistence or recrudescence of this older way of relating (see the comments on separation-individuation in this chapter).

ternal stress, and senility can all impair the reality orientation and the defensive capabilities of the ego.[3]

Whereas the id operates by way of the primary process and in accordance with the pleasure principle, the ego functions by way of the *secondary process* and in symphony with the *reality principle*. As is the case with "primary process," "secondary process" refers to both a mode of cognition and a manner of handling feelings and impulses. The former requires little description since it is the *modus operandi* of our conscious adult intellects. Such thinking is verbal and syntactical, logical, linear, goal-directed, and capable of taking into account information from a variety of sources and modifying its course of action accordingly. It operates in accord with the reality principle in that it strives to be as faithful a representation of the real world as possible. This last process is known as its *reality testing* function. Reality testing means the ability to distinguish between stimuli of internal origins and those of external, to differentiate between fantasy and reality. Our internal representation of the world never corresponds point by point with reality, but is always colored, to different degrees, by our history and preoccupations. Nevertheless, with the exception of extreme stress or fatigue, intoxicated states, and dreams, the reality testing of most of us is reasonably intact. This ability is lost in psychotics, who may mistake the internal auditory representation of a parents' voice for an external process in the environment or may allow a projected fantasy to influence their relationship to a real person in the world. Reality testing is, by and large, a learned affair. The foundation for impaired reality testing is laid by parents who themselves distort reality and who teach their offspring to do so. This can also involve telling a child that he does not really feel what he says he feels, that his parents are not actually doing what he has seen them doing, that the love he does not feel is really there, that the person who is abusing him is not actually doing so, and so forth.[4]

The secondary process method of handling the driving forces is also intimately familiar to the consciousness of the mature adult. It too operates in concert with the *reality principle*. That is, although it aims at

---

[3]Later analytic theoreticians, such as Heinz Hartmann, do not believe that all of the ego's energy is derived from the id. They posit a sphere of primary, and not merely secondary, autonomy within the ego. Freud viewed the mind as an hydraulic, closed system with finite quantities of instinctual energy flowing from compartment to compartment. To give to the ego or superego is to remove from the id, and vice versa. Operationally, this is a useful idea. Every therapist knows that people whose "mental energies" are tied up in conflict or who are in the grip of intense affect seem to have less left over for the ego's reality-oriented functioning. Nevertheless, if this idea is *reified*, to mean that the functioning of the cortical substrate of the ego is fueled by sexual hormones, it becomes incorrect.

[4]See page 41.

the reduction of tension as much as does the id, it takes into account the requirements, possibilities, and limitations of the environment. It is capable of binding forces and tolerating a little present pain or frustration in the interest of adaptation or at the prospect of greater pleasure in the future.

The ego is the home of such free will or conscious volition as we possess. It is also the headquarters of the *defense mechanisms*—those devices, ranging on a continuum from consciousness to (mostly) unconsciousness. It is their responsibility to hold back from conscious awareness and access to the motor apparatus those feeling-toned fantasies that run counter to the demands of current reality or of the superego. The keystone of these defensive maneuvers is, of course, repression. Defense mechanisms can also be directed against perceptions from the external world. Perceptions from outside which excite some sort of conflict or pain within the psychic organism itself can be selectively inattended to or replaced by wish-fulfilling, reality-denying hallucinations. Such a process is often subserved by addiction to drugs or alcohol. In the next chapter I shall elaborate upon the role of the defense mechanisms in psychopathology and shall enumerate, define, and exemplify the major ones.

Earlier in this section I introduced the idea that we are composed of the internal representations of numerous people who were once, or still are, in the external world. At this point I wish to return to this concept and flesh it out in relationship to the ego, especially to that function known as the *self*, that congeries of representations of ourselves formed from interactions with a variety of objects. Otto Kernberg and other contemporary ego psychologists[5] have taught us to conceptualize the internal representations, or depictions, of the interactions between the self and its object as a tripartite constellation. This consists of a picture of 1) the *self* and 2) the *object*, colored in by 3) the *affective tone* of the

---

[4]It is thus best to conceptualize disturbances in reality testing along a continuum. For instance, the normal-neurotic, in day-to-day transactions with his fellows, may act at times as if his boss or colleagues were harboring expectations or evaluations of him similar to those of his father. The neurotic, in the heat of a transference neurosis, may feel intensely that his analyst is feeling and acting toward him as did his father, but he will know, in some corner of his mind, that this is merely his own interpretation. The borderline, in a transference psychosis, by contrast, "knows" that his therapist is in fact feeling and acting toward him exactly as did his father. The schizophrenic carries this still further and may be convinced that his therapist actually *is* his father.

[5]"Id psychology" refers to the earlier phase of psychoanalysis in which the predominant interest was the vicissitudes of the "instinctual drives." In *Group Psychology and the Analysis of the Ego* (1921) and *The Ego and the Id* (1923), Freud laid the foundations for *ego psychology*, the concern with the reality-orienting and defensive operations of the ego.

interaction. In the next section we shall examine the developmental process in the formation and representation of self and objects.

The main point is that part of the ego, both conscious and unconscious, known technically as the *self*, including the "self-image" and "self-esteem," is largely determined by how our environment has acted upon, and reacted to, us. Simply put, *we view and esteem ourselves as others have viewed and esteemed us.*

All this is best conveyed by metaphor. Think of the self-esteem as a balance, on one end of which is placed each and every negatively toned (frustrating, angry, hurtful, fearful, rejecting) interaction with parents, while on the other is settled the positively toned (affectionate, concerned, and need-satisfying) interactions with them. Every time a small boy with a bat and ball is turned away by his father, every time a child is physically or emotionally abused, a contribution is made to one side of the scale. Every time a parent engages in warm and loving face-to-face interaction with the child, conveys positive expectations of him, acknowledges and rewards his achievements, takes appropriate steps to protect him from danger, or firmly but kindly guides his socialization, an increment is added to the other. By the close of early childhood, the so-called "formative" years, each scale tips one way or the other, and the direction inevitably, almost irrevocably, determines the human being's self-esteem and achievement for the rest of his life. This prototypical self-esteem functions as the foundation upon which we lay, the screen through which we filter, others' and our own evaluations of ourselves for as long as we live. If the balance leans in the positive direction, we have a solid sense that we are lovable and worthwhile upon which to build concrete achievements. These achievements in turn redound upon the self-esteem and a beneficent circle is set in motion. If, however, the scale tips toward the opposite pole, we feel unlovable and worthless and we achieve accordingly. We behave in such a way as to elicit the untoward reactions we both expect and fear, and fail to appreciate data that run counter to our self-concept. All this reinforces our negative self-image and a vicious circle is initiated. Or, we might achieve mightily and yet feel worthless, incompetent, and unlovable inside.

Once such a mechanism is set in motion, insight-oriented psychotherapy, in which the patient not only gains insight into the origins of his damaged self-esteem, but eventually internalizes the therapist's consistent esteem of him, is usually the only hope. In the next chapter I shall describe some patients in whom self-esteem looms as the central problem. Indeed, there is considerable evidence that such disorders form much of what the modern therapist sees.

The ego is the agent with which the psychotherapist negotiates. All interactions, whether with the patient's id or superego, are mediated through the ego. It is our ally in the psychotherapeutic process, the patient's one avenue out of the prison of historical determinism. It is the structure whose power all forms of psychotherapy ultimately strive to support. As Freud said, "Where id [and superego, he might have added] was, there shall ego be."

## PERSONALITY DEVELOPMENT

The impact of childhood on adult character has long been recognized. "As the twig is bent, so the tree will grow," goes the cliché. It took Freud, however, to remind psychiatrists of this common knowledge and to systematize it and found it on a scientific basis. From psychotherapeutic and investigative work with adult neurotics he inferred certain truths about childhood development in all of us. Although he never worked directly with children himself,[6] his theories of maturation have been amply documented by those who have.

Most broadly, and in the ideal, development moves from childish to adult modes of operation, from unconsciousness to consciousness, from primary process to secondary process, from pleasure principle to reality principle, from dependency to autonomy, and from determinism to free will. Freud conceptualized psychopathology as *the persistence into adulthood of infantile ways of coping*. The psychotherapist is concerned, simplistically, either with those who have failed to grow up or with those who, having tasted the fruits of adulthood and found them bitter, have returned to the safety of childhood.

Dynamic psychiatrists believe that traumata in childhood play a crucial role in the development of psychiatric disorders in adulthood. Freud stated emphatically that there is a childhood neurosis behind every adult one. Other investigators failed to realize this simply because they never took detailed histories of their patients' childhood development. Freud gave trauma the central place in his developmental theory of psychopathology. *Trauma* refers to either inappropriate and excessive gratification or deprivation and active abuse. A trauma can be a single, isolated event like the death of a nurturer or, more commonly, a series of repeated events like inadequate mothering or sexual abuse.

Freud believed that the traumata of early life played a role out of all proportion to their apparent significance because of the immaturity of the infant's means of coping with reality and strong affect. The same event e.g., the death of a parent, that could be mastered with mild to moderate difficulty at the age of 30 would be devastating at three. Freud (1939, pp. 184-185) expressed it eloquently in a biological metaphor:

> It seems that neuroses are acquired only in early childhood (up to the age of six), even though their symptoms may not make their appearance till

---

[6]He analyzed, through the patient's father (also an analyst), a phobic child known to posterity as "Little Hans."

much later. The childhood neurosis may become manifest for a short time or may even be overlooked. . . . There is no difficulty in accounting for this aetiological preference for the first period of childhood. The neuroses are, as we know, disorders of the ego; and it is not to be wondered at if the ego, so long as it is feeble, immature and incapable of resistance, fails to deal with tasks with which it could cope with later on with the utmost ease. In these circumstances, instinctual demands from within, no less than excitations from the external world, operate as "traumas," particularly if they are met halfway by certain innate dispositions. . . . The damage inflicted on the ego by its first experiences gives us the appearance of being disproportionately great; *but we have only to take as an analogy the differences in the results produced by the prick of a needle into a mass of cells in the act of cell division (as in Roux's experiments) and into the fully grown animal which eventually develops out of them* [my italics].

Trauma leads to the *fixation* of a certain amount of psychical energy (fantasies, fears, and affects, for all practical purposes) in the stage at which it occurred. Hereafter one may move forward, but there remains a weak spot at the point of trauma. Stressors in adulthood, sufficiently similar to the early ones, can lead to a *regression* to the phase of fixation or to the one anterior to it.

There is considerable evidence that, as Freud thought, the nature and timing of these early traumata are specifically related to the form of psychopathology in adulthood, e.g., that oral trauma is particularly important to schizophrenia, anal trauma to obsessive-compulsive disorder, and oedipal trauma to hysteria. Nevertheless, I advocate thinking in terms of the child's *development as a whole* (from 0 to 18) rather than casting about for whoppers from the oral, anal, or oedipal periods that polarized him, once and for all, toward psychopathology. The foundation for adult character (including its psychopathological manifestations) is laid, not by events in any given period of two or three years, but by the total pattern of life experiences in childhood and adolescence. Indeed, as I shall emphasize later in this chapter, personality continues to be formed by life history subsequent to adolescence. If it did not, how could psychotherapy itself stand any chance of working? In short, it is the *style of interaction* between the child and his parents (and significant others), throughout all the periods, in which you are interested.

Freud posited five stages of psychological development, whereas Erikson, who reformulated them from a more psycho*social* point of view, cited eight. I shall refer to the terminology of both men in this account, as well as draw on the work of Margaret Mahler on separation-individuation, Harry Stack Sullivan on latency, and Daniel Levinson on adult development.

Freud termed this process psycho*sexual* development since he believed it was largely the story of the evolution of the libidinal drive. He felt this drive, which is not to be confused with genital sexuality *per se* and which Fenichel has more aptly termed "organ pleasure," moved from a preoccupation with the oral to the anal to the genital zones. He referred to these as *erotogenic* or *erogenous* zones and referred to the libidinal drive associated with the oral and anal regions as the "component instincts." It was only in the phallic or, more accurately, in the even later *genital* period that Freud thought the component instincts were brought together in subservience, as foreplay, to genital sexuality. Perversions and neuroses result when there is a fixation at, or regression to, these pregenital modes of sensual satisfaction. Such fantasies are consciously acted out by perverts, whereas in neurotics they remain unconscious, though still influencing behavior, as symptoms.

It is less important to cleave to Freud's notions about the ultimate (e.g., instinctual) nature of that which develops than to grasp a general idea of the regularities in the process itself and of problems that can arise at points along the way. Most importantly, one cannot understand adult psychopathology (or personality in general) without reference to childhood. Dynamic psychiatry, to reiterate, is the study of *mental experience*, that which is symbolically mediated and potentially communicable from one person to another. This experience, as I stated earlier, arises in some as yet inexplicable way from the *interaction* between *body* and *world*. Mental experience includes our experience of our bodies, our worlds, and the interaction between the two. We can currently speak to the ultimate nature of the biological substrate of *mind* (e.g., the organization of mental experience) no more than we can speak to the ultimate nature of its environmental one. As dynamic psychiatrists we are concerned, not with sorting out the purely biological components in our fantasies, feelings, and fears, but with our *experience* of *body-in-world*.[7]

Rather than viewing this development as nothing more than the unfolding of biologically predetermined processes and instinctual drives, one should conceptualize it as the evolution of the organization of the forces within the individual and of his relationship to the environment—as that which results from the interaction between biological maturation and experience. As I have mentioned previously, none of our impulses, even the most biologically based ones, exists apart from internal representations of the objects toward whom they are directed; conversely, none of the objects in the external world "exists" for us

---

[7]In combating premature attempts to correlate phenomenology with neurobiological happenings, Sullivan (1953, pp. 82-83) enjoined us to "recognize that what we know comes to us through our *experiencing* events, and is therefore always separated from anything really formed or transcendentally real by the limited channels through which we contact what we presume to be the perduring, unknown universe. So if a person really thinks that his thoughts about nerves and synapses and the rest have a higher order of merit than his thoughts about signs and symbols, all I can say is, Heaven, help him!"

apart from the manner in which they impinge upon our bodily sensory apparatus. Dynamic psychiatry takes equally seriously the body and the world as the places in which we live.

In line with this, when I use terms like the "oral," "anal," and "phallic" *zones*, I am referring, not to depots where certain quantities of component instinct are stored but, like Sullivan, to the organism's *zones of interaction* with its environment. The "polymorphous perverse" pleasure of infantile sexuality is derived from the exercise of these zones. Similarly, when I refer to the "oral," "anal," and "phallic" *modes*, I am alluding, like Schafer (1976), not to different patterns of flow of libido, but to the infantile human's particular ways of *desiring* and of *experiencing* and *interpreting* the body and its relationship to the environment.

Initially, all our perceptions of self and world are organized in the categories of basic bodily sensation and primitive bodily need. Our first experiences of self and world, even before we are able to differentiate the former from the latter, are *physical sensations* such as sights, sounds, smells, alimentary processes, pain, and sensations of warmth, cold, and our mother's skin. As we progressively differentiate between outside and inside, we paint pictures of self and world which are at first representations of our *bodily experiences of them*. Our prototypical image of self, for example, is intimately bound up with our experience and perception of our bodies. As Freud phrased this, the ego is first of all a "body ego." Upon this foundation of the representation of one's physical being (and derived from it) are laid all our subsequent characterizations of self, no matter how "decorporealized," no matter how abstract and ethereal, they may ultimately become. Indeed, things like physical aging, the loss of body parts or functions, and weight gain or loss will affect our self-image until the day we die. Similarly, the fashion in which the world *impinges upon our body* and it upon the world is the bedrock upon which is built—no matter how sophisticated and abstract it eventually becomes—our image of world.

To some extent, these early body-based modes of perceiving, organizing, and interpreting the experiences of self-in-world continue, more or less unconsciously, throughout our existence. For example, the conscious sense of well-being in the infant is inseparable from and dependent upon the absence of physical pain and the presence of sensations of nipple-in-mouth, gastric fullness, and warm body contact with mother. Conversely, his sense of despair is inseparable from the presence of painful stimuli or the sensation of gastric emptiness and the absence, when he desires it, of mother's warm body. Adults continue, unconsciously, to associate contentment and despair with these infantile modes of categorizing experience. Depressed persons describe themselves as "empty," "drained," "isolated," "alienated," "out of contact," "cold," "in pain," and "hurting" without recognizing that, unconsciously, they mean this in the quite *literal*, bodily sense as well as in the more abstract, "decorporealized" sense. By contrast, secure and satisfied people depict themselves as *"full* of joy," "in *touch* with the surroundings," "experiencing the *warm glow* of contentment," and "comfortable," equally unconscious of the enduring infantile bodily associations to these happy states.

The obsessive-compulsive favors expletives like "shit" or "crap" without realizing that, unconsciously, he is literally tossing turds, not words, about the room as both gifts and missiles. Alternately, when he is verbally withholding, it is unconsciously feces, as well as feelings, with which he refuses to part. Such behavior is intimately bound up with infantile dominance-submission, expulsion-retention issues in which tasks like the mastery of bladder and bowels play a paradigmatic role.

Men preoccupied with issues of masculine self-esteem use phrases like "I want to be one of the big dicks," "she had me by the balls," "he made me feel small," or "I got screwed," without recognizing that unconsciously they perceive and interpret all their interactions along the lines of sexual battles in which one is the castrater and one the castrate, one the rapist and one the raped.

In short, part of the dictum from Chapter 1 (that we live concurrently in past and present) is that we experience, again simultaneously, our self-in-world in two modes: an earlier, more purely bodily based one (corresponding to primary process) and a later, more abstract and dematerialized one (equivalent to secondary process). For example, a person may be seeking sympathy on one level and looking for breast milk on another; a sculptor may be fashioning a Greek goddess from clay on one level and playing with feces on another; a man may be arguing with his boss on one level and fighting for his penis on another; a woman may be longing for the magical interpretation from her male therapist on the one hand and desiring to possess his penis on the other. Although it is easy to identify the continued operation of these childhood modes of desiring and categorizing of experience as they manifest themselves in the symbols current in songs, literature, advertising, slang, swear words, jokes, or figures of speech, one will never have more than an intellectualized appreciation of them unless he has been in therapy long enough to experience them in himself and has carried a long-term insight-oriented treatment to completion.

## The Oral Phase

Freud called the earliest stage of psychological development the *oral* stage because the infant's primary zone of interaction with its surroundings is through the mucosa of its oral cavity and alimentary canal and the epithelial surface, or skin, of its body. Erikson has termed this period that of *basic trust versus mistrust* to convey the profound degree to which the early mother-infant interaction determines the human's subsequent attitude toward, and expectations from, his environment. Both men believe that this period lasts about 18 months.

Because no infant can give us a coherent verbal account of his dawning experience of self and world, much that I shall present about his perception and internal representation is by necessity inferential and speculative. Nevertheless, these hypotheses have to some extent been supported by observation of children and by work with adult schizophrenics and borderlines who, we posit, regress to these earlier modes of representation and experience.

The newborn infant lives almost exclusively in the unconscious, has no sense of himself nor of his mother as separate and distinct entities, and operates entirely by the primary process and in accordance with the pleasure principle. He is, as he has been facetiously called, an "id with a mouth on it." Mouthing, gastrointestinal sensations, and bodily contact are his sole modes of interaction with the world. They are simultaneously his primary sources of pleasure, the dawning manifestations of infantile sexuality.

In his lack of a clear-cut internal representation of self or mother, much less of the *distinction* between the two, the infant exists in a state of oceanic oneness with his universe. He lives in a half-waking, half-sleeping, objectless, subjectless blur of sights, sounds, and bodily sensations. Since there is not even the most rudimentary conceptual differentiation between inside and outside, it is meaningless to speak of reality testing at this stage. We opine that the severe disorientation of schizophrenia is, in some respects, a hearkening back to this experience. This infantile state of nirvana is what Freud called primary narcissism and what Mahler terms the normal *autistic* phase.

Gradually, after four to eight weeks, the infant begins to paint the dimmest internal portraits of himself and of the objects in his environment, though there is still no sense that he and mother are not somehow melded into a single omnipotent system. In other words, these pictures are of the *interactions* between the undifferentiated self and the undifferentiated object, rather than of a separate and distinct self interacting with an equally separate and distinct object. This is known as the *normal symbiosis* of infancy. Over the next days and weeks the infant grows increasingly attentive to his environment. There is growing evidence that he can respond differentially to stimuli from outside and to those from inside, though the ability to distinguish between the two (reality testing) remains rudimentary. Furthermore, insofar as he relates to mother as a separate object at all, it is as various *part-objects*: a smile, hands, a breast. Insofar as he has an image of self (which, at this stage, is equivalent to *body*), it is as a jumble of unintegrated parts and sensations. In short, he has *integrated* the body parts of himself into a coherent representation of self no more than he has integrated those of mother into a coherent representation of object.

It is assumed that at times when mother is unavailable and needs present themselves, the infant resorts to hallucinatory wish-fulfillment as a temporary means of meeting his needs. We assume that the halluci-nations of adult psychotics are in part a reactivation of this primeval mode of satisfying one's wishes.

At the same time that he begins to have a dawning awareness of his apartness from mother, he is yet unable to *hold* an internal representa-tion of her for any length of time. Because of this there arises the first danger situation: *losing the loved object* (which at this stage would be tantamount to losing the self). Fear of this eventually leads the infant to repress his frustration-born rageful responses to mother and to conform his behavior to her demands—to become educable, in other words. This education, which forms the early nucleus of his ego and superego, also occurs by means of identification with the mother and with her differen-tial reward of desired behaviors and punishment of undesirable ones. Schizophrenic adults, whose preponderant traumata have occurred at this age, likewise have a deficient ability to hold in mind the representa-tions of important others. This accounts in part for the schizophrenic's extreme vulnerability to separation.

Genuine separation-individuation begins from four to six months of age. We surmise that this comes about, in part, because of the infant's differential experience of his own body and because of inevitable frustra-tions at the hands of his mother. As for the first, the infant learns, as Sullivan (1953, p. 14) said, that his body, as opposed to the objects around him, both feels and is felt: "The mouth feels the thumb, and the thumb feels the mouth; that is self-sentience." As for the second, he discovers that certain objects (such as the breast) do not always appear regardless of how much he may wish for them, whereas others (such as his thumb) are available at will.

The generalized smile becomes the specific and preferential smiling response for mother and is a sure sign that the infant recognizes her as an object unlike all others and that bonding between mother and child has occurred. In the following months there is increasing *differentiation* between the infant's representation of self and that of mother. The *integration* of the various perceptions of self and object seems, however, to lag behind.

In what is termed the *preambivalent* mode of object relations, the infant melds together the pictures of mother taken in positively toned interac-tions with her into one composite photograph, the "good mother," and those of her from negatively toned interactions into another, the "bad mother." In other words he is incapable of comprehending that the same human being may be tender and gratifying at one moment and depriving, punitive, and anxiety provoking the next. At the same time that he forms two representations of mother, he forms two representations of self: a "good me" from his positively tinged contacts with her and a "bad me" from his frustrating, rageful, anxious, and hurtful ones. In other words, the infant's sense of self, his *identity*, comes from how he is responded to by others quite as much as does his sense of the world. We come to know ourselves, in other words, through our reflections in mirrors and in others.

If our contact with nurturers is reasonably satisfying, we form a benign and optimistic image of self and environment. If our parents have responded to us as worthwhile, we feel basically worthy and expect the environment to react to us as such. If, on the other hand, the preponderance of our interactions with early nurturers are malignant and frustrating, we feel basically unworthy and expect our world to react to us as such. If the early negative experiences are intense and frequent enough, we remain unable to integrate the good and bad mother on the one hand, and the good and bad self on the other, into coherent representations. In "borderline" and schizophrenic disorders, there is a persistence of this "splitting" mechanism, where it becomes used to ward off the anxiety secondary to conflict.

If one does not believe that the formation of a coherent sense of self and world is this great a struggle, let him watch his own child's reaction when he teases him by calling him by another name or plays the bogeyman or makes faces for a bit too long. "No, I'm Billy," he will angrily and nervously call back in the case of the former and "Daddy? Daddy? Stop! Stop!" in the latter. Young children cannot yet joke about something as precariously established as their sense of self and of others.

Let me illustrate regression to the *preambivalent* mode in two patients, both schizophrenic. The first developed a pattern of lying on the floor in front of the radiator following angry outbursts at me. From his fetal position and associations it was plain that he was acting out a partly conscious, partly unconscious, fantasy of returning to the womb. Its purpose was, he later said quite succinctly, to "go back to a time before I could both love and hate my parents." He regressed to this preambivalent state as an attempt to avoid his rage at the loved objects and his fear of their destroying, or being destroyed by, him.

The second was a young woman who was incapable of tolerating the pain and disillusionment attendant upon recognizing that it was one and the same mother who both suckled and abused her. She had in some respects never moved beyond this preambivalent phase and in others had regressed to it. This patient addressed me by one of several names, depending on how she happened to feel about me at the moment and on whether I seemed to be in a depriving or gratifying mood.

It took me some time to appreciate that she was not merely speaking metaphorically, but that she perceived me, quite literally, as different human beings.

In this dawning stage of the separation-individuation process, when the infant is beginning to be cognizant of the mother as a separate object (or conglomeration of part objects) whose presence and absence he cannot control, he adopts a variety of *transitional objects*, toy furry animals, pieces of clothing, dolls, and so forth, designed to represent the mother in her absence. My own son carried a blanket which he called "Ga Ga." They need such objects because they are still unable to hold the representation of mother in mind. That such objects continue to be cherished by many children well into the fifth and sixth years attests to the fact that the ability to fix an image of the other in mind is a slow and gradual process. These "security blankets" are called *transitional* objects because they are midway between the actual mother and the internal representation of her. They are not "out there" as much as the real mother and yet not "inside" as much as a stable mental representation of her. They are also *transitional* in yet another sense: they represent in part the mother and in part the self (since they not only take on the smell and soil of the self but are totally manipulated, as is a body part, by it).

By eight to nine months the integration and differentiation of self and object have proceeded to the point that mother's image has some distinctness in the infant's mind, although he remains unable to retain it for any length of time. This is the time of *stranger anxiety*, when he is painfully and acutely aware of the difference between Mom and not-Mom. The fact that this anxiety is markedly alleviated when mother enters the room shows that the fear is as much one of losing the mother as of the stranger himself.

The time from 10 or 12 to 16 or 18 months has been termed by Mahler the *practicing subphase* of the separation-individuation process. The infant's motor power has improved greatly and he is actively exploring his world. What Winnicott calls the "good enough mother" allows him the space and independence he needs and yet conveys the calm assurance that out of sight he is not out of mind, and that she will function as a solid and stationary home base. We have all seen young explorers alternate, in ever-widening arcs, between moving out and checking back to home base. This refueling is necessary because his ability to keep in mind a picture of mother's friendly interaction with him is still deficient. The subsequent phase of separation-individuation will be examined in the section on the anal phase.

It is now appreciated that one other important facet of the development of a distinct and integrated representation of self, gender identity, has proceeded quite some distance by the end of the oral period. Indeed, there is much evidence that if the boy is responded to as a girl, and vice versa, a firm foundation for later gender identity disturbances can be laid as early as the second year of life (see Stoller, and Kernberg).

Freud believed the oral phase was characterized by a particular constellation of virtually universal fantasies, among them the wish to devour the nurturing object, to incorporate it quite literally and not merely psychologically. In fact, there is a devouring quality to the neediness of the young infant, and any mother who has breastfed a child has felt the aggressiveness, as well as the affection, in this need. In severely regressed psychotics we sometime see the resurrection of these primal cannibalistic fantasies. It is the fear of losing the mother that causes the young child to repress these incorporative fantasies—fantasies born of both affection and frustration-induced rage. As discussed later, it is posited that this internalized and repressed rage, if it is sufficient, can serve as the foundation for a depressive disposition in adolescence and adulthood.

It is crucial that the psychotherapist understand the vicissitudes of the oral phase and of the separation-individuation process since traumata in this period assume great importance in adult character formation and psychopathology. Indeed, dynamic psychiatrists believe that significant traumata in this earliest of all stages can lead to the most severe disturbance in adulthood: the schizophrenias; borderline, schizotypal, narcissistic, antisocial, and addictive character disorders; and the depressive psychoses. Less severe but significant oral traumata (deprivation or overindulgence) are associated with a particular personality type, the "oral character," distinguished by issues of dependence versus independence, excessive reliance on outside injections for the maintenance of a positive self-esteem, self-centeredness, difficulty tolerating deprivation and postponing gratification, tendency to react to frustration with overwhelming rage, tendency toward substance abuse, devouring needs that often wear the objects out, a difficulty giving to and nurturing others, and a proneness to depression.

It should be emphasized, however, that merely because persons with these disorders and character types seem to have experienced more early trauma than those with neuroses, their entire character structure and psychopathology cannot be explained solely with reference to the oral period. After all, they continue to be reared, throughout all the stages of development, by the same family and social system that presented them with their first traumata. Inadequate or malignant parenting, and maladaptive reactions thereto, do not cease at the end of one stage but proceed, in varying degree, through all of them. Hence, most patients' psychopathology has multiple roots in eras extending from infancy to adolescence and early adulthood. Most schizophrenics, for example, have not only "oral" but "anal" and "phallic" pathology as well. This is true in part because damage in an earlier phase of development interferes not only with functioning in that period but with one's ability to successfully negotiate the tasks of succeeding ones.

I shall now discuss more explicitly what can go wrong in this primal stage of human psychological development. Mothers have received a good deal of bad press from psychiatry. They have been blamed for a host of problems in their offspring from schizophrenia and depression to delinquency. The faultfinding has centered heavily on their role in the traumata of the oral period. There is both truth and falsity in such claims, and in the interest of equity we must attend to both. In addition, one cannot overlook that in recent years fathers have become accountable as well.

First, it is true that the vulnerable and impressionable infant does not come into this world fully formed, but that he must be molded by his environment, and in the majority of instances it is the mother who models and conditions his behavior. Hence, she cannot help but have a tremendous impact on his unfolding biological potentialities. However, it is also true that infants differ biologically among themselves. Some are more, some less, attentive; some are more, some less, irritable; and some are more, some less, responsive to affection. Also, circumstances differ from mother to mother and, at times, over the course of one woman's motherhood itself. For example, being the mother of a third newborn at a time of marital and economic strife is quite different from being a mother of one or two children during marital and financial equilibrium.

Second, it is true that deficient nurturing, physical and emotional abuse, poor role modeling, and faulty conditioning can form a matrix upon which subsequent psychopathology is laid. However, it is also true that no mother ever willfully and systematically set out to warp her child. Mothers "mother" as they were mothered. There is nothing more fascinating than going back several generations in the family of a schizophrenic and seeing the same tragic mistakes being passed down the line. The clinician must allow his patient, as he discovers the errors that were committed on him, to hate and blame these parents and to feel entitled to do so. However, at the same time the therapist must apply his knowledge of historical determinism to the patient's parent as much as to the patient himself, and suspend moral judgment. Indeed, many if not most of these mothers could as well have been his patients as their children. A mother cannot give unto others if she has not been given to. If a mother was a deprived child herself, every demand of the infant will set off a chain of hurt, frustration, and rage going back to childhood, all of which will further interfere with her ability to care for the infant.

Third, to be logically consistent, if we blame the mothers for the pathology of their offspring, we must give them some of the credit for such coping skills as these children possess, as well as for those of their nonschizophrenic children. Fourth, as discussed subsequently, good mothering is an almost impossible task. Not one but a series of evolving behavior patterns is required of the mother who would be in synchrony with her child's development. Patterns of mothering appropriate to a four-month-old are grossly inappropriate for the burgeoning toddler. Some mothers do quite well in one stage but then, for some reason or other, are unable to make the shift required in another.

The disturbances of early life center around deprivation, active abuse, and overindulgence. Deprivation is by far the most common, particularly if one includes loss under this category, but I shall begin with the category of overindulgence and move on to those of deprivation and abuse.

A mother may be oversolicitous for a variety of reasons including a reaction formation against unconscious resentment or out of an attempt to make up for inadequacies in the mothering she herself received. This presents no problem in the very early phase in which mother and child exist in an undifferentiated amalgam. Indeed, an optimally attentive mother, whose supplies tightly interlock with her infant's needs, is ideal in this stage. Many therapists feel that most adult schizophrenics have been denied this infantile paradise and feel they must, after a fashion, go back and get it with the therapist: the therapeutic symbiosis. Later on, however, if the mother keeps up this behavior then the infant experiences insufficient frustration to adequately differentiate himself from her. Some of the usual coping mechanisms for dealing with frustration and anxiety and for obtaining mother's presence will develop late or not at all. A humorous story about a five-year-old who had never spoken illustrates this second point. One day at dinner, he surprised the whole family by blurting out, "The soup's cold." When the astonished mother asked why he had not talked before, he said, "Everything was all right until now!"

Often such overindulgence depends upon the child meeting certain of the mother's *conditions*: that he fulfill her need to feel wanted and appreciated and that he deny his own autonomy, independence, and any anger that develops toward her. Such conditions, tolerable to the infant and young toddler, soon become insufferable to him. The mother, in the practicing subphase, must be an interested and receptive fueling station, but she must give the toddler free rein. If she is anxiously and oppressively hovering, he will come to view the world as a dangerous place and will form a low opinion of his own abilities. The mother, on her part, will begin to get something she did not bargain for and which will seem like the most heinous ingratitude—his rage. The child must then either repress this anger and sacrifice his individuality or battle with her and risk losing the loved object.

More usual than wholesale overindulgence is indulgence in some areas and deprivation in others. For example, food or toys may be showered upon the infant as a substitute for affection and parental time. This leads logically to the category of deprivation, which is responsible for the overwhelming majority of problems arising out of early childhood. I shall be referring to the deprivation, not of food, but to a special class of nutrients—affection. If the deprivation of cuddling and rocking is early and severe enough, as Rene Spitz found in his study of a Mexican foundling home, it can be as lethal as the deprivation of biological nutrients. Many of these otherwise well-fed infants became lethargic and apathetic, and simply gave up and died. Spitz termed this response *anaclitic* depression. Less severe deprivation may not lead to death, but can form the foundation for lifelong depression, low self-esteem, and pessimistic expectations of the world.

Deprivation which begins in the oral period usually does not stop there, but extends throughout childhood. The emotionally deprived child feels hurt and angry. He may internalize this anger rather than direct it toward the parents and risk abuse or a further loss of nurturance. Eventually he comes to feel they must be avoiding him for good reasons—that, in other words, there must be something wrong with *him*. He must be bad and getting what he deserves. He grows to expect that others will treat him likewise and will handle himself accordingly. All this ties in intimately with my comments in the previous section on self-esteem.

Children respond to such deprivation in one of two ways. They either internalize their rage, become depressed, and resignedly withdraw or else they throw tantrums and become terrors in order to receive attention. It may seem incomprehensible, but children prefer negative attention to none at all. This can be documented again and again. Of course, this latter behavior does not get them their desired results either. Either behavior pattern, carried forward into adulthood, guarantees the continued frustration of their emotional needs.

I shall describe two cases in which early deprivation played an important role:

> F. was a 17-year-old schizoid male. From my interviews with him and the social worker's interviews with his mother, a good deal of information about the early mother-child interaction was obtained. First, it is important to note that the mother herself was handed over to a series of nannies by her own rich and socially self-conscious mother. She was quite consciously aware of the deficiencies in the mothering she herself had received and was determined to make up for this with F. During her pregnancy she read every child care manual she could obtain. By the time F. arrived she was "in an utter state of anxiety." She cleaved to those manuals which advocated rigid regimentation of feeding and sleeping schedules.

Infants can perceive, or "resonate" with, a mother's anxiety in a number of ways. There is nothing mysterious about it. They can feel her muscular tension and rigidity, the rapid throbbing of her heart, the perspiration, and so forth. The content of adrenaline and other stress-related neuroendocrines rises in the breast milk. Soon they learn to recognize by sight and sound the tense and drawn facies, the altered gait and posture, and the change in tone of voice that herald the onset of the bad, anxiety-laden nipple. The infant's anxiety, as Sullivan (1953) said, opposes the operation of need-satisfying behaviors such as suckling, and this leaves the infant with frustration on top of anxiety. The mother is likely to respond with still more anxiety and a vicious circle is set in motion. The infant thus learns that the tensions of anxiety, as opposed to those of the purely biological needs, are unmanageable, largely because the person who would otherwise respond to those tensions is herself creating them.

Right away F. reacted to her anxiety and to the rigid schedule with anxiety of his own manifested in colic, irritability, and feeding and sleeping difficulties. This was a horrible blow to the mother's self-esteem. After all, she was going to right all the wrongs of her own mother. F. could literally throw her into "hysterics" by leaving a handful of carrots on his plate. F. was patently refusing to meet his mother's needs for receiving affection and feeling wanted and successful. She concluded that he was a "difficult and unaffectionate" infant and withdrew from him. Photographs of her at this time show her in a rigid, automaton-like posture holding her child virtually at arm's length. Predictably, a vicious circle was set up in which her withdrawal increased his irritability and sleeping and feeding problems until finally, when he was ten months old, she did to him what her own mother had done to her and brought in a nanny. Her resentment toward F.'s surrogate caretakers assured that, by the time he was four, three nannies had come and gone. She was now ready to take him back, but his reaction to that was predictable. The broken mother-son bond was never repaired.

F.'s father, for his part, had lost his favorite uncle shortly before F.'s birth. He had consciously-unconsciously decided that F. was supposed to become a carbon copy of the extraverted old man. Anything F. received from his father was dependent upon F.'s denying his own needs and individuality in order to be like the dead great uncle. When it soon became apparent that he neither wished to, nor could, fill the dead man's shoes, his father lost interest. This foundation of early deprivation and rejection led F. to mistrust the world. Would-be friends and nurturers were pushed away as having "something up their sleeves." Rather than risk repeated rejection, he withdrew from others. He became a cold and aloof child with a rich and increasingly bizarre fantasy life. At the same time that he secluded himself in his room he had a paradoxical need to periodically check and make sure his parents and sisters were still at home, since his painful experiences and insecurities from infancy had left him with an impaired ability to hold a representation of self or object in mind. Indeed, he literally could not describe himself to me without looking in a mirror or describe his family without seeing their photographs.

F. overcompensated for his intensely negative, unconscious self-esteem with a variety of conscious, grandiose ideas about himself.

Once the infant has developed, from resonance with mother, the capacity to experience anxiety, it becomes the vehicle for much of his subsequent socialization. The parents wittingly and unwittingly use it to transmit their particular view of what constitutes enculturation. The child learns, as Sullivan (1953, p. 152) said, on the "anxiety gradient"—"that is, learning to discriminate increasing from diminishing anxiety and alter activity in the direction of the latter." Too much anxiety, however (that which results from extremely forbidding gestures on the part of the parents), and social learning actually is impaired. The child splits off, as did F., many of his needs and large segments of his interpersonal experience to form what Freud called the "repressed unconscious" and what Sullivan termed the "not me."

The next case is that of Ms. Y., a 30-year-old unemployed cosmetologist, who presented with the chief complaint, "I don't have any feelings. I feel blah and like nothing inside."

It soon became apparent that her central problem was an incredibly low self-esteem and sense of worth, with the concomitant notion that she was unentitled to hold feelings about her past. She was the product of an unplanned pregnancy. Her mother was a vain and self-centered sometime fashion designer who blamed her daughter for the lack of success in her own career. Her father was a professor who, when he was not away on trips or at the office, was by himself reading. The patient responded to the lack of attention with temper tantrums which earned her verbal or physical abuse and got her locked in her room. The combination of disinterest and abuse left her feeling bad and worthless. Because none of her interests in school, socializing, or recreation was encouraged, she never developed any friendships or special talents. When she would begin a task, it would seem insurmountable to her and she was never encouraged by her parents to keep at it, but was allowed to drop it at a moment's notice. Consequently, she never developed social and academic skills nor achieved, despite better than average intelligence and appearance, in these areas. This fed back to decrease an already virtually nonexistent self-esteem.

Gradually, as a result of treatment, she became aware of what had contributed to her low self-esteem. This was accompanied by a great deal of pain and anger. Eventually she stopped seeing herself as unlovable, worthless, and incapable. She moved out of her parents' house and made some tentative social steps that were rewarded by her environment. She completed a refresher course in cosmetology and obtained a job. These achievements reinforced her self-esteem, and a beneficent circle was set in motion. Her last step was to accept the fact that her parents were never going to acknowledge their role in her problems. When she tried to discuss it with them, they told her much the same thing she heard when she was a child: "We provided you with every opportunity and it's not our fault you didn't take advantage of it. You were a difficult child from the start. No one could get close to you." In the psychotherapy chapters we shall have ample occasion to return to Ms. Y.

## The Anal Period

Freud called the period from 18 months to 2½ or 3 years the *anal period* because he viewed the anal area as the primary erotogenic zone, or path for the discharge of libidinal drive. The child was posited to derive "organ pleasure" from the retention and discharge of feces and from the cleansing and wiping of this area by self and mother. Certain adult character types and neurotics (the obsessive-compulsives) continue to preserve a greater than usual interest in this area.

Although there is some cogency in Freud's theorizing about the role of the "instincts" in the anal phase, I believe that here, as in the other stages, it has been much exaggerated. There is more to be gained by looking at the *interaction* between the psyche (including whatever is instinctual in it) and its environment than by speculating about the ultimate nature of its mental forces. Because of this there are perhaps some advantages to Erikson's name for this period: *autonomy versus shame and doubt.*

This is a phase of newfound autonomy for the infant. His improved speech and motor control make him an infinitely more effective engine in the world. Separation-individuation proceeds apace with what Mahler calls the subphase of *rapprochement* (18 to 24 months). During this time the toddler acts out his *ambi*valence about separating from mother. You observe the "shadowing and darting" phenomenon. The toddler comes toward mother and then runs away when she approaches. The shadowing of mother expresses his continued insecurity and need for protection. The darting manifests his longing for independence and desire to be chased, as well as the fear that his as yet precarious sense of self might become reabsorbed in that of the mother. Fear of losing a fragile sense of self, of fusing with the object, can become a motive for withdrawal in schizophrenic and borderline adults. As one young man put it, "I want to be with people but I'm afraid to. When I'm with X, I start laughing and gesturing like him. I don't want to. I can't help it. I can't stop it once it starts. . . . My head gets filled up with other people's ideas and I can't have my own thoughts anymore."

Although the point of *object constancy*, the ability to hold a fully integrated picture of the absent mother in mind, is not yet attained, the child has improved sufficiently in this area that it is not so much the loss of the mother herself but rather that of her *love* that he fears. Thus, the danger situation of the oral stage, which is loss of the loved *object*, is replaced by loss of the loved object's *love*. Fear of this loss is the motive that leads the toddler to renounce his infantile omnipotence and take account of the feelings and demands of others.

The mother, in turn, capitalizes upon this fear by making her previously (relatively) unconditional tenderness contingent upon the toddler's performance of socially desirable behavior. He must learn to postpone the gratification of some impulses and to curb others altogether. In particular, he must develop appropriate ways of discharging and binding anger (an important affect at this time), and he must renounce certain pleasures such as those associated with the manipulation of the anus and the fingering, smearing, and smelling of feces. These latter desires can persist in the consciousness of some adults as perversions, and in the unconsciousness of certain obsessive-compulsive characters and neurotics, and can become consciously reactivated in the regressive states of still others in severe cases of schizophrenia.

Toilet training is the case in point in the civilizing of the young savage. Whereas previously he could soil himself and others with impunity, indeed with pleasure, he must now restrict the relief of these tensions to the appropriate time and place. He must also learn to part with a piece of himself in the interest of others. (Some children become quite anxious about seeing something fall out of them and fear that they too may swirl down the toilet. Freud saw this as a precursor of castration anxiety, to be treated in the next section.)

Dynamic psychiatrists dwell on toilet training not because it possesses some magical significance, but because the interactions between parents and child around it are often characteristic of their contact around many other tasks of socialization as well—tasks extending throughout all the phases of development. Is there, for instance, such a perfect fit between the parents' style of reward and punishment and the needs of the child to relieve his tensions, win their approval, and avoid losing their love that he learns with a minimum of trouble for all? Do the parents value his achievement sufficiently for him to value it himself? Do they have their own needs or the child's more in mind? Does, for example, mother's self-esteem depend on Johnny's being the youngest toilet-trained child on the block? Does she take his failures so personally that she communicates to him that her well-being depends on when and where he deposits a few lumps of smelly brown substance? If so, then he may become frightened or he may come to feel he has a mighty instrument with which to control her if he chooses. Some children learn to use the retention and expulsion of urine and feces as a weapon in battles for control with their parents. Is the child harshly punished when he fails, but ignored when he succeeds, such that he eventually feels the best he can ever do is avoid a negative response? Is he shamed or battered unmercifully into compliance? If the parents are hasty and hard-driving in toilet training and the other tasks of socialization, never giving the child a sense of restful satisfaction in his work, then he will be likewise to himself.

This stage forms the germs of the child's superego. It is the time when he first learns that some of his wishes may clash with those of the environment. Focusing on the paradigmatic role of toilet training, Freud called this sphincter morality. If the parents have been overly severe and have reacted to the child's excrement with disgust and loathing, then he begins to form a sense of his body and its processes as somehow bad. If such parental attitudes continue throughout the subsequent oedipal period, then there develops a firm foundation for conflicts over natural bodily processes. No part of the body or its functions is inherently disgusting. Disgust is a socially acquired emotion.

Freud believed that those with problems in the anal phase of development were particularly likely to develop into obsessive-compulsive, or "anal," personalities or neurotics in adulthood. The former is a character type in which qualities like orderliness, obstinacy, and parsimony predominate. Freud saw many of their characteristics, like orderliness and cleanliness, as *reaction formations* against underlying desires to be quite the opposite. "Every obsessional has his dirty drawer," as the psychiatric humorists say. Among these unconscious trends may be strong interests in defecation, the anus, and other bodily parts and processes that, in his conscious life, the obsessional considers disgusting. In some, these unconscious preoccupations may manifest themselves in coprolalia: the frequent use of swear words with anal and fecal connotations. Not occasionally, one will find, after many sessions of treatment, that the prim and proper obsessive character has a number of secret scatological rituals, e.g., anal masturbation or delight in the smell of flatus and feces. These are to be understood as adult survivals of the anal-erotic modes of pleasure-seeking of early childhood.

Obsessional individuals have remnants of the heightened ambivalence so characteristic of the anal child. Intense love and hatred toward the same object will jostle one another uncomfortably. Like the anal child, the compulsive adult is often preoccupied with issues of control of self and others, of power in other words. Obsessive-compulsive neurotics are caricatures of the character style. What were *ego syntonic* (not unpleasurable or ego alien) personality traits in the obsessional character become *ego dystonic* (unpleasurable and not sensed as integral parts of the self) *symptoms* in the obsessional neurotic. For example, what was exaggerated cleanliness in the former becomes the symptom of compulsive hand washing, perhaps a hundred times a day, in the latter. The meticulous attention to detail in the former becomes checking and re-checking the figures in one's checking account a hundred times in the latter.

An example of a person with traumata and fixations dating from the anal period is the case of Mrs. B., a middle-aged divorcée who presented with psychosomatic bowel symptoms in an obsessive-compulsive character structure:

> She had been raised by a rigidly perfectionistic and coldly disciplinary mother and an aloof and barely less obsessional father. Her mother actually began toilet training at six (!) months, changing her diaper on the hour, every hour. From the time the child became capable of controlling her sphincter she had frequent problems with constipation, which was both an indirect way of rebelling against the mother and a way of getting her attention by enemas and laxatives. She described the "tremendous relief, the freedom" associated with her evacuations, with obvious pleasure. Her preoccupation with the anus was an erotic one, as well as a way of defending against genital sexual impulses. Her intestinal symptoms disappeared with marriage and the attendant sexual gratification and with the birth of a child. Some time after she had discovered her husband's infidelity and divorced him for it, the symptoms recurred while she was working in the department store of her sister and brother-in-law, who were obsessional, depriving carbon copies of her parents. This time, however, it was diarrhea, not constipation, from which she suffered. Several times she defecated in her pants at work, both defending against her considerable rage at her parents and parent imagoes (sister and brother-in-law) and surreptitiously expressing it ("shitting all over their place").

In Chapter 3 these common personality types and symptoms are discussed further.

## The Phallic, or Oedipal, Period

Freud termed the years from 3 to 5½ or 6 as the *phallic* phase of psychosexual development.[8] Libidinal drive which had previously cathected (invested) the mental representation of the bodily surface as a whole, the oral cavity and alimentary canal, and the anus, now begins to center around the mental representation of the genitals. This is the time when the sexes begin to compare genitals. Because, in the course of these comparisons, the penis is the most conspicuous object to both sexes and because Freud believed the girl's sexuality centers around the clitoris (the embryological homologue of the penis) rather than the

---

[8]Freud also posited, at various times, a *urethral* stage existing in the interface between the anal and phallic. It was characterized by pleasure from the retention and release of urine. Sublimated urethral erotism in adulthood was supposed to produce intense ambition.

vagina as a whole, he termed this the phallic phase.[9] Erikson, focusing again on the psycho*social* aspects of this time, called it the stage of *initiative versus guilt.*

The separation-individuation process culminates in this period with the establishment of the ability to 1) paint a faithful picture of the object which includes both its "good" and "bad," its gratifying and depriving, aspects, 2) paint a faithful picture of self which integrates both "good" and "bad" aspects, 3) store moving pictures of the interaction between the integrated self and the integrated object, 4) differentiate between the portraits of self and those of objects, and 5) fix all this in mind in a permanent gallery whose existence does not depend on the physical presence of the object or the reflection of self in others and mirrors. The early separation-individuation process comes to a close by the end of the oedipal period, but we continue to touch up the photographs of self and others, to make them sharper and more accurate representations of reality, throughout latency, adolescence (when there is a recrudescence of many of the separation-individuation issues of childhood), and early adulthood. Indeed, to some extent this process continues throughout life.

The phallic phase is the time of the famous Oedipus complex, a constellation of *sexual* and *aggressive* fantasies about the objects in one's environment (e.g., the parents). Seen by many as a preposterous notion, I believe that it is, on the contrary, a "common sense" idea. Many philosophers and writers before Freud anticipated this notion. E. R. Dodds (1951), the well-known classicist, cites evidence from ancient writers that frankly oedipal dreams were common in antiquity. Of course, there was the famous Oedipus play of Sophocles. Denis Diderot, the eighteenth-century French encyclopedist, wrote, "If the little savage were left to himself, preserving all his foolishness and adding to the small sense of a child in the cradle the violent passions of a man of thirty, he would strangle his father and lie with his mother" (in Freud, 1916–1917, p. 338). Many nineteenth-century physicians and sexologists commented on various aspects of childhood sexuality. Popular songs ("I want a girl just like the girl that married dear old Dad") and swear words (mother f___er) take account of this phenomenon.

Anyone who does not believe in childhood sexuality is best advised to watch his own children. Infant boys have erections and very young children, particularly in the phallic stage, fondle and finger their genitals with manifest delight. Every father has felt what can only be called "coquettish" behavior in his little girl. At times such behavior expresses

---

[9]Freud's idea of the clitoral orgasm as being the earlier, i.e., phallic, form of feminine sexuality while the vaginal orgasm was its later and mature form has been dealt a serious blow by Masters and Johnson.

both the desire and the defense against it. During her oedipal years my daughter would get my attention by hitting me and then fleeing, screaming "Don't you get me, Daddy. You stay away from me, Daddy. I don't like you, Daddy." Children are preoccupied with displaying their bodies and looking at those of others: the "doctor game." They are intensely curious about where babies come from and about what Mommy and Daddy do in bed, a place where they will often end up in the middle of the night. In their play with toy miniature persons, onto which they project desires and fears of which they are not consciously aware or do not know how to verbalize, there is further evidence of the Oedipus complex. When my daughter was four she liked to take the toy Daddy and daughter on boat rides, leaving the Mommy and brother on shore, when she did not throw them into the water!

Those who do not believe in the aggressiveness of children are urged, here again, simply to listen to and watch them. The small child who screams, "Mommy, take baby back to the hospital" or "throw him in the garbage can" means, quite literally, what he is saying. The slightest frustration can evoke an "I hate you Mommy" or "I wish Daddy would go away and not come back." Children act out violent fantasies with their dolls, toy animals, and soldiers, and in play with each other. They can tell stories whose gore puts anything in Grimms' to shame. Boys of oedipal age take great delight, as did my own, in pummelling their fathers—an expression of oedipal aggression as much as of affection.

Other evidence for the Oedipus complex comes from the analysis of adults. Recall, for example, the precipitous marriage of Mrs. A. Here again, it seems common sense that one's lifelong relationships with important members of the same and opposite sex will be ineluctably influenced by our countless interactions with the prototypical representatives of these sexes: mother and father. There is ample cross-cultural evidence that the Oedipus complex is universal in human ontogeny owing to certain constants in biological endowment and social structure (e.g., the documented ubiquity of the biological parents-child family unit).[10] It does not seem radical to suggest that the child's biologically based affectionate and sexual drives, and the aggression that results from the frustration of them, will take as their objects whomever is available in the environment. Since the most important persons in the first years of life are the biological parents or, in the event of their absence, parent surrogates, they will inescapably receive the first investments of affection, sexuality, and aggression.

The sexual and affectionate currents are never invested equally in both parents. Inevitably one receives more than the other, usually the

---

[10]For numerous examples of the cross-cultural evidence for the Oedipus complex see my recent book *Freud and Anthropology: A History and Reappraisal* (1982).

mother in the case of the boy and the father in that of the girl.[11] The same-sexed parent then comes to be viewed as an intruder and rival and receives a considerable deposit of the child's aggression.

Having painted the broad strokes, I shall brush in the details. The development and resolution of the complex are less complicated in the case of the boy, and I shall begin with him. The mother, toward whom his sexuality and affection are supposed to be directed, is the first caretaking and nurturing object and she receives his incipient sexual and affectionate currents as a matter of course.[12] This is the time of infantile masturbation to unconscious oedipal fantasies which may form the basis for conflicts over masturbation in adolescence and adulthood. It is then only a case of these feelings and fantasies unfolding themselves until they butt up against the presence of the father. When they do, considerable anger, accompanied by conscious or unconscious murderous fantasies, will develop toward him. The young rake eventually abandons his designs on mother for three reasons: 1) out of fear of retaliation by, and physical injury at the hands of, the father, which includes *fear of castration,* the third danger situation in the scale of development; 2) out of the love that always, at least to some extent, existed for father and the fear of losing him; and 3) out of hurt and anger over the mother's refusal to play along.

Let me return briefly to the first reason. Freud felt that castration would be a specific fear of the small boy for at least two reasons: 1) because he was likely to receive such threats from a parent, maid, or nurse, e.g., "if you don't take your hands out of your pants I will cut it off"; and 2) because, having observed that girls do not possess a penis, he concludes that it is possible to have had one once and then to lose it. Through the analysis of adults, we know that castration anxiety does play a large role in the lives of many men and can manifest itself in a variety of ways from inhibitions of assertiveness and competitiveness and avoidance of public speaking to sexual problems. I encourage you to understand the term "castration anxiety" as referring not only to the specific fear of genital injury itself, but to the fear of physical injury and mortification in general.

In any event, the outcome of the Oedipus complex in the normal situation is that the boy abandons, or more likely *represses,* his aims for

---

[11]Incestuous fantasies for siblings of the opposite sex occur both as primary impulses in their own right and as displacements of those from the parent.

[12]Freud generally considered affection as a derivative of sexuality, as aim-inhibited libido, although in places he implied that the two were somehow separate and that the affectionate currents were even older (1912, p. 180). The sexual currents were then posited to attach themselves to the objects of affection.

mother and replaces them by a (conscious-unconscious) *identification* with the father. As Freud expressed it, he "abandons an object cathexis for an identification." In other words, he chooses to become *like* the father rather than to possess the mother. This identification with, or incorporation of the characteristics of, the father is responsible for a good deal of the small boy's ego and, especially, superego. As to the former, he will adopt, for better or worse, many of the father's mannerisms and coping skills. As for the latter, he will adopt the father's repertoire of "thou shalts" and "thou shalt nots." Freud thus thought the superego was the heir to the resolution of the Oedipus complex, and that its benignity or harshness, its laxity or rigidity, bore a one-to-one correspondence to that of the father in his interactions with the child. Freud also believed that a certain amount of the aggressiveness in the superego was an internalization of the son's aggression toward the father.

In the case of the little girl, all this is more complex since, like the little boy, her embryonic affectionate and sexual impulses are also directed toward the first nurturing object—the mother—and her aggressive impulses toward the person with unlimited access to her—the father. When the mother refuses to indulge her fantasies she turns, in frustration and anger, to the father who, if he is sufficiently accepting, becomes the new object of her desires. The complex then proceeds as in the case of the boy, except that the sexuality is directed toward father and the aggression toward mother, with the eventual abandonment (or repression) of father as a sexual object and identification with mother.

Freud felt there was one other reason the little girl abandons her mother as the primary object: her discovery, from comparison with boys, that she does not possess the organ with which to make love to the mother. In her fury she blames her mother for this "omission" and turns to the father. Freud felt this was the basis for what he considered to be the universal, mostly unconscious, penis envy of women. He believed that the desire for a penis was replaced by the desire to have a baby, which then becomes the unconscious surrogate for the penis. It is, of course, hard to divorce any consideration of this idea from its sexist implications, but I believe that it should be judged on the basis of the data and not on its potentiality for political misuse. I have seen evidence for its importance in some women but not in others.

I shall cite two examples. The first I observed in the interaction between a five-year-old boy and girl in a day-care center.

> They were both "going potty" and the latter pointed to the former's penis and said, "What's that?" He replied, "My tinkle." She then looked down at her own genital and said "This is mine. Do you wish you had one like it?" He responded, "No, do you wish you had one like mine?" She said, "Yes."

The other example is that of an adult woman whom I had in treatment for several years.

> She was preoccupied with what she considered men's inordinate pride in their genitals, what she called their "power tool." She would describe, with ill-concealed pleasure, episodes in which any of her numerous sexual partners was impotent. On several occasions she demolished paper chains (which she had a habit of making) following arguments with boyfriends. Eventually she described an adolescent fantasy, after seeing her brother naked, of chopping off his member. Her sense of castration had been heightened by a number of operative procedures on her urethra in childhood. Her resentment of males was increased by the fact that her brother received much more attention from her parents than she, leaving her feeling that there were distinct advantages associated with the possession of a penis. In addition to her hatred and envy of the penis itself, she resented it as the symbol of a male-dominated society which had, in reality, blocked her advancement at several turns.

Today we know that the counterpart of penis envy in women, breast or womb envy, can also occur in men. There are many cases of men driven by envy of the gestational capacity of women and laboring under the influence of unconscious pregnancy fantasies. Artistic or literary creativity in some men has the unconscious significance of bearing a child.

Freud taught us that, in both males and females, for every "positive," or typical, Oedipus complex, there is also a "negative" or "inverted" one. This means that, in the case of the little girl, there remains an unconscious remnant of that early attraction for mother and hatred of father. In the case of the boy there exists a rudiment of unconscious sexual and affectionate, submissive desires for father and resentment toward mother. These passive-submissive "feminine" desires for father and those who unconsciously represent him remain among the most strongly repudiated psychical trends in the male sex. Freud felt there is a remnant of bisexuality in all of us and that the most platonically affectionate relationships between persons of the same sex are in part a sublimation of frankly sexual trends. Manifest homosexuality can result from an especially powerful negative Oedipus as well as, as we shall see, from the need to defend against an especially powerful positive one.

Much can go wrong at this time. As is true in the other stages, the parent must achieve a balance between inappropriate gratification and extreme deprivation. The parent of the opposite sex must not be seductive or overly responsive at the same time that he or she acknowledges the budding sexuality of the child. To reject the child for it would leave him or her feeling bad about a normal bodily function and would permanently damage his masculine or her feminine self-esteem. For example, the father must show the little coquette wearing mother's makeup that he is pleased with her femininity. Were he to scream at her to remove it, he could adversely affect her feminine sexual identity and self-confidence and make her feel bad for wanting to be a woman attractive to the opposite sex. He would lead her to feel men do not appreciate that sort of thing. Were he to become flirtatious in turn, he would intensify her oedipal fantasies and cause her to harbor unrealistic expectations concerning their fulfillment. The mother as well must nurture and foster her son's incipient manliness without being teasing or provocative. If the parent of the opposite sex goes too far in the direction of either stimulation or inhibition, a number of problems can result: impotence and frigidity, broken marriages and affairs, and homosexuality.

There are, of course, degrees of overstimulation and overindulgence, such as incest, exhibitionism and fondling, parental indiscretion in love-making, teasing, and the appearance that father and mother are not getting along and that perhaps one of them is "available." Outright incest results when one parent, usually the mother, is so conflicted about sexuality herself that, in order to avoid it, she unconsciously hands her daughter over to the disturbed father. Such activities leave the girl with guilt over the satisfaction of her oedipal longings and her trespass against mother, as well as resentment and mistrust of father, who upon one level she knows is abusing her. There is resentment as well toward mother, who was supposed to protect her both from her own sexuality and from father's. The resultant mix of supercharged incestuous strivings, guilt, resentment, and mistrust can lead to permanent inability to form a lasting or satisfactory relationship with any man, each of whom unconsciously represents yet another incestuous object.

In the case of the boy, it is much rarer that manifest incest occurs. Nevertheless, there is a good deal that the mother can do that would approximate it. If, for instance, father is physically and emotionally absent most of the time, the frustrated mother may, unconsciously, take her son as a sort of surrogate spouse, e.g., putting him in her bed and smothering him with physical affection. If this behavior leads to other forms of teasing and sexual provocativeness, then she will supercharge her young son's desires. This is painful for him on at least two accounts. First of all, she is not prepared to follow through on what she has implicitly promised, leaving him with a sense of rejection and worthlessness as a man. Second, there is a good deal of guilt over these strivings and over trespassing on father's domain, as well as fears about father's reaction (castration anxiety). The small boy needs to know that daddy is there to protect mommy and him from his sexual strivings. If this is not the case and mother is seductive, then the small boy's fear of his own sexuality may lead to a permanently impaired sexual functioning. At the least, he may be unable to direct both affectionate and sexual currents toward the same woman because that would resemble too closely the dangerously longed-for situation in childhood. In other words, that woman would unconsciously represent his mother, thereby stimulating a host of guilt-laden unconscious associations. This can lead to a situation like that in the well-known eighteenth-century play, *She Stoops to Conquer,* or in what the Latins call the "Madonna-putana" complex in which the man has one woman whom he loves only in the affectionate sense and a mistress whom he loves in the purely sensual. Or, he might be able to establish some semblance of a sexual-affectionate relationship with a woman, which he sooner or later sabotages out of an unconscious sense of guilt. Oedipal conflicts in men can also lead to complete inhibition of feelings toward women and lifelong sexual dysfunction. Many cases of impotence result from guilt feelings over sexual strivings for a woman who signifies, unconsciously, the mother.

In extreme cases the combination of maternal seductiveness and paternal withdrawal can lead to homosexuality in men. (If one substitutes "girl" for "boy" and "father" for "mother," then this scenario also accounts for a good deal of homosexuality in women.) The small boy becomes so frightened by his (largely unconscious) incestuous fantasies for mother that he identifies with her, rather than retaining her as a sexual object. This is facilitated by the absence of the father, with whom he would normally identify. This unconscious identification with mother leads him in adolescence and adulthood to seek out sexual partners who unconsciously represent his boyhood self. He than lavishes on them the sex and affection he would like to have received from mother— a sort of vicarious satisfaction. Thus, like the normal boy, he resolves his Oedipus complex by *identification,* but of a very different sort. This is the case of homosexuality as a defense against heterosexuality.[13]

Overseeing or overhearing the parents in intercourse is a classic augmenter of oedipal issues. This is termed the *primal scene* and is much more common than one might imagine. Whether it has occurred or not, there will be *primal scene fantasies:* conscious and unconscious daydreams about what mommy and daddy do together in bed. I have treated adult patients who eventually recall childhood anxiety attacks and insomnia

---

[13]I am not implying these are the only dynamics of homosexuality. I had one patient who was literally institutionalized into it by his older brothers. I have both seen and heard tell of male and female homosexuals whose primary dynamic seemed to be the need to deny that the opposite sex had anything worthwhile to deliver. Such people are almost invariably gravely disappointed in childhood by the parent of the opposite sex. Sullivan (1953, p. 258) spoke of the increased likelihood of homosexuality in the delayed preadolescent who develops his chumship late and with a person who has already entered adolescence.

associated with noises from the parental bedroom. Oftentimes what mommy and daddy do together is imagined as a violent act. An hysteric under hypnosis described, in the voice of a small child, the primal scene she witnessed as "Daddy beating Mommy."

As for the opposite pole, that of inhibition, it can lead to severe conflicts as well. If the parents overreact to the manifestations of the child's sexuality, he will be led to believe that sexuality is "dirty" or "bad." If the small child's hand is violently slapped away from his genitals and he is informed "nice children don't do that," if his flirtatiousness is harshly repudiated, or if curiosity about sexual issues brings overwhelmingly negative reactions, then he will internalize these inhibitions to the detriment of the expression of his sexuality in adulthood. If the parent of the opposite sex participates heavily in this "repression," then his masculine or her feminine self-esteem and sense of attractiveness will be markedly impaired.

At this point I want to emphasize that the "Oedipus complex" is only seen directly in exotic cases like Oedipus who slew his father and slept with his mother or in psychotics whose repressions have failed so completely that they consciously relate such fantasies. (It is mostly *unconscious* even in children of oedipal age.) Otherwise, it is *inferred* from the data, from its *derivatives*—patterns of behavior with the opposite sex, dreams, parapraxes, the transference relationship with the therapist, and so forth. In other words, the Oedipus complex is invoked as the most parsimonious, or economical, explanation for the data at hand.

A good example is the case of Mrs. A., whose precipitous marriage was an enactment of unconscious oedipal fantasies. Her father's alternately teasing and rejecting behavior did not confine itself to her oedipal period, but extended throughout latency and adolescence. This included using her as a confidante, and at times a facilitator, in his extramarital affairs, complaining to her about her mother's frigidity, holding her in his lap until well into her teens, patting her bottom, and so forth. She found it quite striking, when telling me about it, that at the time she did *not* consciously recognize it as titillating. She was aware only of extreme discomfort and of the fact that she nevertheless sought out, or allowed herself to be put in, these situations.

Another woman's Oedipus complex was manifested in depression and suicidal ideations which followed, like clockwork, each encounter with her divorced father and his mistress. Witnessing her recently available father with another woman aroused her unconscious incestuous strivings at the same time that his frustration of them stirred up considerable rage. Her depression and suicidal ideation resulted from anger turned in on the self and self-punishment out of guilt over her desires. In another woman the compromise between her incestuous wishes and superego injunctions against them expressed itself in a chain of affairs with men "who just happened to turn out to be homosexual," thus removing the danger of sexual intercourse with a father imago.

Another blatant example of the data from which such a complex is inferred is that of the man who had several broken marriages and affairs with slightly older women with hair coloring, complexion, and figure similar to those of his mother. When speaking of his current wife at times he even slipped and said "my mother." His seeking out a woman resembling his mother was an expression of his unconscious incestuous desires, while his sabotaging of the relationships was in deference to his guilt feelings.

Other common examples are those people who are only attracted to persons who are already "attached." One woman had a series of affairs with married men, thereby acting out her sexual feelings for her father and her aggressive ones for her mother, as well as insuring there was little possibility of having to face the guilt feelings attendant upon a permanent relationship. Predictably, she developed a passionate attraction for her therapist who she knew was a married man. The whole conflict then played itself out in the therapeutic relationship (transference) whose historical roots were interpreted by the therapist. Or the aggressive pole of the Oedipus may be the primary one acted out. This is often the case with intensely competitive men, out to triumph over a variety of father figures with the unconscious prize being the acclaim of mother. Dreams, where one's inhibitions are at their lowest, may occur in which a man is having sex with a figure suspiciously similar to the mother or is beating a man resembling his father. The complex can even manifest itself culturally. Myths, fairy tales, and all sorts of literature can express oedipal themes. People can use cultural material to express and/ or defend against such fantasies. Adoration of the Virgin Mary can be a safe way for certain men to indulge oedipal strivings. In the next chapter I shall describe the culturally provided means for expression of, and defense against, our unconscious strivings. In a psychotic woman I once treated, the complex manifested itself in conscious fantasies of intercourse with Jesus, which were followed by the fear that she would be punished for these by the death of her mother (which was also, of course, what she secretly wished for; see the discussion of compromise formation in Chapter 3).

Freud termed the Oedipus the "nuclear complex" of neurosis and, indeed, in the better adjusted patients whom we see it *is* the predominant area of conflict. It continues in importance not merely because it remains in the unconscious continually pressing for satisfaction, but because the person seeks out partners with whom he can recreate *in reality* a situation that resembles that from his childhood. Recall the case of Mrs. A., in whom oedipal conflicts were kept alive not only because of factors within her psyche but because of factors without it as well, i.e., that she had married a man who behaved like her father. We have only to look at ourselves and our neighbors to see how we strive, in our own marriages, to recapitulate those of our parents. (Recall the anniversary phenomena I described in Chapter 1.)

We shall see that conflicts from the oedipal period are associated most closely with the hysterical personality and hysterical neurosis, and with the more highly developed neuroses and character disorders of adulthood. More often than not, oedipal issues are inseparably intertwined with preoedipal ones (especially dependency and emotional nurturance) as well.

One particularly baneful result of disturbed parenting in these early years is what Sullivan (1953, p. 214) termed the "malevolent transformation." This can occur when the child discovers that the expressed need for tenderness brings, not satisfying physical and emotional intimacy, but anxiety-provoking or even physically painful responses. Under these circumstances, the child associates the perceived need for tenderness with the anticipation of anxiety or pain. He feels that he lives among enemies and behaves toward them accordingly. A vicious circle is then set in motion in which his malevolence makes it less likely he will receive, from his parents or anyone else, that which he urgently, but now unconsciously, desires. This is another way of formulating what has been known for centuries: that those who are treated unlovingly tend to become unlovable. (Recall Ms. H. who exhibited a relatively benign species of the malevolent transformation.)

Freud believed that one's *character*—one's particular style of *adaptation*, of establishing equilibrium among the forces within one and between these and the pressures of the environment—was virtually fixed by the close of the oedipal period. We now appreciate that the situation is much more complex and that character formation proceeds well into adulthood. Nevertheless, these early *formative* years *do* form a matrix of possibilities and limitations with which one's subsequent development must take account.

## Latency

The years from five or six until puberty were termed by Freud the latency stage because of the *relative* quiescence of the sexual impulses during this time. Erikson, focusing on the tasks of enculturation, called it the age of *industry versus inferiority*. Sullivan divided it into two eras: the *juvenile* and *preadolescent*.

How much the latency period is biologically, and how much culturally, determined is a moot point. The ethnological evidence suggests that in some cultures the manifestations of sexuality at this age are much more intense than in ours. Probably the latency stage is a biological potentiality of which some cultures make more use than others; the repression of sensuality at the close of the Oedipus is more heavy-handed in some societies than in others.

Latency is a time of rapid development of the ego functions. The child learns information and skills crucial to coping with life in the real world. This occurs for at least two reasons. First of all, since this is an era in which the child is less buffeted about by the demands of sexuality, he has more energy to spare for academic and social learning. That there is some relationship between all this and the slumber of sexuality is proved by the rapid decline in school performance often seen in children with the onset of puberty. Second, researchers like Piaget have documented that tremendous maturation of the cognitive apparatus occurs at this time and that the child is able to grasp and manipulate concepts far beyond him before.

From the standpoint of socialization, in particular, the latency period is anything but an uneventful interlude between infantile sexuality and puberty. In the wake of Freud's brilliant discoveries about the importance of early childhood, the formative role of the latency years has been underestimated. One must now learn to compete, compromise, and collaborate with the group in a socially acceptable way. The child is confronted with a paradox: at the same time that he is becoming more of an individual (with a more differentiated and integrated self-representation) he must learn to set aside his individual interests for the good of the group. Under favorable social circumstances, as Sullivan (1953) said, much of the warp and idiosyncrasy acquired in the parental home is open to remedy. Conversely, subjection of an already damaged child to ostracism, stereotyping, and ridicule could make bad matters worse.

Whereas the oedipal child is likely to have friends of the opposite sex, in latency there is more emphasis on what Sullivan termed *"chumship,"* close relationships with age mates of the same sex. Indeed, each sex is usually treated contemptuously by the other. Minor episodes of homosexuality may occur which have little or no impact on one's eventual sexual orientation.

Chumship becomes particularly developed in the latter half of latency (from about nine or ten), which Sullivan called the "preadolescent era." One's chum is defined as a person of intense importance to one and whose needs and sensitivities are taken into account nearly as much as one's own. This is the training ground for adult intimacy, empathy, and altruism. The validation of one's personal worth in a successful chumship may even help, Sullivan posited, to undo the effects of a previous malevolent transformation.

From the integration of two-group chumships, *gangs* often develop. Here one learns not only to participate in hierarchical interactions with a leader, but to see oneself through the eyes of others. Prior distortions in self-world view and idiosyncratic symbolizations tend to move, in response to group scrutiny, closer to consensually validated norms.

This is a time of the blossoming and ripening not only of socialization and ego functions, but of the superego as well. The superstructure of this agency is built upon the foundation laid in the anal and oedipal periods and continues to carry, to a large extent, the form established by the interactions with parents during those early years. Although it is unlikely that its rigidity or flexibility, malignancy or benignity, or rewarding or punitive nature will be altered in any fundamentally qualitative way, it undergoes a good deal of remodeling at the hands of teachers and peers.

The development of the superego, like that of the ego, is in part dependent on the maturation of the biological substrate of the cognitive apparatus. Growth in the cognitive underpinnings is required to be able to recognize another's point of view and feelings—to empathize, in other words. Similarly, the progressive *abstraction* of the early personifications in the superego, the transformation of mother's or father's voice into abstract moral commandments, is dependent upon the development of the cognitive apparatus that occurs at this time.

In this period the danger situation is less that of castration or of loss of the object or its love than that of *superego condemnation*. The condemnation of the superego is a painful state accompanied by guilt and lowered self-esteem and, for that reason, we strive to avoid it. In other words, we have *internalized* the moral arbitration of our parents and it is now our censure, as much as theirs, that we fear.

Latency is the time of many of the childhood neuroses and dysfunctions that the psychiatrist sees. The former may manifest themselves in ritualistic obsessive-compulsive behaviors, phobias, and other symptoms, and the latter in disorders ranging from hyperkinesis, truancy, and enuresis to frank psychosis. Certain events, such as family relocations, can be more traumatic for the peer-oriented latency child than for his younger, family-centered counterpart.

If the social, moral, and academic learning of this time is deficient, then the child will face the internal and external demands of adolescent and adult development with an impaired adaptational apparatus. He will not have the capability to bind, sublimate, and appropriately fulfill the upsurge of sexual and aggressive energies and fantasies of adolescence.

## The Genital Stage

Freud, retaining his emphasis on psychosexuality, termed the culminating point of infantile development the *genital* stage. One who has reached this pinnacle is termed the "genital personality." This is viewed more as the *ideal* than the norm and, more than any of the other stages, expresses Freud's value judgments about what is desirable. This is the point at which the various component instincts should pay fealty to the supremacy of the genitals. Pregenital sexuality must limit itself to fore-play (kissing, mouthing, cuddling), while genital intercourse should become the "be all and end all" of the sexual encounter. At this point one is able to fuse his sexual and affectionate currents and direct them toward a member of the opposite sex. It is supposed that one has attained a good deal of autonomy, a stable and secure sense of the self and the world, an internally regulated self-esteem, a good deal of ability to control and direct one's impulses, and a degree of empathy for, and concern with, the welfare of important others. *Arbeiten und lieben,* the ability to work and love, was Freud's most succinct characterization of the genital personality.

What Freud termed the genital stage has been subdivided into four stages by Erikson and, as discussed subsequently, into more than that by Levinson, a theoretician of adult development. Erikson termed the early years of the genital phase, what is usually considered the time of adolescence, as the period of *identity versus role confusion*, thereby em-phasizing the separation-individuation issues which reappear at this time.

Emotional turbulence is of course the norm, not the exception, in adolescence. Because every adolescent is a little "crazy" by adult stan-dards, it is difficult to diagnose with any certainty at this time! Even so, more severe psychiatric disorders first manifest themselves in adoles-cence and early adulthood than at any other time. This is because ego deficits and conflict-laden areas that were unapparent earlier, when fewer demands were placed on the personality, now become apparent with the increased exactions of society and of the sexual impulses. A much-cherished latency-age equilibrium, established by a precarious ego over relatively weak sexual and aggressive forces, can be upset almost overnight by the violent torrents of the drives in puberty. Great strain is put on the ego to juggle the claims of the id with those of the superego and reality. One is called upon to become increasingly inde-pendent of the family of origin, to interact in more mature ways with members of the opposite sex, and to develop some workable compro-mise between forging an individual identity and following the demands for conformity. This is a time, as Sullivan said, when the three great needs (for self-esteem and freedom from anxiety; for emotional intima-cy; and for sensual satisfaction) are intricately intertwined and yet not always compatible.

There is a recrudescence of the oedipal sexual and aggressive fantasies which, generally, are displaced onto one's peers and teachers. Thinly disguised oedipal dreams can occur at this time. Unresolved issues from the oedipal stage make themselves felt. Conflicts over unconscious incestuous fantasies may lead to guilt over masturbation or inhibited behavior toward the opposite sex. In the task of mediating between the demands of id and superego, an adolescent may become excessively hedonistic or ascetic with, not uncommonly, the same adolescent oscillating violently back and forth between these two poles. Occasionally, the adolescent deals with troublesome unconscious incestuous feelings by avoiding, fighting with, or pushing away the parent of the opposite sex. Paradoxically, if the parent takes such behavior at its face value, the adolescent may feel rejected in turn.

If there is a recrudescence of oedipal issues, there is also a resurrection of the control issues of the anal period and the independence versus dependency issues of the anal and oral phases. No one can be more obstinately withholding or defiantly expulsive than an adolescent. No one can shift more quickly to and fro between the most obstreperous independence and the most abject dependency. His central fear is of the latter and, rather than acknowledge his intense dependency strivings and fears of growing up, he often engages in "pseudoindependent" behaviors (up to, and including, running away), actions that implicitly cry out to the parents for control. Paradoxically, although he may react angrily to the parents' "clamping down," this is often precisely what he wanted all along, and he may ultimately feel reassured and cared for. Pill popping and other self-destructive behaviors are often unconscious attempts to get parents to notice their children's problems. Like the pregenital child, the adolescent frequently gives two communications, the classic "double message," one with his mouth and another with his behavior. He may badger his parents for financial independence and then overdraw his account so they have to bail him out. He may interdict mother from his room and then forget to set the alarm so that she is constantly forced to drag him out of bed. He abhors being told what to do and yet leaves his clothes around the house so that he invariably is reprimanded.

Continued identity formation and consolidation are crucial issues in adolescence. "Who am I?" is the central question. Erikson (1963, pp. 261-262) defines identity as "the accrued confidence that the inner sameness and continuity prepared in the past are matched by the sameness and continuity of one's meaning for others . . ." Although the broad strokes of one's identity have been laid down by age six, and although the limitations and possibilities of this outline cannot be ignored, the details of this portrait are yet to be touched in. In adolescence the picture of self becomes increasingly integrated and differentiated, and gradually less dependent on the reactions of the environment for its definition and esteem. This self-representation must also incorporate the rather drastic bodily changes in puberty. One's body image must change from that of a child to that of a mature adult.

Those with an amorphous and ill-defined representation of self and with a low self-esteem may remain excessively dependent on the environment for their sense of worth and who they are. Throughout life they may parrot the style of whatever person or group they want to be with and may never relate as an integrated and differentiated self to an integrated and differentiated object. Poorly defined and integrated representations of self often accompany correspondingly vague and unintegrated representations of objects. Thus, in addition to being particularly vulnerable to taking on the qualities of others, the person with an inchoate sense of identity may have as much problem recognizing that his own needs and preoccupations may not also be those of others. When this extends to the attribution of one's unconscious, warded-off impulses to others, we speak of *projection,* a reality-distorting defense mechanism that we shall examine in Chapter 3.

The vague, playful, rapidly shifting occupational fantasies of childhood must become sharper, more stable, and more reality-oriented. For many adolescents, particularly those from middle- and upper-class families, this is a time of what Erikson has called "psychosocial moratorium," in which one can still try out various occupational and social identities before making a commitment "for real." College and military service fulfill such a purpose for many. Erikson, Levinson, and others have stressed the crucial role of vocation for one's identity and self-esteem.

We now appreciate that personality growth and development do not stop at age six or even 16, but that they continue throughout the entire life cycle. Freud was so intent on combating the hitherto almost exclusive focus on adulthood that he went to the other extreme and dismissed most of adolescent and adult development as a recapitulation of themes from childhood. Erikson has termed this the "originological fallacy," i.e., collapsing the motives and meanings of rich and complicated present-day behaviors entirely into their infantile dynamics. One would be engaging in this fallacy, for example, if he explained the meaning of, and motivations for, my practice of the psychiatric profession solely with reference to the infantile factors I outlined in Chapter 1.

Adolescence and adulthood are not simply perennial resurrections of the conflicts and modes of adaptation of childhood. Although the trials and tribulations in the adolescent's relationship with the opposite sex and with authority figures are in some respects replays of the earlier oedipal ones, they also have important new features peculiar to this age itself. Although there are similarities in the task posed the oedipal child and that posed the adolescent, everyone would agree that there are crucial differences as well. Adolescence can be adequately explained with reference to the oedipal period no more than the latter can be exhaustively understood with reference to the preoedipal. By now Freud has established the case for childhood determinism sufficiently that we can safely shift the balance a bit in the other direction.

Erikson and Levinson have accomplished some of the most sophisticated work on adult development. The former conceptualizes three more stages after that of adolescence. The first of these, *intimacy versus isolation,* concerns the task of relating to a member of the opposite sex in a lasting way, not merely on the basis of one's own needs, but with a mature recognition of the individuality of the other as well. Erikson (1963, p. 266) defines what he calls the "utopia" of genitality as follows:

1. mutuality of orgasm
2. with a loved partner
3. of the other sex
4. with whom one is able and willing to share a mutual trust
5. and with whom one is able and willing to regulate the cycles of:
   a. work
   b. procreation
   c. recreation
6. so as to secure to the offspring, too, all the stages of a satisfactory development [i.e., the possibility that they too can achieve the 'utopia' of genitality]"

Erikson's next stage, *generativity versus stagnation,* refers to the period in which one must establish himself occupationally and socially, as well as establish and guide the next generation. It is concerned with issues popularly styled "productivity" and "creativity." The last of his eight stages is that of *ego integrity versus despair.* He defines the former as "the acceptance of one's one and only life cycle as something that had to be and that, by necessity, permitted of no substitutions . . ." (p. 268). Accompanying this are a new and different sort of love for one's parents, a sense of one's place in the overall continuity of generations, and a realistic acceptance of one's mortality. Despair, by contrast, is the feeling that "the time is now too short, too short for the attempt to start another life and to try out alternate roads to integrity" (p. 269).

Levinson, who has studied the life cycles of many contemporary and historical persons, speaks of the development of the *life structure* in adulthood. By "life structure" he means the pattern or design of a person's life at any given time. This pattern is best defined in terms of the important *relationships* between oneself and his world (the latter including persons both living and dead; places; ideas; vocation; and political, religious, and ethnic systems). To be satisfactory, a life structure must be both *viable* in society and *suitable* to the self.

These patterns, and the relationships within them, are not static over time. Levinson has identified what appear to be regularities in the evolution of the life structure from adult to adult.[14] As in the stages of childhood development, a failure to negotiate successfully the tasks of an earlier period can affect one's development in a later stage. The adult life cycle breaks down into a series of "transitional" or "structure-changing" periods alternating with more stable "structure-building" periods. These transitional periods tend to be much more stressful than the structure-building periods, and the therapist might suppose that one's reaction to any given external event would depend to some extent on whether one is in a structure-changing or structure-building period. He should also know that death and rebirth symbolism is common in times of transition.

He divides adulthood into three *eras:* early, middle, and late adulthood. The first era is from approximately age 17 to 45. It is subdivided into an early adult transition, early adulthood, and the mid-life transition. The first task of the early adult transition, roughly from age 17 to 22, is to modify and terminate relationships extant from the child and adolescent period and to reappraise and refashion the preadult self. The second is to make preliminary forays into the adult world and explore its possibilities, to imagine oneself as a participant in it, to consolidate an initial adult identity, and to make and test some preliminary choices.

Early adulthood proper is partitioned into *Entering the Adult World*, the *Age Thirty Transition*, and *Settling Down*. In the first subphase one must make and test out some preliminary commitments to occupation, love relationships, friendships, values, and life style. One has two primary and somewhat antithetical tasks: to explore the possibilities and keep one's options open and yet to become more stable and responsible. During this subphase and the one that follows, one of the most important tasks is forming what Levinson calls the *Dream* and giving it a place in the life structure. The Dream is a vague vision or sense of self-in-an-adult-world. It is an image of the relationship between self and the world in all its components—occupation, achievement, status, family,

---

[14]Levinson's published work to date has dealt only with men. His current project on adult development in women (the results of which will soon be published) so far supports the idea that these same eras and stages apply to women as well, though the issues they face and their manner of negotiating them are of course not identical to those of men. The impact of the recent sociocultural changes on women must be borne in mind by every therapist. Never before have so many women had so many options, and yet prejudices against women are far from dead in many areas. At the same time that new possibilities and responsibilities have arisen, many of the old responsibilities remain. Often women are subjected by their families and society to intense and conflicting double messages and expectations about independence versus dependency, assertiveness versus submissiveness, competitiveness versus passivity, career versus homemaking and childbearing, and so forth.

home, friends, leisure, community, and political, religious, or philo-sophical ideals and practices. At the start it is poorly articulated but, as time goes on, it must become more well defined and realistic. Those who build a life structure around this dream, says Levinson, have a better chance for a sense of personal fulfillment and happiness than those who do not. In later life one has to reappraise the Dream, identify its magical aspects, and modify its place in the life structure.

The *Age Thirty Transition* provides the opportunity "to work on the flaws and limitations of the first adult life structure, and to create the basis for a more satisfactory structure with which to complete the era of early adulthood" (Levinson, p. 58). It is a time in which issues that "should" have been faced in the early adult transition, but were not, can be confronted and worked on. The provisional quality of the twenties is ending and life is becoming more serious. There is the recognition that if one is going to make major changes they must be made soon, or never. Of course people differ widely in the type of life structure they form for themselves in this period but one thing appears certain: the life structure at the end of the Age Thirty Transition is significantly different from that at the beginning. The therapist should know that, for *most* of Levinson's 40 contemporary subjects, this transition was a time of *moderate to severe emotional distress.*

In the first two subphases of early adulthood the mentor relationship is often one of the most important elements. This is a relationship with a person roughly a half generation older, who functions as teacher, spon-sor, counselor, and exemplar, and who supports and facilitates the realization of one's Dream. It is important to know that mentoring relationships are more likely to end in strong conflict and bitterness on both sides than to die a natural death or become a modest and warm friendship.

"*Settling Down,*" or building a culminating life structure for early adulthood, begins for most between 31 and 34 and ends at about 40. Having wrestled more or less successfully with the dilemmas of the Age Thirty Transition, having questioned more or less adequately the first adult life structure, one makes his choices and begins to implement them. Upon this foundation he erects a life structure with one or two components in the center (usually career and family or other interper-sonal relations) and others radiating out toward the periphery.

The person enters the "Settling Down" subphase on the bottom rung of the social-occupational ladder of the senior adult world. He wants to climb that ladder[15] as far as possible. He seeks both to follow the way of his heart and to be affirmed and acknowledged by society, two goals that are not always compatible. In men the second half of this stage is so

---

[15] See page 80.

distinctive that Levinson has given it a special name: "Becoming One's Own Man." Research to date suggests that women go through a similar phase of becoming one's own woman. One is beginning to arrive, to feel and be acknowledged as competent and senior at one's craft, to establish oneself as a certain type of parent, spouse, friend, and a valued member of the tribe, and to speak confidently and with one's own voice. The completion of Settling Down is often capped by a "culminating event," which may be a social, occupational, or other success (or failure). For most people this period seems one of moderate or flawed success rather than total triumph or abject defeat.

The *Mid-life Transition*, the bridge from early to middle adulthood, is another stage in which most of Levinson's subjects reported moderate to severe turmoil. This is a time of review of one's accomplishments and aspirations. "During a transition period—and especially in the Mid-life Transition—the neglected parts of the self more urgently seek expression and stimulate the modification of the existing structure" (Levinson, 1978, p. 61). In the case of men this often involves shifting some of the attention from career and status toward family, friends, and feelings.

In some the life structure that results from the questioning during the *Mid-life Transition* is markedly different from that which came before, whereas in others there is mostly a deepening and enriching of the relationships that existed before. Some enter middle adulthood (45 to 65) with a sense of satisfaction and anticipation, others with a sense of defeat. These former are "less tyrannized by the ambitions, passions and illusions of youth," "more deeply attached to others and yet more separate, more centered in the self."

The time from age 50 on has been less thoroughly studied by Levinson and others so it is impossible to speak with the same assurance of any regularities in the development of those years. Levinson describes an *Age Fifty Transition*, spanning the years from 50 to 55, with functions in some ways similar to those of the Age Thirty Transition. In it one can review and modify the life structure established in the mid-forties. It can be a time of crisis for those who changed too little in their Mid-life Transition. From 55 to 60 there is a second structure-building period in middle adulthood. This period is analogous to the Settling Down of early adulthood. The Late Adult Transition, the time from 60 to 65, terminates middle adulthood and forms the basis for starting late adult-

---

[15]Some have suggested that, in feminine development, the image of the *lattice* is more accurate than that of the ladder in that many women seem to be devoting roughly equivalent amounts of energy to several tasks (career, family, community, and so forth) simultaneously, or alternately, within the settling down life structure. Many men, by contrast, seem to be climbing a more single-minded career ladder in which their devotion to career all but precludes their development in other important areas (especially family and emotional life).

hood. It too is a period of significant development and marks a major turning point in the life cycle.

Levinson's most important message for the psychotherapist is that he should not view the static adult character structure as the norm and the fluid and evolving one as pathological. Indeed, he believes that in adulthood, as in childhood, stasis can lead to more problems than mobility. "No matter how satisfactory a [life] structure is, in time its utility declines and its flaws generate conflict that leads to modification or transformation of the structure" (Levinson, 1978, p. 54).

By teaching us that we continue to develop throughout the life course, adult development theory provides a useful corrective to any "originological" tendencies. The interaction between human psychobiology and the environment, in some as yet incomprehensible way, leads to demonstrable periods, or seasons, in the lives of us all. Each of these stages poses somewhat different tasks, opportunities, and burdens. Each calls upon us to make and place our bets—wagers that determine the capital with which we confront the next turn of the wheel.

Our childhood history provides us with a more or less strong or weak foundation upon which to erect our adult life structures. It ensures that no two of us will approach adulthood with the same possibilities, options, desires, and range of conscious volition. It ensures that infantile meanings and motives will participate in all of our important adult behaviors, often sufficiently to override current and conscious considerations. Nevertheless, hemmed in by our history as we are, we do *choose*, within the limitations it has provided us, for conscious and unconscious, current and historical reasons, and each of us lives with the joys and tribulations of his decisions. The story of adult development is the saga of these choices and of our more or less adaptive and creative coming to terms with the tasks posed by our histories and current environments. Dynamic psychiatry is the science which seeks to broaden these options and to improve this coming to terms with past and present (recall footnote 8, Chapter 1).

## SUGGESTED READINGS FOR CHAPTER 2

Aichorn, A.: *Wayward Youth*. New York, Viking Press, 1971. A 1925 classic on adolescence by one of Freud's early disciples.

Blos, P.: *On Adolescence: A Psychoanalytic Interpretation*. A somewhat advanced text. Difficult reading, but well worth the effort.

Erikson, E.: *Childhood and Society*. Revised Edition. New York, W.W. Norton & Co., Inc. 1963. His groundbreaking work on the relationship between psychological development and society.

Erikson, E.: *Identity, Youth, and Crisis*. New York, W.W. Norton & Co., Inc. 1968. An important collection of essays on identity formation and adolescent development.

Fraiberg, S.: *The Magic Years*. New York, Charles Scribner's Sons, 1959. Delightfully written primer on childhood development.

Freud, S. (1900 [1899]): *The Interpretation of Dreams.* Standard Edition of the Complete Psychological Works of Sigmund Freud,* Volume V, Chapter VII. London, Hogarth Press, 1953. The chapter which broaches the topographic model and the theory of the primary and secondary process.

Freud, S. (1905): *Three Essays on the Theory of Sexuality.* Standard Edition, Volume VII. London, Hogarth Press, 1953. Freud's exposition of psychosexual development, of the concepts of fixation and regression, and of the relationship between all this and adult psychopathology.

Freud, S. (1921): *Group Psychology and the Analysis of the Ego.* Standard Edition, Volume XVIII. London, Hogarth Press, 1955. This work and the one that follows are the *Ur*works of ego psychology. The concepts of ego, and ego ideal, as well as those of identification and character formation, are here expounded.

Freud, S. (1923): *The Ego and the Id.* Standard Edition, Volume XIX. London, Hogarth Press, 1961.

Kernberg, D.: *Object Relations Theory and Clinical Psychoanalysis.* New York, Aronson, 1976. A good review of the previous work in object relations theory and an exposition of the current thinking on the matter. Difficult reading, but repays the effort.

Levinson, D.: *The Seasons of a Man's Life.* New York, Ballantine Books, 1979. Well worth reading. Contains Levinson's theory of adult development and material from interviews with 40 men.

Lidz, T.: *The Person: His and Her Development Throughout the Life Cycle.* New York, Basic Books, 1976. Justifiably popular exposition of human development throughout the life span.

Mahler, M., Pine, F., and Bergman, A.: *The Psychological Birth of the Human Infant.* New York, Basic Books, 1975. Contains her seminal work on separation-individuation.

---

*Hereafter referred to as "Standard Edition."

# 3

# Conflict, Character, and Psychopathology

Having hewn out the stone, let us build the edifice—the dynamic theory of character and psychopathology. Central to this presentation are the concepts of *unconscious conflict, signal anxiety, defense, compromise formation, history, transference, overdetermination, adaptation, and atavism.*

First, I want to reemphasize that there is a continuum between psychopathology and normality. The healthiest among us exhibit pathological behavior at times, just as the most disturbed are capable of moments of health. *Mental health,* most broadly defined, is a state of equilibrium among one's mental forces and between these forces and the environment. It is, in other words, a state of optimum adaptation, "adaptation" being defined roughly as the ability to meet one's needs for satisfaction of the basic bodily demands, affiliation, and the preservation and promotion of self-esteem without violating those of one's neighbor. Implicit in the concept of adaptation is the possession of a certain flexibility in the appraisal of, and action upon, the kaleidoscopically changing situations that confront us from day to day.

Psychopathology, on the contrary, is a state of disequilibrium, or conflict, among the internal forces and/or between them and the environment. It is a special case of maladaptation already referred to as *atavism,* the persistence of once adaptive, historically based modes of behavior into the present where they are no longer appropriate. Atavistic behavior is stereotypic and inflexible. Because the person is not usually aware of either the behavior patterns or from whence they come, he is not capable of modifying them appropriately when circumstances command.

Character, pathology, dreams, and parapraxes—those entities which I discuss in this chapter—are all manifestations of, or attempts to come to terms with, unconscious intrapsychic conflict and its attendant anxiety. I shall begin with an elucidation of conflict with reference to its most classic expression, the neurotic symptom, and then discuss the other categories under consideration. Clinical examples follow each theoretical presentation.

Unconscious intrapsychic conflict is ubiquitous. All of us are beset by it from time to time. If it is sufficiently frequent, or severe, or our means of dealing with it are sufficiently maladaptive, we are in danger of falling prey to one of the psychopathological labels. In conflict an unconscious affect-laden fantasy, disagreeable to the demands of superego or society, threatens to rise into consciousness, raising the possibility it might then be translated into *action*. The unconscious ego experiences this as an imminent *danger situation*, the dangers ranging, as we have seen, from loss of the loved object through loss of the object's love and castration to superego condemnation. In order to prevent the feared response from superego or society, the ego generates *anxiety* which *may or may not* be perceived by the *conscious* ego. This anxiety, or *signal anxiety* as it is called, is unpleasurable and, since the psyche moves toward pleasure and away from pain, in accordance with the pleasure principle, a *defense mechanism* is *unconsciously* set in motion to ward out of awareness the offending impulse and to remove the need for anxiety.

If the defensive maneuver is successful, a certain equilibrium is established, albeit at the cost of the continuous expenditure of the psychic energy necessary to maintain the repression and at the cost of, in the case of the more reality-distorting mechanisms, an adaptive relationship with the real world. When the defense mechanism fails, a *symptom* results. A symptom is a last ditch stand against the unconscious impulse; it is a final attempt to establish some sort of internal equilibrium and adaptation to the outside world. A symptom is a *compromise* between the unconscious impulse striving for expression and the defense against it. Dream elements, many character traits, neurotic styles, and parapraxes can also be understood, as I shall demonstrate, as *compromise formations*. In other words, a symptom is simultaneously a *disguised gratification* of the warded-off impulse and a *defense* against it. Insofar as it is the former, it is the example of a failed repression, or the "return of the repressed." Insofar as it is the latter, it functions as a sort of poor man's defense mechanism.

The following are two cases of failed defenses and compromise formation: one in a man with pronounced ambivalence toward his wife, the other in a compulsive woman who was deathly afraid of acknowledging her dependency and anger (in part because both were associated with a fear of rejection).

Mr. O. set out, unbeknownst to his wife, to repair her long-damaged and much-cherished heirloom necklace. He was planning to surprise her with it on their anniversary. Unfortunately, on his way to the repairman he lost half of it! His decision to fix the jewelry was itself a reaction formation to a considerable unconscious aggression toward his wife, an aggression that prevailed in the end. What started out as a respectable reaction formation degenerated into a troublesome symptom.

Ms. Q. began the session by telling me about her previous psychiatrist, Dr. C., whom she left because he had criticized her, asking her to slow down what he called her "pressured" speech. Implied in this, of course, was a concern that I would do the same. She then nervously told me about another incident in his office. She had an obsessional fear of fires and was compulsively scrupulous about dousing her cigarettes. On that particular occasion, she had just put out a cigarette in the ashtray. Noticing it was full, she decided to empty it for Dr. C. She carefully poured the ashes into a folded bit of paper and deposited them in the waste basket. Lo and behold, within seconds there was a roaring fire in his office, which she of course assiduously put out! After the end of our session she returned almost immediately to my office, having had the obsessional fear that she might not have doused her last cigarette! Her behavior with both Dr. C. and me was *symptomatic*. It reflected a *compromise* between the unconscious desire to harm us (for a variety of reasons into which I shall not go) and the defense against it. It was also a way of getting herself back into my office which she did not, unconsciously, want to leave.[1]

Before resuming the discussion of conflict theory itself, I shall elaborate on the concept of *anxiety*. Both Freud and Sullivan, the most creative psychoanalytic revisionist, agree on the centrality of anxiety in psychopathology. Indeed, an impulse is repressed or leads to a symptom not because of the impulse *per se*, but because it leads to the production of anxiety. To the degree that the defensive maneuver or symptomatic behavior is "successful," this "signal" anxiety is both diminished and remains unconscious. In other words, one can (therapists included) be anxious and yet consciously *un*aware of it. Later in this chapter I shall provide an example of a resident whose anxiety, even though (or rather

---

[1]This is also a good example of the symbolism in symptomatic behavior, the fire representing anger and, as would become patent later, an even more strenuously repressed sexuality. Similar symbolism expresses itself in everyday parlance: "aflame with sexual desire," "the heat of passion," "mad as fire," "hot with sensuality." Pay particular attention to the point at which cigarettes are lighted within a session since, in addition to being a nonspecific response to the heightened tension of fear or neediness, they often manifest sensuality or aggression.

because) she was unconscious of it, markedly influenced her behavior with a patient.

When the defense or symptom is unsuccessful, the signal anxiety (which is always unconscious) becomes experienced consciously as the well-known affect "anxiety." It is crucial to remember that anxiety, whether experienced in a crowded airport or in a closet, is always an *interpersonal* phenomenon. If people are not physically present, it is at least related to (conscious and unconscious) feelings and fantasies about, or memories or anticipations of, interactions with people. In this sense there is no such thing as "free-floating anxiety," for it is always connected to an object or objects.

When anxiety occurs within the context of a real person or persons, it bears some relation to conflict-laden feelings and fantasies about these people and those whom they unconsciously represent. In such a situation, even though the primary objects of our anxiety may be historical, internalized ones, the anxiety still affects our relationship with the flesh and blood ones before us. Anxiety invariably disturbs our interaction, our communication, with the other person. If it is overt, then he is likely to become anxious as well—anxiety having a markedly contagious effect. Since it is unpleasurable, the two parties withdraw from one another. It has, as Sullivan (1953) said, a "disjunctive" effect on the relationship.

Even if the anxiety is unconscious and hidden from the view of ourselves and the other, however, it still is likely to disturb the interaction. It may, for instance, be warded off by symptomatic behaviors that distance people, such as bizarre psychotic behavior or neurotic rituals. Or, so much energy may be expended in keeping the impulse and its concomitant anxiety unconscious that we are distracted, unable to attend to and communicate effectively with our partner. Furthermore, pronounced anxiety has an effect on learning and recall resembling that of a blow on the head:

> [It produces] a useless disturbance of the factors of sentience which immediately preceded its onset, a phenomenon which is so striking that in later life the great problem of psychotherapy is very often centered on this very matter of getting the patient to see just when anxiety intervened, because that area is disturbed in such a way that it is almost as if it had not been (Sullivan, 1953, p. 152).[2]

The symptom's binding of the anxiety secondary to unconscious intrapsychic conflict is referred to as its *primary* or *paranosic* gain, and is of course the main reason (or reinforcement value, as a behaviorist would say) for its maintenance. Often, concrete advantages concerning external reality arise *after the fact* of the symptom, such as decreased demand

---

[2]See page 87.

for responsible adult behavior, increased attention, or disability payments. This is known as *secondary* or *epinosic* gain. Even though it arises subsequent to the formation of the symptom, it can contribute, as well, to its maintenance. Indeed, we shall find that it is more the rule than the exception that any given symptom is determined from several different directions, expresses and defends against several trends, and serves several different purposes (*overdetermination*). Since symptoms occur within an interpersonal context, they can also be understood as *veiled, symbolic communications* to particular persons in the environment. In fact, we shall see that Freud conceptualized both the neurotic symptom and the dream symbol as *disguised* communications of unconscious desires. Shortly I shall describe an hysterical symptom that served as an oblique communication of one man's complaint to his wife.

The other crucial aspect about present-day conflict is that *it originates in childhood*. All conflict is originally between the inner and outer worlds, but as this outer world becomes incorporated, the conflicts tend to become internal ones. The behavior of one's parents, who are more or less faithful representatives of the sociocultural norms as well as of their own idiosyncratic needs, interacts with the nascent personality, itself the result of biological endowment and its still earlier experience with parents, to produce *intrapsychic conflict*. Owing to certain biological and social structural universals shared by all human beings (e.g., we all have bodies and are reared in family units composed of at least a parental male and female), there are some conflicts shared by virtually all of us. However, because of manifold differences in the day-to-day experiences encountered by each of us in our separate families and subcultures,

---

[2]There are some differences, but many points in common, between Freud's and Sullivan's theories of anxiety. Because some writers, such as Fromm-Reichmann, prefer Sullivan's terminology to Freud's, I shall briefly outline it here. From experience with the forbidding, anxiety-provoking gestures of the parents in response to certain of his behaviors, the child develops the *self system*. The self system is an organization (mostly unconscious) of that experience which has been associated with anxiety and diminished self-esteem at the hands of the parents. Damage to self-esteem is, for Sullivan, the preeminent danger situation. The need for security is the need to protect the self-esteem and to avoid the anxiety that would accompany its injury. Fantasies or feelings that run counter to the consciously acceptable view of one's self (the *good me*) and which are associated in the self system with past experiences of anxiety periodically threaten to rise into consciousness. The self system responds to this by activating one or more of the *security operations* which split off from awareness the offending impulses or direct them into socially acceptable channels. Sullivan saw the self system as relatively fixed by the close of childhood, though he believed it was open to influence at the threshold of each of the succeeding developmental eras (the juvenile, preadolescent, early adolescent, and late adolescent) and through psychotherapy. Apart from anxiety, *loneliness* was, for Sullivan, the other fundamental affect. He felt its dysphoria often leads people to seek out, despite considerable anxiety, interpersonal contact.

there are significant differences in which types of conflict are most important, as well as in the patterns and editions of the universal ones. Because of our idiosyncratic personal histories and constitutions, not only the conflicts but the *ways of coping with these conflicts* differ. Because of modeling of parental coping mechanisms and parents' differential reinforcement and punishment of certain attempts at adaptation, and because of personal creativity and cognitive-motor endowment, each person's favorite defensive maneuvers and ways of coming to terms with the environment vary.

Once established, these ways of adapting to the inner and outer worlds, our character styles and symptoms, become relatively fixed for a number of interrelated reasons: 1) They are largely *unconscious*, even though the most untrained observer, perceptive grandmother, or best friend could often point them out to us; 2) these patterns are ingrained and habitual and there is a certain economy of expenditure in allowing our behavior to follow along old and timeworn paths; 3) those who unconsciously represent our parents, siblings, and other early signifi- cant others (e.g., imagoes) stimulate dormant unconscious impulses directed toward those originals, thereby calling into operation the old tried and true defensive maneuvers; 4) because we unconsciously expect these imagoes to behave toward us as did the originals, in anticipation, we react to them with the same repertory of defense mechanisms that were developed in our contact with the prototypes; and 5) our behavior toward these imagoes often ensures that they will in fact react to us as we fear and we may end up actually needing our defensive maneuvers in the present—the classic neurotic self-fulfilling prophecy. In addition, some people have an uncanny knack for spotting those in the environ- ment who will treat them as did the originals, thereby bringing alive the past in the present (recall Mrs. A.).

## CONFLICT IN A SYMPTOM NEUROSIS

I shall illustrate the points raised thus far with a lengthy clinical example:

A fundamentalist Missouri lay minister, Mr. T., who had always been dominated by his father and who was psychologically battered down by him or "preached to" whenever he tried to assert himself, married a woman much like his father—in fact, a woman chosen for him, like his career, by this man. As time progressed, her nagging, domineering, and depriving behavior began to stir up years of pent-up, unconscious rage. In other words, his wife's behavior *in the present* was functioning as the precipitant for intense aggression with roots extending into the remotest past. These aggressive impulses ran counter to the patient's superego which told him it was wrong to want to kill one's father and wife; they ran counter to his expectation that his father, a large man, would have beaten him up and that his wife would have left him. In other words, the current aggression toward the wife, based on that toward the father in childhood, brought up three *danger situations:* condemnation by the superego, loss of the loved object and, to some extent, physical injury (castration). This was a case in which there was conflict between an id impulse e.g., aggression, and the social and superego forces opposing it. The ego, as we shall see, elected to take the side of superego and reality against the id.

The ego responded to the imminence of these dangers with signal anxiety, which was, of course, unpleasurable and mobilized *repression* which, in the case of our patient, failed. The offending fantasy continued and threatened to rise into awareness. A *symptom,* a conversion reaction or hysterical paraplegia, resulted. It must be emphasized that this whole process was *unconscious.* The patient was not malingering and was convinced his disability was organic. Indeed, it had occurred shortly after he had overturned his car, so there appeared to be a basis for it in reality. It was such a convincing paralysis that it persuaded a competent neurosurgeon to perform an operative procedure! He was quite insensitive to pin prick and other noxious stimuli over the affected area and there was no sign of power in his legs. He showed the conversion hysteric's characteristic relaxed resignation (*la belle indifférence*) toward his disability. This symptom was a *compromise formation.* It removed any possibility that the patient would become aware of, or act upon, his aggression. At the same time, it obliquely expressed his anger by forcing his wife to become the breadwinner and to wait on him hand and foot, and by subjecting her to his fecal and urinary incontinence in bed. It was overdetermined in the sense that it also met his needs to be dependent and to receive attention, absolved him from the necessity of performing sexually (about which he had previously had some anxiety), and expressed his most deeply unconscious desire of all, to submit to the father (a derivative of his negative Oedipus). The secondary gain was his absolution from adult responsibility and the reception of disability payments.

The "choice of symptom," his "coping" mechanism, was itself *historically based.* In childhood he had witnessed his mother develop similar symptoms as her way of dealing with anger toward, and frustrated needs for affection from, her husband, the patient's father. An aunt also had had conversion reactions. As a child, the patient was frequently too sick, usually with a variety of vague gastrointestinal complaints, to go to school. On such days he received a good deal of pampering from his grandmother as well as some of the little bit of nurturance he received from his cold and domineering father. His tendency to resort to hysterical and psychosomatic symptoms was thus *atavistic* in the sense that it was an adaptive response (granted, to an inappropriate situation, but adaptive nonetheless) in childhood, but not in the current adult reality in which he was forced to make his way. Or, more accurately, it was an attempt, albeit a miscarried and ill-advised one, to adapt both to his historically based internal conflicts and to the present-day reality of his relationship with his wife. Nevertheless, the symptom did succeed in keeping the conflict unconscious and in binding the anxiety attendant upon it. Indeed, he was a singularly placid individual. The decision was made to remove the symptom through hypnosis. While in a deep trance he was told that he would see, upon an hallucinated movie screen, a scene of great importance to his paralysis. In

a moment he informed us that he saw his wife standing there and upbraid-
ing him on several counts. When asked what the problem was he said,
"She's screaming at me. I can't stand it. *I can't stand up to my wife* [one of
the symbolic communications of the symptom]." When asked repeatedly
how he felt, he began to admit to a little anger which, in the course of a
few minutes, became a towering rage. As this man's previously placid face
quivered and contorted with rage and (now quite conscious) anxiety, and
as he cursed his wife, the power began slowly to return to his legs. He was
then told that in waking life he would become conscious only gradually of
his repressed aggression toward his wife. He was then awakened and
pushed his wheelchair back to the ward, where he was treated to the
astonishment of patients and staff alike.

Unfortunately, the story did not end here. What followed was a
powerful illustration of my point in Chapter 1 about facilely tampering
with a patient's cherished, though in many respects maladaptive, equilibrium.

With hypnosis we sliced through this man's manifold resistances to becoming conscious of his murderous rage toward wife and father. We
bypassed the slow and painful process of first dealing with his fears of
facing this material such that he would become aware of it only as he was
capable of integrating it with the rest of his conscious self-image. His
unconscious did not listen very well to our suggestion that he would only
become consciously aware of the aggression as he was capable of handling
it. As these powerful affect-laden fantasies moved closer to consciousness,
as well as anxiety over conflicts around sexual performance and homosexuality that had previously been bound by the symptom, this hitherto
monument of tranquility became a "nervous wreck." This previously
passive man had several violent outbursts toward his wife, which she took
quite badly. Indeed, not only his internal equilibrium, but that in his
marriage, was upset by his increased "assertiveness," as he called it. In a
frantic, of course unconscious, attempt to defend against this upsurge of
feelings, he soon developed a *substitute symptom*, an illusion. When he
looked in the mirror he saw, not his own face, but that of a man with long
white hair and beard, bright red lips, and sharp teeth. He became so
frightened he refused to look in the mirror, stopped shaving, and let his
beard grow. Gradually, in face-to-face psychotherapy in full consciousness, we became aware of the meaning of this new symptom. His first
thoughts upon initially seeing the face were "It's my father; no, it's me."
In a later session he commented "The face looks like Santa Claus with
sharp teeth." Then he recalled that he first remembered seeing his father,
who was absent in World War II when the patient was a toddler, during
the father's Christmas furlough. "He came and brought me candy and
then disappeared as fast as he came. Maybe I never forgave him for it."
Thus, one underpinning of the new symptom was a small boy's longing
for, and disappointment in, his father: "Santa Claus with sharp teeth."

The other underpinning was more recent and related to his wife. He
recalled that the face also resembled that of a picture of Judas Iscariot that
he and his wife had seen in some religious gardens, interestingly, on their

honeymoon several years before! The patient had referred to himself as the "betrayer" of his own masculinity vis-à-vis his wife and father. Thus, the illusion was intimately related both to frustrated needs for affection in childhood and adulthood, and to anger about this and about being dominated. It was largely a projection of his own unconscious rage at wife and father. Since he grew a beard, like the figure, and even wondered for a time whether he should hang himself, like Judas, he was also secondarily identifying with the illusion and those whom it represented and thus reinternalizing much of the rage he had projected. (Internalized rage, anger turned on the self, leads, as we shall see later, to depression.) As he became affectively and cognitively aware of this conflict (which, incidentally, also played itself out in his relationship with me) and its current and historical roots, the illusion disappeared and his anxiety and depression resolved. He became more appropriately assertive with his wife and she was helped to deal with this through marital therapy.

This case also illustrates the principle of *overdetermination*, or *multiple function*, as Waelder has renamed it. This principle states that each symptom, or almost any normal behavior for that matter, is determined from several different directions, expresses several different trends, and serves several different purposes. This was well illustrated by both symptoms of our hysteric. The hysterical paralysis was determined by current and historical conflicts over aggression (as was the illusion) and by a deeply repressed need to assume a submissive attitude toward the father and his imago (wife).

Another fascinating example is the woman whose symptomatic eating binges represented: a way of dealing with a constellation of rage, hurt, and low self-esteem related to current rejections (being left by her father and my going away on vacation); an attempt to deal with unresolved feelings about prior deprivation and rejection precipitated by the current ones; an identification with her mother who ate when she had argued with the patient's father and when he withdrew from her; an attempt to receive the attention of an otherwise indifferent mother who would lecture her at length about her weight; a substitute for genital sexual pleasure over which she was too conflicted to engage in; and the acting out of an unconscious fantasy of being impregnated by the therapist (based on an underlying oedipal one) and, simultaneously, defending against the possibility of intercourse with him by gaining weight and trying to make herself unattractive to him.

Both these examples illustrate that the symptom has a function within the current interpersonal context quite as well as in the intrapsychic one. The former is, however, particularly well exemplified in the case of Susan, a girl of latency age with a penchant for holding her feces for weeks at a time and then explosively plugging up the family toilet with them. Quite apart from the (quite consciously) sensual pleasure associated with this, it served to energize her depressed, isolated, and emotionally unexpressive parents. She was simultaneously expelling her unconscious aggression toward them and getting them together, however briefly, around her problem. She was pleading that they drop the pretense that "everything is all right around our house" and recognize that they were all suffering immensely. Unfortunately, they did not understand her message and shifted the problem onto the pediatrician.

## CHARACTER, CHARACTER NEUROSIS, AND CHARACTER DISORDER

Before progressing to other examples of conflict, I shall define some terms. We have just examined one of several ways of dealing with, and manifesting, conflict, the symptom neurosis. The *symptom neuroses* (hysteria, phobias, obsessive-compulsive disorders) are characterized by discrete phenomena (hand washing, private ritualistic behavior and persistent unwanted thoughts, avoidances) which are not viewed as integral and acceptable parts of one's identity and which are, with the exception of conversion hysteria, quite uncomfortable (*i.e., ego dystonic*). All symptoms are, as we have just seen, *compromise formations* between an affect-laden fantasy striving for expression and those forces that oppose it. They are miscarried attempts at adaptation, at reestablishing some sort of equilibrium within the self and with its environment.

*Character traits*, on the contrary, are viewed, if they are recognized consciously at all, as integral parts of the self and are quite comfortable to one (*i.e., ego syntonic*). When character traits are working, the person is in relatively little pain even though aspects of his character may make life difficult for others. The term *character* refers to the total assemblage and pattern of character traits, to one's particular and enduring style of balancing the forces within and harmonizing them with the environment. It is our idiosyncratic way of dealing with the conflict that is ubiquitous to life, of obtaining a modicum of gratification for the drives, and of meeting the demands of society for a measure of productive work and consideration for our fellows. Character results from the interaction of biological endowment, personal creativity, and what we have learned and modeled from our parents. Like symptoms, character traits are compromises between: the forces of repression and those striving for expression; the injunctions of society, superego, and ego ideal; and the pressures from the id. Character traits can be classified according to whether they are closer to the side of expression or repression in this compromise. They may be perpetuations of the original id impulses in more or less modified form, or they may be sublimations of them or reaction formations to them. They may take great account of the demands of superego and society and little of those of id, or vice versa. The criminal character expresses his aggressive and sexual id impulsions in barely modified or unmodified form. The hard-driving businessman, self-centered in the pursuit of his own advancement, neglectful of the feelings and needs of friends, colleagues, and family, and constantly teasing his secretaries, is expressing his aggressive and sexual impulses in more modified form. The saccharine-sweet, oversolicitous personality may be still another way of dealing with id impulses. The rigid and methodical character, perhaps even manifesting itself in carriage, mannerisms, and posture, might defend against a host of bumptious fantasies and affects.

The presentation of Mr. E. reflected a character style that was built around conflicts over intimacy. He would seek people out and yet carried his obese body in a slouched and slovenly manner. He was unkempt, looked down at his navel, spoke in a rambling and subvocalizing mumble, and was tardy when he did not forget his engagements altogether. His behavior was thus a compromise, expressing the desire for closeness at the same time that it distanced and alienated others as a way of avoiding a number of unconscious dangers associated with intimacy. Another man's character expressed itself in his manner of taking leave of me. He would spring from his chair right on the 50-minute mark, never allowing me to call time, then rush to the door without looking at me and say, not "good-bye," but "I'll see you next time." This sort of behavior was characteristic of his interactions with others as well and reflected strong reaction formations against dependency. Still another patient dealt with the same strivings in an opposite way, with a virtual inability to bring a conversation or a letter to a close, much to the chagrin of his friends and acquaintances.

When character shifts toward the pole of antisocial behavior, it is termed a *character disorder*. This is characterized by ego syntonic character traits which are quite comfortable to the practitioner, but run counter to the interests and well-being of his fellows and, ultimately (because of their reaction to him), run counter to his own. The psychopathic or delinquent personality, the individual who discharges his id impulses and their derivatives in virtually unmodified form, is the classic example of this sort of behavior. He is in little intrapsychic conflict and has little capability or desire to bind and inhibit his antisocial fantasies and to deal with frustration and mental pain. Not his behaviors themselves, but the social consequences, are experienced as painful.

When, by contrast, character moves toward the pole of neurosis, it is termed a *character neurosis*. The *character neurosis,* as opposed to the symptom neurosis, is not characterized by discrete, ego dystonic behaviors, but by *behavior patterns* which no longer function successfully as means of adapting to the external world and of maintaining internal equilibrium. One might say that the patient's entire repertory of behavior is his symptom. Thus, these behavior patterns—compromise formations, like symptoms—*begin* to become a bit ego dystonic. The person begins to suffer and, quite often, to become aware of how his behavior makes others suffer. This form of neurosis now seems more common than the discrete and well-defined hysterical, phobic, and obsessive-compulsive neuroses of Freud's day.

The continuum between character, character neurosis, and symptom neurosis is best illustrated with reference to obsessive-compulsive behaviors. In the previous chapter I referred briefly to the orderliness, obstinacy, parsimony, ambivalence, and preoccupation with power and control that characterize this personality type. Its caricature would be the cold, methodical, and efficient scholar or accountant. The primary purpose of such a behavior style is to ward off *feelings* that accompany, or arise in reaction to, conscious and unconscious fantasies.

In his repertory of defenses, *isolation, intellectualization, undoing,* and *reaction formation* are particularly prominent. All these are described in more detail later in this chapter. Isolation refers to the separation of the ideational and affective components of a fantasy. In practice this usually involves the conscious awareness of the idea, while the feeling connected with it is relegated to unconsciousness. In the first chapter I gave the example of the man who was aware of his parents' divorce in his childhood but not of his feelings about it. Or, one could have fleeting murderous thoughts, but without the rageful and guilty feelings associated with them. Intellectualization is closely related to isolation in that its primary purpose is to use thinking to keep feelings at bay. Undoing functions to absolve the obsessional of guilty feelings over (mostly) unconscious unacceptable fantasies and feelings. Often it is preceded by *doing*, which expresses the very impulse that undoing wards off. For example, he tells a sadistic joke on a neighbor and then undoes it with apologies and praise. He expresses an unconscious desire to be rid of his family by checking the oven to make sure the gas is turned off, first turning it on, then flipping it off. I have already described reaction formation.

The obsessional has to feel in control of everything, particularly his own feelings and his relationships with others. He has great trouble with intimacy lest he lose control of his warm and dependent desires and become so enamored of other persons that they can control him. His interaction with early caretakers has been of such a nature that he is left with a good deal of hatred, as well as love, toward them. The fear that this hatred will become mobilized, along with the love, becomes another reason for avoiding close relationships.

Obsessive-compulsive character styles are resistant to change because they are usually effective in keeping feelings and fantasies at bay. Furthermore, the obsessional is often a highly efficient machine who is much rewarded by his employers. For example, the meticulous and officious bookkeeper who checks and rechecks the columns of numbers is simultaneously keeping a host of feelings at bay and pleasing his boss.

The problem is that this bookkeeper cannot shut off his behavior at five o'clock, if indeed he allows himself to go home that early, but carries it out the door with him. He brings the same cool, calculating "efficiency" to his interactions with spouse, friends, and children.

The compromise quality of much of his behavior is best illustrated with reference to aggression. His busy, no-nonsense, driven, and mechanical quality often makes life miserable for others at the same time that it defends against his desire to do so. Nevertheless, although his style may interfere with the well-being of family and friends and although, at the same time that it protects him from much pain, it robs him of much pleasure, he is usually comfortable with it.

Like all other character styles, this one originates in childhood through a combination of personal creativity, learning, and modeling. It takes shape and persists because it is *adaptive.* Let us consider the example of a small boy (who became Mr. X.) whose father was a workaholic intellectual.

> Central to this child's dynamics were the father's physical and emotional absence and the mother's overprotectiveness and smothering seductiveness. The result was a child of six who was 1) frightened of his closeness to mother, guilty about his supercharged feelings for her, and angry at her both for not indulging the desires she had stimulated and for curbing his freedom, and 2) angry and resentful at, and hurt by, the father's lack of attention to him. In short, the behavior of this child's parents produced considerable ambivalence toward both of them. The boy dealt with these conflicting feelings by developing his natural cognitive abilities. He would read and perform calculations for hours, keeping sex, affection, anger, guilt, and hurt at bay. This intellectual activity was also a way of resolving his oedipal issues and feelings about his father's absence by identifying with him. Such activity was positively reinforced by the mother and much of the little attention he received from the father was related to this. Later it was rewarded by parent surrogates at school. Thus, this character style of intellectualization and isolation was reinforced from *two* directions: the reduction of internal tensions and the praise of the environment. It was quite *adaptive* given that the boy was psychologically battered down when he expressed his feelings toward father and mother, and given that his behavior was rewarded by both school and parents. It was, in other words, appropriate to the situation in childhood.

> However, when the boy left home and encountered children and adults who were not like his parents, he no longer needed to fear that they would react to his feelings as did the parents. Nevertheless, he unconsciously expected that they would, so he continued his style right on into his marriage where he became quite as absent and coolly intellectual toward his wife and children as was his father toward him (atavism). There was every reason to believe that his own children would replicate the cycle.

If such a person's behavior becomes extreme enough, causes enough pain in his environment, and begins to fail in its defensive and adaptive functions, and if the person himself begins to be uncomfortable with it, self-conscious of it, and begins to view it as something that persists at considerable cost to himself and others, we can call it an obsessive-compulsive *character neurosis*. In Mr. X. it progressed to that point.

> The aggressive, sexual, and dependent fantasies this behavior was designed to ward off began to move closer to consciousness. His perennial hard-driving, ambitious, and competitive style began to get out of hand at work and to antagonize his colleagues and supervisors. His wife became resentful of his aloofness from her and his ever-increasing absorption in work. On his part, the bitterness to her (largely based on that toward his mother) began to surface. The children began to throw tantrums to make their father notice them, when they did not mope about the house or withdraw by themselves. Mr. X. became increasingly aware of the malignant effect he was gaving on family and friends and was uncomfortable about it. Furthermore, the years of frustrated dependency needs for the father, and anger and hurt over the father's rejection of him, began to surface. Mr. X. began to feel anxious, depressed, and needy. His personality style was becoming *ego dystonic;* there were things about himself he did not like and wanted to be rid of. He recognized he was robbing himself of the enjoyment in life. Mr. X. entered treatment, which was quite a task in itself for this man who strongly needed to deny his needs for others, and duplicated his neurotic style of behavior in his relationship with the therapist, who unconsciously represented his mother and, especially, his father. In order for this man to change, it was necessary for him to come to terms with a wealth of hurt, neediness, sexuality, rage, and guilt. Eventually he lost the need for his outmoded, historically determined behavior style and became more accessible to the feelings and needs of himself and others, to the benefit of all.

In an obsessive-compulsive *symptom neurosis*, by contrast, the picture is dominated by discrete, ego alien, ego dystonic thoughts and behaviors. Like many character neurotics, Mr. X. did indeed have certain symptoms, but they occurred only occasionally and were never of central importance. For example, he would occasionally have fleeting hostile thoughts about various family members, following which he would tap on wood four times. He would at times check and recheck the oven to make sure it was turned off before leaving for work. He would occasionally feel a compulsion to count the number of words in a line of print he had just read. His meticulous cleanliness at times approached the level of a symptom and it alternated, interestingly, with a variety of scatological behaviors.

Since I have already described a symptom neurosis (hysteria) in some detail, I shall only mention briefly the obsessive-compulsive symptom neurosis, which is less common than the corresponding character neurosis. The best example is Freud's case of the Rat Man. The Rat Man had a variety of issues, most especially related to ambivalence toward his recently deceased father and, to a lesser extent, toward his current girl friend. Freud (1909, pp. 189-190) describes these latter:

> One day, when he was out with her in a boat and there was a still breeze blowing, he was obliged to make her put on his cap, because a command had been formulated in his mind that *nothing must happen to her*. This was a kind of *obsession for protecting*, and it bore other fruit besides this. Another time, as they were sitting together during a thunderstorm, he was obsessed, he could not tell why, with the *necessity for* counting up to forty or fifty between each flash of lightning and its accompanying thunder-clap. On the day of her departure he knocked his foot against a stone lying in the road, and was *obliged* to put it out of the way by the side of the road, because the idea struck him that her carriage would be driving along the same road in a few hours' time and might come to grief against this stone. But a few minutes later it occurred to him that this was absurd, and he was *obliged* to go back and replace the stone in its original position in the middle of the road.

This last, incidentally, is an excellent example of both doing and undoing and compromise formation. The unconscious hostile wish is defended against by removing the stone and the wish itself is expressed in replacing the stone. This case is full of other obsessional thoughts and compulsive actions, and the reader is advised to read it in full.

Mr. Y. serves as an example of a character disorder:

> He was raised in a slum by an alcoholic father who frequently deserted the family for weeks at a time and by a mother who brought a series of lovers into their small apartment. When the patient was born his mother already had two small children underfoot. Her pregnancy with him had been an unwanted one, and he was deprived and abused from the outset. In addition to being physically and verbally abused by the mother, he witnessed a great deal of overt display of aggression between the parents and sexuality between the mother and her lovers. The patient soon learned not to express his needs and frustration-born hurt and rage to the parents for he was then battered down even more unmercifully. Self-restraint was not modeled to him by the parents, who were themselves openly involved in a number of illegal activities—drug selling, prostitution, stealing. From the parents he also learned to excuse his own problems by blaming them on others (a form of rationalization known as "externalization"). There was much animosity between him and his siblings, the older of whom usually got the better of him.

> This early history had left him, by age six, with several intense conflicts. First of all, there was the tension between the desire to express his dependent needs and his knowledge that he would be pushed away, or worse, for them. Second, there was the conflict between his desire to beat up his parents for their misuse and deprivation of him and his knowledge that if he attempted it he would be "taken to the cleaners," as he said. These first two conflicts were more or less conscious, although eventually parts of them became more or less repressed. The third conflict, over his

sexual strivings for his mother, was almost entirely unconscious from the outset. Her affairs and sexual exhibitionism were supercharging his oedipal fantasies, all the more so because of the absent father. He was not aware of his incestuous desires for her but only of his extreme discomfort at the sights and sounds in the maternal bedroom. He displaced the feelings onto his sister, with whom he often engaged in childish sexual play. The fourth issue was his shaky masculine identity caused by the virtual absence of a father with whom to identify. The primary characteristics he would adopt from this father were his physical abusiveness toward women, his alcoholism, and his thievery. After all, this is what his father had taught him being a man was all about.

In latency, adolescence, and adulthood Mr. Y. developed a variety of behaviors designed to deal with the residue of feelings bequeathed to him by his past. In order to obtain the family and father he never really had, he joined an adolescent street gang led by a boy about 25 years of age (father imago). He was also able to act out his sibling rivalry vis-à-vis his fellow members in the competition for the leader's attentions and sexual favors from the "women's auxiliary." His tough "macho" style was in part an attempt to cover up his underlying shaky sense of masculine identity. Involvement in gang rapes and muggings allowed him to *act out* his unconscious incestuous desires toward his mother and conscious aggressive fantasies (in reaction to deprivation and rejection) toward both parents. He continued in this behavior until apprehended and imprisoned.

Mr. Y. illustrates many of the principles involved in understanding the character-disordered, psychopathic, or antisocial individual. First, historical factors played just as large a role in his behavior as in the neurotic's. Second, he was not without unconscious intrapsychic conflicts, but they were much less prominent than in the neurotic. For example, impulses that were quite conscious and comfortable to him, like patricidal fantasies about the father, would have been deeply unconscious and conflictual in the neurotic. His incestuous fantasies were unconscious and conflictual like those in the neurotic but, unlike the latter, he *lacked control* over the expression of the *derivatives* of these fantasies. In other words, he translated what would have remained conscious or unconscious derivative *fantasies* in a neurotic (e.g., of having intercourse with a middle-aged woman) into *action* (actually raping these women). Third, his behaviors were not ego alien or uncomfortable to him. He was causing much pain to others but experiencing little himself. When a twinge of hurt about his parents' behavior toward him or a dawning sense of deficient manhood overtook him, he would drown it in drugs, drink, or violence. He went to his psychiatric consultation not out of a sense of inner hurting or remorse and any motivation to change, but because the authorities were forcing him to feel uncomfortable, with the threat of an extended prison sentence. Were this external pressure removed and were he released from prison, his discomfort would cease and he would return to his old behaviors.

## SYMPTOMATIC ACTS, PARAPRAXES, AND JOKES

Virtually any behavior can function symptomatically (to both express and ward off affect-laden fantasies, and to bind anxiety), from the most blatant phobia or obsessive-compulsive ritual to the practice of one's very livelihood itself. Under the rubric "symptomatic acts" are included parapraxes, bungled actions, and what are usually called mannerisms or habits.

### Symptomatic Acts

Symptomatic acts include bungled actions and those habitual and absentminded gestures of which we are all capable. An example of the former is portrayed in the following case.

> The patient came in with a large bandage on his thumb. When I inquired about it, he informed me he had "accidentally" hit it with a hammer the weekend before. His wife had been "nagging" him for weeks about putting up some kitchen shelving. Partly as a way of obliquely expressing his considerable dissatisfaction with her, he had been taking his "own sweet time" about it. On Saturday she "hit" him with it again and, exasperated, he got his tools and began work. Within minutes he had hurt himself and lost no time in showing his thumb to his wife. It was not difficult for the patient himself to realize, within minutes, that he really wanted to smash her, not himself, and that hitting himself was a way of both defending against, and punishing himself for, this desire, as well as a way of "getting at her," by throwing his wounded thumb up in her face and by ensuring he could not complete the cabinets. "Maybe I should have gone back to work and gotten her to hold the nail!" he quipped as he left off the topic.

That familiar class of individuals that I would call the "klutzy saints"—those who cover your suit with the cup of tea they are graciously offering, who bring you gin when you ask for vodka, who light your chin instead of your cigarette—are past masters of the symptomatic act. They are simultaneously defending against and expressing their unfriendly intentions.

The following is a good example of the second type of symptomatic act.

> Mrs. O. was beginning to develop a strong, but as yet unconscious, erotic and dependent transference to me. This, coupled with a great (but largely unconscious as well) ambivalence toward her husband, manifested itself in a constant playing with her wedding ring. She would move it off her finger, thereby expressing the desire to throw her husband over for me, and then replace it, thereby undoing the unacceptable wish. The to and fro motion of her finger in the ring was also a symbolic expression of what she wanted to transpire between the two of us. Eventually all this became conscious and was expressed verbally rather than being symptomatically acted out.

## Parapraxes

Parapraxes, or slips, were considered by Freud under the rubric of the "psychopathology of everyday life." He elucidated their mechanism in a book of the same title, in which he also makes one of his strongest statements about the ubiquity of psychic causality. Slips, as much as symptoms, manifest unconscious intrapsychic conflict. A miscarried action results when two intentions run counter to each other. For example, when we mispronounce the name of a person we dislike or one who unconsciously reminds us of someone whom we dislike, the conscious intention to say his name correctly is opposed by the unconscious one to insult him. Or, to reconceptualize this in terms of conflict theory, the unconscious wish to insult him (and those whom he represents) is associated with any of a number of danger situations (loss of love, castration, superego condemnation, and so forth). The ego generates signal anxiety, and a defensive maneuver is set in motion. In the case of the parapraxis, this is a distortion or disguise of the insult unconsciously intended. The word that results is a hybrid between the unconsciously intended one and the correct pronunciation, reflecting the compromise between the forces of expression and those of inhibition. This is humorously illustrated by a slip a patient made one day. Speaking of her ex-boyfriend's wealthy new girlfriend, whom she detested, she mistakenly referred to her as Mitch rather than Martha. She caught her error almost immediately and laughed, "I guess I meant to say 'Martha, that rich bitch.'"

Often, the "commonsense" explanation for a slip is that "I was fatigued, preoccupied with something else, drank too much," and so forth. This is true only to the extent that fatigue, conscious preoccupations, and alcohol may facilitate, by weakening one's inhibitions, the entry of forbidden material into consciousness. Furthermore, fatigue or alcohol do not affect the *content* of what emerges. The same is true of "habit," which is often invoked to "explain away" a parapraxis. For example, the patient who said "I forgot our last appointment because we had changed the time to Tuesday and I was used to coming on Wednesday" was only half right. The patient was a highly intelligent man with an excellent memory. His work required him to keep tabs on an ever-changing round of appointments. In his case, "habit" was functioning as a vehicle upon which his unconscious aggression toward me (in part in reaction to my changing his hour) got a free ride.

I shall provide four more examples: three from patients I was treating, the other from a psychiatric resident I was supervising.

Central to Mrs. R. were dependency-independence issues. She was finding a number of convenient excuses to avoid making the separation from her widowed father with whom she was living in a far from harmonious state. When she finally did move out and set up in her own apartment, she

experienced considerable loneliness and turmoil. Eventually she attempted suicide and was admitted to a short-term inpatient unit. When, after
the first two days, her anxiety had subsided, she said to me, "I'm ready to
leave, I'm glad this ward only keeps you 7 *weeks* [days] to 14 days." This
statement reflected, of course, her unconscious ambivalence about being
discharged.

In another case a patient of mine who was contemplating quitting therapy
because "it wasn't going anywhere" returned almost immediately to my
office to retrieve his hat. However, he did not bring his hat that day in the
first place! This is an instance of a *paramnesia* which led to a symptomatic
act—his return to my office. It was an epiphenomenon of his deeply
repressed desires to be back in my office and dependent on me. Another
patient, scrupulously careful to pay me at the end of every session rather
than waiting for my bill at the end of the month, miswrote the check for
"sixteen" rather than "sixty" dollars, thus expressing her unconscious
ambivalence about the fee.

The following example comes from an observed resident interview.

The psychiatric resident was interviewing a 40-year-old mother of three
children who was separated from her husband of 20 years. This woman,
like her husband, had served a prison sentence for conspiring in what she
strongly implied, but would not come out and say directly, was the sexual
abuse of their children. She attributed most of her problems to her husband, toward whom she said she could never assert herself. "I don't have
any backbone and let him push me this way and that. I gave in to what he
wanted so I could keep my swimming pool and the good life." A litany of
the problems others had caused her continued for the next half hour, and
she did not permit the resident to get a word in edgewise.

After this observed interview, the resident commented that she had felt
extremely warm and physically uncomfortable in the room. When one of
her fellow residents asked about the ethnic background of the patient, it
suddenly occurred to her that *she had forgotten the patient's name.* Upon a
little reflection it became apparent that this amnesia, like her discomfort
and flushed feeling in the interview itself, was symptomatic of an unconscious conflict. On the one hand, there was anger at the patient over her
misuse of her children (the resident was herself a mother) and refusal to
own the role she played in her problems and on the other a professional
superego which told her, "It's not all right to feel angry at a patient."[3] The
ego generated signal anxiety at the prospect of superego condemnation,
and the emerging anger was repressed.

In the interview she was conscious only of her physical discomfort (which
she initially blamed on the chair and the air conditioning, both of which
were in fact no different from usual). She was conscious of *neither* her
anxiety (although her fidgetiness was plain to her colleagues and me) *nor*
the conflict that produced it and led to her forgetting the patient's name.
In other words, she wanted to push out of awareness the name of the
person whose behavior was stimulating her discomfort.

---

[3]See page 102.

## Jokes

Freud maintained that there is a good deal of truth in jokes and that we often betray our underlying sentiments through them. In his 1905 classic on wit he explained the joke as a temporary release of inhibitions against the expression of sexual and aggressive drive derivatives. He conceptualized the laugh as a manifestation of the temporary saving of psychic energy (counter-cathexis) otherwise required to maintain the repression. You will find that your patients, like your friends, express much truth in their jokes. One patient, with the wish-fear for/of dependency and intimacy, said, only a few days after learning of my impending vacation, "This is a five-day paper [meaning a notice of intent to leave the hospital within five days]. No, only joking, it's a copy of a letter to a friend." This was the closest he could then come to dealing with his feelings about my leaving. The joke, like the symptom, is a compromise. It is both a defense against a more direct expression of the unconscious impulse as well as a veiled satisfaction of it.

## DREAMS

It was, of course, Freud's 1899 *magnum opus* on dreams that inaugurated the history of psychoanalysis. Because the internal resistances against the emergence of unconscious material weaken in sleep, we have conscious access to memories and fantasies from which we are debarred in waking life. For this reason, Freud called dreams the "royal road to the unconscious." It is a central dictum of Freudian dream theory that one must assume personal responsibility for what appears in his dreams. This brings to mind the anecdote about a prim and proper middle-aged spinster who dreamed she was abducted into the woods by a rough-looking rogue. When he tossed a blanket on the ground and threw her upon it she asked in terror, "What are you going to do with me, Sir?" He replied "That depends on you lady, it's your dream!"

---

[3]This is not true of course. All therapists have feelings toward their patients and it behooves them to know what they are. We are interdicted from *acting* on these feelings, but we can use them nonetheless. Often they are valuable clues to the patient's intentions toward us. Frequently there is an inextricable interaction between what the patient is attempting to induce in us and our own psychodynamics. An excellent example is the middle-aged resident who found himself making critical comments to the patient, a young woman of his same religious group, about her aimless, promiscuous, and irresponsible life-style. Her direct and indirect attempts to make him act as a father impinged upon his father countertransference to her and adversely affected his technique. He was, by the way, unconscious of this whole process at the time. Had he been aware of his paternally judgmental and protective response, he would have had some important information not only about himself but about the role this young woman was inducing him to take.

Nevertheless, even in sleep our resistances, or the *dream censorship* as they are called, continue to operate. For this reason a dream element, like a symptom, is a compromise between unconscious fantasies striving for expression and the forces opposing them. A dream, in other words, is just as much a manifestation of conflict as is a neurosis. It is usually only in the dreams of psychotics, prepsychotics, and small children that socially unacceptable unconscious impulses regularly express themselves unabashedly. Otherwise, dreams are *disguised* fulfillments of an unconscious wish. The dream is the nightly craziness in all of us and, by the fantasied satisfaction of ungratified desires and the working through of tensions, it serves a cathartic and cleansing function that helps us preserve our sanity during the day.[4] These disguised gratifications also discharge tensions that would otherwise lead to the dreamer's awakening. Thus, one of the primary functions of the dream is, as Freud said, to preserve sleep.

This disguised expression of unconscious strivings, the dream of which the patient is aware and reports to the therapist, is called the *manifest content*. Its unconscious underpinnings are dubbed the *latent content*. The *dream work* is the process which disguises the latent content sufficiently that it can escape the censorship, rise into consciousness, and still not, in most circumstances, disturb sleep. The primary process mechanisms, such as displacement, condensation, and symbolization, constitute the tools with which the dream work fashions the disguise. *Secondary elaboration*, which strives to meld the whole into some semblance of a coherent tale, also functions in the service of disguise. If the dream work is successful, the impulse receives a measure of gratification *and* sleep remains undisturbed. If not, and the latent content begins to manifest itself too blatantly, then one of the various danger situations arises and the ego responds with anxiety that awakens the dreamer— the nightmare, or *anxiety dream*.

In addition, dreams can be important diagnostically and prognostically. As a rule, the more distance there is between the latent and manifest contents of the dream, the healthier the dreamer, or at least the stronger his ego and its defensive capabilities. Sparse disguise of the latent content may indicate a previously unrecognized psychotic or prepsychotic state. Jung described an apparently healthy young man whom he declined to analyze after the latter reported a dream, in the first meeting, of an idiot smearing feces inside a sumptuous palace. I recall an attractive young woman, an executive secretary, who astonished me by re-

---

[4]It is well known, both by many schizophrenics and by their therapists, that several nights of apparently dreamless sleep can be a harbinger of an exacerbation of the psychosis. This can be used as a barometer for medication dosage adjustments.

porting, after only a few sessions, a dream in which her sister's head was sitting in the dishwater and in which she stabbed it and removed it to the counter, from whence it gazed at her reproachfully. That was my first indication that I should soften my attempts to get her to deal with her anger, proceed more cautiously, and give greater respect to her defenses.

Like neuroses, dreams and their elements are overdetermined and have roots running all the way from childhood to recent reality. (One can never completely interpret a dream, said Freud.) Processes and events with which the waking mind is concerned carry over into sleep where we continue to mull over them at an unconscious level. These concerns from the day before, for example, a rebuke from the boss, are called the *day residue*. They are not sufficient in themselves to produce a dream unless they enlist the aid of deeply unconscious strivings— conflicts with father and other early authority figures, in this case. To use Freud's analogy, current concerns function as the broker while historical, unconscious preoccupations furnish the capital. However, exactly *which specific events* from the previous day will function as the day residue is itself in part a function of the unconscious dynamics of the dreamer, e.g., the rebuke from the boss stimulated a dream only because of the prior father conflict of the dreamer. Furthermore, such historically based conflicts themselves scan current reality for a nidus to precipitate around, and this is what the day residue provides them. In the aforementioned example, a dream might result in which one triumphs over a man representing a composite of father, high school football coach, Army officer, and current supervisor.

In the previous chapter I discussed the primary process mode of operation in dreams and I shall not recapitulate that here. The interested reader can, of course, do no better than to read *The Interpretation of Dreams*, or at least Freud's abridgement of it, *On Dreams*. The use of dreams in psychotherapy is discussed in a later chapter.

The following vignette illustrates the idea of the dream as a manifestation of conflict and a compromise formation.

> Mrs. K. was a 55-year-old married woman whose husband had recently had a severe heart attack and was afraid to subject himself to the cardiovascular stress of sexual intercourse. There is a reasonable possibility that he was impotent anyway. Her husband had become increasingly withdrawn and preoccupied with himself since the coronary, and her symptoms of anxiety and depression dated from that time. She strenuously denied, however, that her husband's illness and withdrawal had anything to do with it. She was not troubled, she asserted, with sexual frustration since she was "no longer interested in that anyway."

> In the second week of treatment she reported the following dream. Her husband was lying on a raft out in the middle of a lake at G., a place where

she and he used to picnic when they were young lovers. The raft floated to the pier and he got out and walked to shore. He looked bedraggled and there was a hole in his finger from which *brown* blood was streaming. In the next scene she had taken him to the hospital and he was hooked up to a cardiac monitor. The rhythm and rate were regular. Suddenly the scene shifted and she was in the next room lying on a bed with an intravenous line in her arm. Her blood was being withdrawn through a complicated system of tubes leading into the adjacent room. Precipitously, the scene shifted back to the coronary care unit and her husband's monitor. The rate and rhythm remained regular. Suddenly there was a power shortage and the lights went out. When they came back on, the monitor showed a flat line EKG. Her husband was resuscitated and then died again. The dream ended with the recovery of his heart beat.

This dream expresses nicely what this woman would never allow herself to acknowledge in waking consciousness: that she was ambivalent toward her husband and dissatisfied with his impotence. The *ambivalence* is nicely expressed, in compromise formation, by putting her husband in the middle of the lake but then bringing him to shore, and by allowing him to repeatedly die and yet be resuscitated in the coronary care unit. The wounded finger, dripping *brown* blood, expresses an uncomplimentary opinion about the state of his penis, while the withdrawal of her own blood expresses the idea that his illness, with its increased dependency, withdrawal, and impotence, was draining the life blood from her. The location of the raft scene at a lake where she and her husband had had better times expresses her nostalgia for a red-blooded, not brown-blooded, partner in sexuality and affection. Nevertheless, this dream, although it may not appear disguised to us, was sufficiently so to this psychologically untutored woman that she remained consciously unaware of her conflict.

The historical roots, upon which I shall not expand, included the loss of her own father to a heart attack when she was a young child. There were fond memories of early family outings at the same lake where she courted her husband. There was also a wealth of resentment toward the father for leaving her at the height of her oedipal period. Since anger, like sexuality, was not "allowed" around her house, this resentment was repressed and turned upon herself. Thus, her present-day conflicts over sexuality and aggression rested upon a foundation from childhood. Her husband's behavior was stressful not only in itself, but because it was resurrecting unresolved issues from childhood.[5]

---

[5]Where one finds strong inhibitions against anger, one usually discovers that either anger was not "kosher" in the early home or else that a situation in which one parent could become violent caused anger to be viewed as a dangerous, even life-threatening, feeling to be avoided at all costs. Conflicts over anger, like conflicts in general, are often manifested by precipitous oscillations between total inhibition and obstreperous expression of the impulses in question.

Before closing this section let me mention one additional, interesting species of dream that was for a time a puzzle to Freud and the early analysts: the *post-traumatic dream*. Such dreams are a repetitive recapitulation of the traumatic experience and affect associated with it. Since they regularly produce the same dysphoric affect, Freud believed they violated the pleasure principle and he used them as a primary rationale for the idea of a *repetition compulsion* capable, in its blind repetitiveness, of overriding the pleasure principle.[6] Most dynamic psychiatrists believe that the post-traumatic dream can be explained without recourse to any mysterious new principle. The pain of the post-traumatic dream is not its primary intent but rather a byproduct of the attempt to work through one's anxiety over the experience. To do this one has to mentally return to the situation and reexperience the strong affect. In part, of course, this results from the unrealistic fantasy of going back and making the events turn out differently this time. If the trauma involves a reaction to the death of a loved one, dreaming about it can of course also be a way of 1) punishing oneself for not having been able to save him, or 2) expressing hostility toward him for leaving us (by putting him back into the situation), or 3) getting him back (because at least we regain him for a while if only in the traumatic situation itself). I treated a young woman whose husband, like the patient's boyfriend in Chapter 1, died in a boating accident. She was not present at the time, though the accident was explained to her in intimate detail. She presented because of a series of dreams in which the accident was recurring, to her considerable anxiety. Two or three sessions of abreacting her sorrow, anger, and guilt feelings and informing her that the dreams did not mean, as she feared, that she was going crazy were enough to cause their cessation.[7]

## CULTURE AND CONFLICT

Cultural institutions can provide us with ready-made modes of release of, or defense against, our unconscious impulses. For example, unac-

---

[6]Often this term is used inappropriately to refer to the tendency to reenact historically based patterns of behavior. Such behavior is quite in accordance with the pleasure principle. It is the unconscious strivings continuing to press for satisfaction, despite the pain they cause other parts of the psychic apparatus. Schur (1969), in my opinion, has debunked the "repetition compulsion."
[7]There can even be what one could only call "pretraumatic" dreams. The best example is the so-called "examination dream." Such dreams occur in anticipation of a stressful situation where one feels one's abilities and self-esteem will somehow be put to a test. Usually they are dreams of similar situations in the past where one emerged successful. They serve to abreact one's anxiety and to remind one of past success. Occasionally, they redepict the past, successfully negotiated experience as a failure; in this case the "pay-off" arises from the relief one experiences upon awakening and recognizing the absurdity of the dream and, by implication, the absurdity of one's current anxieties.

ceptable impulses can be attributed to Satan or evil spirits (e.g., projection), thus sparing us the task of acknowledging them. Often, the same cultural behavior can both express and defend against the same fantasy; in other words, it can function as a compromise formation. Consider the case of the 19-year-old man of Italian extraction, troubled from childhood by the combination of a smothering and seductive mother and an absent father.

> Following a seduction attempt by an attractive college coed, he fled to a monastery in southern Italy where he became preoccupied, among other things, with meditation upon the Virgin Mary. This was a frantic attempt to ward off the upsurge of incestuous fantasies with religious asceticism. Nevertheless, that his adoration of the Virgin surreptitiously expressed, as well as defended against, these fantasies soon became obvious. He wrote religious poetry about Mary in which the mildly erotic metaphors characteristic of much of mystical writing gradually coarsened into lurid descriptions of intercourse with the Virgin. In other words, the expressive pole of the compromise became increasingly powerful until its defensive functions essentially disappeared and the man was psychotic.

The modal conflicts, and ways of dealing with them, can differ somewhat from culture to culture. For example, ethnology teaches us that the particular manner of manifestation of even so universal a conflict as the Oedipus can vary from culture to culture depending on whether the society is patrilineal or matrilineal, to what degree the extended family is present, the manner of the preoedipal nurturing, and so forth. Modes of upbringing in some cultures, like those in which the male child is suckled until seven or eight and in which the father is away for much of this time, may considerably intensify the incestuous drives. Similarly, each culture provides different institutions to assist in overcoming and resolving such conflicts: torturous initiation ceremonies and abrupt separation of the latency-age boy from the mother in some, projection or displacement onto religious institutions in others. Kardiner (1939) has produced evidence that cultures in which the institutionalized patterns of child care are depriving and punitive produce adults with conflictual issues around dependency and independence, frustration-born rage, and basic trust-versus-mistrust.

Different cultures can favor different defense mechanisms. Inn Seok Oh, a Korean-born psychiatrist, believes that reaction formation is particularly common in Oriental cultures, with their emphasis on institutionalized politeness and avoidance of overt hostility. (Perhaps the same could be said of our own South.) The same degree of anger at parents that would be quite conscious in a Westerner is likely to be deeply repressed in an Oriental. Likewise, suppression of both sexuality and aggression is emphasized in these cultures. Sexual matters that would be discussed quite openly in this culture would bring painful embarrassment to the Oriental. An emphasis on aspects of the ego ideal and superego expressed as "duty" and of the ego expressed as "will" and "self-restraint" leads to ways of resolving conflicts between personal inclinations and those of society that are quite different than in contemporary America. Cultures that place a high premium on turning against the self are likely to have a higher incidence of depression and suicide (e.g., Japan). The social stigma in this country, at least until recently, against expressions of anger and assertiveness in women has been cited by some as a prime reason for the greater incidence of depression in females. Projection seems to be a much-used mechanism among individuals in many contemporary preliterate, or so-called "primitive," cultures and among certain religious fundamentalists. Religious rituals can serve as a means of undoing one's unconscious antisocial fantasies and of keeping unwanted thoughts at bay. The long hours of productive labor and frantic pace enjoined by many modern societies can function in the service of isolation of affect and denial of painful aspects of reality. Institutionalized carnivals, festivals, and sporting events can serve as a means of displacing sexual and aggressive feelings from their unconscious objects to more consciously acceptable representatives of them. Myths and fairy tales can function likewise.

## THE DEFENSE MECHANISMS

The reader is by now quite aware of defensive maneuvers and processes. Dynamic psychiatrists today appreciate that virtually *anything* can serve as a defense at one time or another. One affect-laden fantasy can defend against another, as well as being an impulse in its own right—anger against sexuality, sexuality against affection and dependency, and so on. Good examples of the former are the hysterical character who fights with and pushes away a man to whom she is actually attracted and the paranoid latent homosexual who reacts fearfully and aggressively toward those whom he unconsciously loves. A good illustration of the latter is the "swinger," deprived of affection in childhood, who defends against his dependent needs and associated fear that these needs will meet with rejection by "love 'em and leave 'em" behavior. Talking about the present can be a defense against troublesome issues from the past, and vice versa. Focusing on the past or on current reality can be a way of avoiding transference issues toward the therapist, or vice versa.

There can even be defenses against defenses! One patient's heterosexual fantasies before and during the hour functioned to ward off underlying homosexual attractions to the therapist. These latter defended against still more unconscious and ego dystonic, infantile, dependent longings for him. Freud's Dora used reaction formation to ward off her sexual feelings for Herr K., which themselves warded off her homosexual desires for his wife.

Not everything that is defended against has its home in the id. Superego impulsions can be warded off quite as strongly as those of the id. We can project, rather than acknowledge, self-critical and self-accusatory trends onto others and react to them as if they, and not we, are our accusers. A classic example of this is the family members of a recently deceased hospitalized patient who dealt with their largely irrational and unconscious sense that they somehow failed their cancerous relative and could have done more for him by displacing their criticisms onto the hospital (e.g., "it is you doctors who failed him, not us"). Or, to take a similar example, extremely self-punitive superego trends can become projected upon the environment or allayed with drugs and alcohol lest they lead to a conscious feeling of guilt or decreased self-esteem or even, in extreme cases, to one's self-destruction. A good illustration of this is the person with a hypercritical and guilt-inducing superego who projects his own inordinately severe standards onto others and then reacts to them angrily, as if they and not he were placing the unreasonable demands on him.

Certain relatively discrete defensive processes are so common as to be labeled the *defense mechanisms*. They are among the most important functions of the ego. There are a dozen or so of them depending, since there is some overlap among them, upon how they are classified. They are *not* pathological in and of themselves (for this reason they are often called the *mental*, rather than defense, mechanisms) and may in fact be quite adaptive in terms of both internal equilibrium and external reality. The scholar's intellectual preoccupations not only result in publications that bring him tenure, but help him defend against a host of feelings and fantasies as well. This mechanism of intellectualization is also a good example of how each individual uses defensively whatever is constitutionally and experientially at hand. A mentally retarded person or one from a family with no emphasis on learning would hardly have the same access to intellectualization as does the professor.

Defense mechanisms only come to the attention of the psychiatrist when they are associated with problems in adaptation, either because they no longer serve to maintain an internal equilibrium or because they maintain this equilibrium at the expense of serious disturbances in one's perceptions of, and actions upon, the environment. For example, one man's inhibitions against aggression may be so overpowering that they prohibit him from exercising the normal assertiveness and aggressiveness necessary in day-to-day life on the job, at home, and with one's friends. Another's conflicts over his unconscious homosexual tendencies lead him to project them onto others, misperceive their communications, and pick fights with, and insult, them. A middle-aged spinster's projection of her sexual impulses leads her to fear rape from every man she sees and leads her to lock herself up in her house.

In short, the psychiatrist encounters those whose defense mechanisms are either failing, with resultant symptom formation and return of the repressed, or interfering with their enjoyment of, and productivity in, life, or hindering the well-being of others. Defense mechanisms manifest themselves to the clinician in the form of *resistances* to remembering, talking about, or otherwise dealing directly with affect-laden material. Whether the therapist is more involved in dissecting and getting beneath the defense mechanisms, or attempting to strengthen them or substitute new ones for those which are failing, depends upon the particular pathology of the patient. Broadly speaking, as we shall see in a later chapter, psychotherapeutic strategies may be differentiated as to whether they adopt one or the other of these two strategies toward the defense mechanisms.

Strictly speaking, the defense mechanisms are thought of as *unconscious* processes of the ego. However, I urge you to conceptualize them as existing on a *continuum* from consciousness to unconsciousness. Many of us have kicked the dog or yelled at the spouse after an argument with the boss, knowing quite well we were displacing anger actually directed at our employer. At other times we may have done so unawares and yet shamefully recognized what we were doing almost immediately *afterward*, in which case one would have to say the mechanism was preconscious. On still other occasions we have done so unconsciously and have remained totally unconscious of it.

We have all caught ourselves in the act of attributing our own sentiments and preoccupations to others. Who has not offered a trumped-up explanation or rationalization that he does not half believe to excuse his omissions, unfriendly motivations, and mistakes? At times we can bend over backwards to be nice to people we actually do not like. Thus, our own conscious experience gives us some idea of how defense mechanisms operate.

I shall define and exemplify the most commonly encountered defense mechanisms. All of them serve to reinforce the keystone mechanism, *repression*. Repression is the warding off of affects and fantasies that run counter to the aims of society and superego. A certain amount of mental energy, or *countercathexis*, is required to oppose the unconscious impulse's continued cathexis of the internal and external object world. The active forgetting of repression is an *unconscious* process, as opposed to *suppression*, which is a quite *conscious* decision to forget, or not to think about, something.

*Projection* is the attribution of our own unacceptable strivings and affects to others, e.g., the aforementioned latent homosexual who fears a sexual assault from every man he meets or the envious and competitive man who ascribes these tendencies to others. Projection is one of the most socially maladaptive mechanisms, since it leads us to react to others not as they actually are, but as we consider them to be. Often we project around a kernel of truth in reality and then behave in such a way as to induce the other person to treat us as we fear. A good example is the woman who deals with an unconscious dislike of her husband and a desire to "run around" on him by constantly accusing him of hating her and of having affairs. Such tactics may actually lead him to do so, thus giving her good grounds for her suspicion. Paranoids are remarkably skillful at inducing people to conform to their expectations of them.

Closely related to, and in some ways a subspecies of, projection (and rationalization) is *externalization*. This is the shifting of the responsibility for one's own role in the problem. The tendency to blame others for one's plight accompanies the conviction that only others (e.g., the therapist) can rescue one from it. It is common in dependent personalities.

*Projective identification* is a hybrid between projection and identification, but is much closer to the former than to the latter. Thought to be particularly common in the so-called "borderline," it is probably one of the most commonly used defensive maneuvers of all. It is a "poor projection" in which the individual often remains partly aware that the mote in his brother's eye is the beam in his own. He projects his own desires, preoccupations, fears, and affects onto another and then identifies with what is projected onto him. Subsequently, he may vicariously enjoy, empathize with, and/or be revolted by and attempt to control what he has projected onto the other. For example, a mother with partly conscious conflicts over exhibitionistic impulses may alternately vicariously enjoy and rail out against and attempt to control the exhibitionism of her daughter. The same can be true of parents dealing with a host of other boisterous adolescent behaviors. A highly competitive and envious man may project his strivings and feelings onto others and then act in such a way (passive withdrawal or feigned humility) as to minimize what he views as *their* competitiveness with, and envy of, him.

Projective identification is particularly common in marriages. Both partners may be ambivalent about the same issue—frugality versus expenditure in money matters, or how much independence a particular child should have—and yet, each of them projects one-half of this ambivalence onto the other so they can battle it out between, rather than within, themselves. The person engaging in projective identification is often extremely skillful at seeking out someone with preoccupations and conflicts similar to his and then inducing him to take complete ownership of one-half of the conflict. Freud engaged in this defensive maneuver in his relationships with Fliess and Jung, two physicians with scientifically unorthodox, virtually mystical, preoccupations. With his own interests in the occult, telepathy, and certain highly speculative ideas,

Freud was dimly aware of a similar streak in himself, but he was always conflicted and embarrassed about it. He projected these tendencies onto Fliess and Jung, whose mysticism he vicariously enjoyed, while he was at the same time able to continue to consider himself a strict rationalist and positivist. Eventually he fought with them over their irrational tendencies rather than acknowledge that the battle was also raging within himself (Wallace, 1978).

*Splitting* is another of the more reality-distorting, or pathological, defenses. It is particularly characteristic of borderlines, schizophrenics, schizoids, and schizotypal personalities. It arises in the child who has developed—in response to situations in which he was repeatedly deprived, rejected, and abused—overwhelmingly intense rage toward the internalized representations of the parents and negative feelings about his own self-worth. Partly out of an attempt to preserve his precariously few internal representations of a loving parent interacting with a contented and beloved child, in order to prevent their destruction by the predominant representations of negative interactions, the borderline splits apart and keeps separate the one from the other. It is as if he said "that mother who beat, deprived, and deserted me, an unloved and unlovable infant, cannot also be the one who gave birth to, nurtured, and protected me, the loved and lovable child." An extreme example would be the schizophrenic mentioned in Chapter 2 who reacted to me as if I were two or more separate individuals, depending on whether I seemed giving or depriving. Less extreme examples are those patients who view you as all-knowing and all-loving on one day, and as stupid, depriving, and malicious on the next. Although they frequently retain some conscious awareness of their widely disparate attitudes toward you (and, by implication, toward themselves), they seem to be unable to *affectively* appreciate that the devil at whom they are enraged today was the lovable saint yesterday.

*Primitive idealization,* as Kernberg refers to it, or "idealization as a defense against scorn," as Searles calls it, is in some ways a species of reaction formation. It is a way of avoiding coming to terms with an overwhelming sense of disappointment in, and rage toward, parental figures and their current and transference representatives. The basic fear is that the rage will destroy whatever love and goodness there is in themselves and in the world. It is not uncommon that the same patient will oscillate between totally idealizing you and utterly devaluing you. When this occurs you have splitting. In addition, frequently one parent or person in the patient's life is idealized, while another is scornfully devalued, when in fact neither of them is so totally devilish nor so totally angelic as the patient has depicted him.

*Denial* is, after projection, the most reality-distorting mental mechanism. This involves the refusal to apprehend, or come to terms with, an important piece of the real world. It is common in children where it is not to be confused with lying! The best example I have observed was in a stubborn two-year-old. Dragged to the potty, he kept insisting he did not have to defecate, even while the stool was passing from his anus! Denial can take place simply by literally or figuratively turning one's head the other way, either through 1) involvement in recreational pursuits, workaholic behavior, drugs, and alcohol or 2) substitution of a wish-fulfilling, reality-denying fantasy for the offensive perception of reality. A case of the former is the man who immersed himself in work and alcohol as a way of not acknowledging his wife's recent death. Examples of the latter are the adolescent girl who hallucinated the voice of her recently deceased father and the man who dealt with his financial and occupational failures with fantasies of wealth and prestige. Denial, like projection, is especially prominent in paranoid and schizophrenic disorders.

The next four mental mechanisms—isolation, intellectualization, reaction formation, and undoing (or ritualization)—can occur in all types of character and psychopathology, but they are particularly common, as we have already seen, in the obsessive-compulsive neurotic and personality.

*Isolation* is the separation of a feeling from the idea or memory belonging to it. This may involve the conscious awareness of the idea or memory, but a lack of awareness of its affective charge or significance in the patient's emotional life. Recall the example of the man in Chapter 1 who well remembered his parents' divorce when he was ten but did not appreciate its significance to his problems then or now. Or, one might be consciously aware of one's feelings but not of the fantasy or memory to which they are connected. One may know he is morose and irritable but not realize this is related to the therapist's recent announcement of an impending vacation. Isolation is also exemplified in fleeting unacceptable fantasies which occur without the affect appropriate to them, almost as if they were not our own thoughts: the thought of stabbing a friend, throwing a baby out the window, shouting an obscenity in church, and so forth. Isolation of the affect normally appropriate to situations is essential for certain facets of many professions—the surgeon in the operating room, for instance.

The classic example of isolation is Freud's case of the Wolf Man. He had lost his sister, ostensibly unimportant to him, months before and did not have much reaction to her death. Sometime later, while touring, he visited the tomb of a poet and burst into tears. This was quite unaccountable to him since the poet had been dead for generations. Only later did he realize that his father had often compared the sister's verse to that of the great poet. Seeing the tomb had opened the flood gates to a torrent of unresolved grief.

We call this "isolation" because at one point he had consciously in mind the *memory* of his sister's death but without the affect appropriate to it, while at another he experienced the *affect* but unconnected to the idea of the sister's death. It was only later that he was able to connect the two.

*Intellectualization* is a defense mechanism in its own right, but it can often subserve the process of isolation of affect. This is the use of one's cognitive faculties to keep objectionable affect-laden fantasies at bay, e.g., the student who studies constantly to ward off sexual fantasies. Obsessional neurotics and character types can vex the therapist with their ability to use intellectual insight into their dynamics defensively to avoid feelings and to label issues in order to bring them to premature closure. *Rationalization* is a special kind of intellectualization in which, rather than acknowledge one's true motives and feelings, one explains them away. Therapists commonly encounter this in patients with all sorts of perfectly good reasons for arriving late or missing appointments—reasons that allow them to ignore those related to feelings about the therapist and those whom he represents.

*Reaction formation* is an especially active way of defending against the unacceptable impulse, by adopting a stance diametrically opposed to it, e.g., the unconscious voyeur who heads up an antipornography campaign, the person who is overly gracious to the unwanted guest, or the former alcoholic who becomes a dedicated AA worker. Extreme and fanatical behavior of any description is often a reaction formation against impulses to do quite the opposite. *Undoing* is a magical attempt to undo the equally magical idea of the damage our unexpressed fantasies may do (i.e., omnipotence of thoughts). An example is the person who knocks on wood after an unfriendly thought. Lady Macbeth's hand washing is a classic example of an attempt to undo the effects of a fantasy that was translated into reality.

*Displacement* is the shifting of an affect or impulse from its original object to another, e.g., the man who displaces his sexual impulses from his mother to an older woman with whom he works, or the woman who takes out her anger at the husband who deserted her on her son who physically resembles him. Guilt feelings as well can be shifted from the fantasies and feelings to which they are most powerfully connected to less troublesome, more conscious ones. Displacement is a primary mechanism of the transference phenomenon, in which the patient displaces onto the therapist a host of feelings and fantasies originally directed toward parents and siblings. Broadly conceived, as the substitution of one set of preoccupations for other more anxiety-laden and unconscious ones, displacement is perhaps the most important defensive maneuver. Displacement, accompanied by projection, is the central mechanism in phobias, the best example being Little Hans, who displaced and projected his aggressive impulses toward the father onto the horse whom he henceforth both hated and feared.

*Turning (anger) against the self* is the most important mechanism in depression. Freud elucidated this process in the seminal paper, "On Mourning and Melancholia." This mechanism serves to bar from awareness our anger at loved ones and turns it on ourselves or, more accurately, upon the internal representations of these persons that exist within ourselves. The result is depression. The woman who becomes depressed after her date stands her up or the wife who cries when her husband argues with, or frustrates, her are excellent examples. Suicide, in which one murders oneself as an indirect way of indulging one's wish to murder the other, is of course the ultimate expression of this defense.

*Identification* is the process of becoming like another to avoid becoming aware of one's sexual or aggressive feelings toward him or acknowledging feelings related to the loss of that other. Examples are the child who identifies with his tyrannical father and turns into a terror himself rather than express his anger at father directly or the homemaker who takes over her husband's business and hard-driving character style after his death. *Negative identification* is a special instance in which one becomes the diametrical opposite of the object of identification. At times one person in the family is held up as someone not to emulate. The son of an atheistic and irresponsible alcoholic who becomes a religious, hardworking, and punctual teetotaler is negatively identifying with the old man.

*Conversion* and *dissociation* are two clearly pathological maneuvers which are characteristic of hysteria. The former is a nonphysiologically based, symbolic physical symptom, such as pain, paralysis, or sensory deficit, designed to reduce the anxiety attendant upon conflict. I have already described in detail a typical case of conversion hysteria. Dissociation is the actual splitting off of an unacceptable part of the personality, a complex of ideas and affects which then behaves, periodically, like an alternate center of consciousness or else is simply repressed and inaccessible to our normal awareness, e.g., split personality and fugue in the case of the former and hysterical amnesia in that of the latter. The woman who recounted the primal scene fantasy under hypnosis had presented with amnesia for the events up through the death of her mother just a few weeks before entering treatment. The actual precipitant turned out to be a sexual advance upon her by her father shortly after the mother's death. She dealt with the incestuous feelings, rage, guilt and disappointment which this aroused by blocking out her awareness of the events leading up to this and her mother's death. Many cases of split personality, some more authentic and more uncontaminated by the investigator's procedures than others, have by now been described. Often, like Thigpen and Cleckley's Eve, a staid and proper individual has a "wild and woolly" alter ego—recall Dr. Jekyll and Mr. Hyde. The "fugue" reaction is a variation in which a person unconsciously abandons his prior identity and relationships and moves to another location, where he takes on a different name and occupation and replaces his old ties with new ones. In such states he often engages in antisocial or imprudent behavior quite out of keeping with his usual personality.

*Negation* is the expression of unconscious material in the form of its negative. For example, when asked whom the woman in his dream seemed to be, the patient replied, "It certainly was *not* my mother" when from the context of his history and previous associations it was plain that it was. This mechanism is easy to see in everyday life: "I *don't* mean to be critical *but* . . . ," *no* insult intended . . . ," "What you said *doesn't* offend me in the *least*," and so forth. We have all observed people loudly and violently remonstrate that they are not angry or tell a snide joke on a friend and then say "only joking of course, I didn't mean anything by it." At other times negation can be expressed positively. Preambles like "to tell the truth" and "frankly speaking" often alert you to a forthcoming misrepresentation or partial truth. Often, content that is negated is fairly close to consciousness and, if we pin the person down, we can get him to own up to it.

*Regression*, as well, can function as a defense mechanism. For example, a man can deal with conflicts over patricidal aggression, aroused by the imminent prospect of career advancement, by becoming less assertive, less responsible and competent, and more dependent at work. A patient may retreat from newly awakened oedipal strivings for her male therapist by regressing to dependent, childlike, and pregenital positions.

*Sublimation* is not, technically, one of the defense mechanisms, but it is closely related to them. Freud deemed it the most adaptive way of dealing with one's antisocial impulses. It is actually as much a discharge and substitute gratification of these strivings as a defense against them. It is the attempt to obtain a modicum of gratification of unacceptable strivings in a way acceptable to society and superego. This mechanism too can operate consciously or unconsciously. All of us have decided to jog, play our favorite sport or instrument, read, or otherwise divert our attentions from quite conscious aggressive or sexual fantasies for inappropriate objects in untimely situations. On a more unconscious level, learning to play the piano (or fiddle) can be in part a sublimation of desires to masturbate. Becoming a surgeon may sublimate aggressive trends. Becoming an orator, politician, preacher, or lecturer can function as a sublimation of sexual exhibitionism. Becoming a psychiatrist can sublimate voyeuristic trends! The list could be extended indefinitely. Usually a therapist is careful about tampering with a patient's time-honored occupational, recreational, social, and religious sublimations and, even if he deems it appropriate to analyze them, tries to avoid implying that he views them as "pathological."

When the defensive maneuvers begin to express as much, or more, of the impulse as they defend against, then they are considered genuine symptoms or compromise formations. For example, the depressive may begin to turn his anger on himself in such a way that he makes life miserable for his family and friends. The pacifist begins engaging in street brawls in the name of peace. The antipornography crusader spends more and more time poring over "dirty" pictures, the better to denounce them of course! The mother reacting against unconscious hostility toward her children may become so solicitous and protecting that she is insufferable to them. It is of course in cases like these that the therapist may enter the picture. We do not worry about the successful and adaptive defense mechanisms, only the failing or maladaptive ones.

## SUGGESTED READINGS FOR CHAPTER 3

Brenner, C.; *Psychoanalytic Technique and Psychic Conflict*. New York, International Universities Press, 1976. Nice presentation of the relation of conflict theory to actual clinical practice.

Freud, A. (1936): *The Ego and the Mechanisms of Defense*. The Writings of Anna Freud, Volume II. New York, International Universities Press, 1967. Classical exposition of the defense mechanisms.

Freud, S., and Breuer, J. (1895): *Studies on Hysteria*. Standard Edition, Volume II. London, Hogarth Press, 1955. The *Ur* work of psychoanalysis. Contains several interesting clinical cases.

Freud, S. (1900 [1899]): *The Interpretation of Dreams*. Standard Edition, Volumes IV and V. London, Hogarth Press, 1953. One of the world's great books.

Freud, S. (1901): *On Dreams*. Standard Edition, Volume V. London, Hogarth Press, 1953. An excellent abridgement of *The Interpretation of Dreams* and probably the one the novice should read first.

Freud, S. (1901): *The Psychopathology of Everyday Life*. Standard Edition, Volume VI. London, Hogarth Press, 1960. A classic application of psychic determinism to day-to-day life and illustration of how conflict theory applies to parapraxes and symptomatic acts.

Freud, S. (1905): *Jokes and Their Relation to the Unconscious*. Standard Edition, Volume VIII. London, Hogarth Press, 1960. Much appreciated by the literary world Applies conflict theory to humor.

Freud, S. (1905): *Fragment of an Analysis of a Case of Hysteria*. Standard Edition, Volume VII. London, Hogarth Press, 1953. The famous "Dora" case.

Freud, S. (1909): *Analysis of a Phobia in a Five-Year-Old Boy*. Standard Edition, Volume X. London, Hogarth Press, 1955. The case of "Little Hans."

Freud, S. (1909): *Notes Upon a Case of Obsessional Neurosis*. Standard Edition, Volume X. London, Hogarth Press, 1955. The "Rat Man" case.

Freud, S. (1911): *Psycho-Analytic Notes on an Autobiographical Account of a Case of Paranoia*. Standard Edition, Volume XII. London, Hogarth Press, 1958. The "Schreber Case."

Freud, S. (1914): *From the History of an Infantile Neurosis*. Standard Edition, Volume XVII. London, Hogarth Press, 1955. The "Wolf Man," perhaps

Freud's best-known case. Freud's five classical case histories are a must for any student of dynamic psychiatry.

Freud, S. (1926): *Inhibitions, Symptoms, and Anxiety.* Standard Edition, Volume XX. London, Hogarth Press, 1959. Freud's ground-breaking treatment of the relationship between conflict, anxiety, and symptoms, and a landmark in the advance of ego psychology.

Mahl, G.: *Psychological Conflict and Defense.* New York, Harcourt Brace Jovanovich, 1969. Full of excellent examples of intrapsychic conflict and the defense mechanisms.

Moore, B., and Fine, B. (eds.): *A Glossary of Psychoanalytic Terms and Concepts.* New York, The American Psychoanalytic Association, 1968. A useful dictionary of commonly used dynamic terminology.

# The Psychiatric Evaluation

# 4

# History Gathering

I shall begin this chapter by presenting the general principles and technique of history taking. In the next chapter I shall discuss the mental status examination and formulation and present sample case material. Chapter 6 will treat the topic of diagnosis in dynamic psychiatry.

## GENERAL CONSIDERATIONS

The single most important differentiating characteristic of the dynamic therapist is his conviction in the importance of history in understanding a patient's character and predicament. Alerting us to the role of the individual's life history is, in my opinion, Freud's most significant contribution to psychiatry. The quality of one's evaluation interviews is the acid test of one's adherence to historical determinism. In these sessions we do not approach the patient "blind," but frame our questions in accordance with what dynamic theory teaches us about psychopathology, the role of history, and certain universal, enduring conflicts and developmental tasks. The theory leads us to ask questions we would not otherwise think of and to make sense of the answers that we receive. Conversely, we only come to appreciate the value of the theory if we obtain sufficient data to make it usable. When we are learning dynamic psychiatry, it is far better to have an in-depth knowledge of a few patients than a superficial acquaintance with many.

The most important preconception with which we approach the evaluation interview, indeed psychotherapy in general, is that a life or set of problems, no matter how chaotic it appears on the surface and in the

121

present, will *make sense* when placed within the context of the patient's historically determined view of himself and of the world, and of his perennial strivings and fears. Human beings, unless they are in the grip of overwhelmingly neurological or organic mental disease, do *not* do things which are nonsensical. If a patient's behavior is not intelligible within the context of current reality, then delve into his past until you find a reality within the context of which it *was* (and unconsciously still *is*) intelligible. Recall my example of atavism in Chapter 1.

The dynamic therapist is engaged in a process that is in many ways closer to history than to science. We are our patients' biographers or clinical historians. Like all biographers, we attempt to get into our subject and see the world from his side. We try to discern lifelong *themes, patterns,* and *preoccupations.* We are concerned with "artistic" matters like the *form, style,* and *arrangement* of the patient's life. Only *after* we have spotted these patterns are we in a position to make causal or motivational inferences about a patient's behavior.

We differ from the ordinary biographer in at least three respects: 1) Our subject is still alive so we can test our hypotheses against his subsequent behavior and responses; 2) we organize our biography within the theoretical framework which I outlined in Chapters 1 through 3; and 3) we are pragmatic biographers, i.e., our aim is not merely to write history but to make it. We help the patient to reclaim his history so that he can free himself from its hold on his present, and so that he will stop imposing historically determined categories of interpretation on his present world and the people in it. This whole process starts in the evaluation.

Therefore, the task of the evaluator is plain: to obtain an exquisitely detailed history of the present and past problems and of the life course. On the basis of this history he makes his *formulation* (or clinical hypothesis) of the historical and current forces, and attempts at adaptation, that conspire to make the patient what he is today. This clinical hypothesis is far from academic because the treatment plan itself follows from it. Initially somewhat vague and tentative, it nevertheless serves as an indispensable map to previously uncharted terrain and is modified and detailed to conform with subsequent discoveries. As I shall emphasize again and again, the formulation is the *real diagnosis* in dynamic psychiatry.

Because I believe it is essential to have a good history and formulation at the outset of treatment, I find myself in opposition to those who advocate the "associative anamnesis"—that is, letting the patient talk, from the beginning, about whatever he chooses, and taking your history as he spontaneously gives it or as the opportunity arises. Adherents of this approach maintain that, within a few sessions, you receive as much historical data as from the other method and that you have this history

within the context of the patient's current and transference preoccupations to boot. This method can work well for experienced therapists, but
for the novice it is taboo. The trainee should glean his history and make
his formulation *first*. In time he will find that he can make a reasonable
provisional formulation after two to three hours of efficient history
gathering. Of course, you must explain to your patients, many of whom
have never experienced a psychiatric evaluation, the rationale for your
history-taking.

I advocate a thorough history and systematic clinical hypothesis at the
outset for at least seven reasons.

First of all, current and recent issues that arise in subsequent sessions
are appreciated sooner and in their proper contexts and full significance
if one has a prior grasp of their history. Fewer relevant current data are
overlooked and less time is wasted.

Second, insofar as the therapist obtains an initial understanding of
what otherwise seems a chaotic assortment of current symptoms and
anxieties, then his *own* anxiety is reduced. Since anxiety, like calm, is
contagious, whatever is good for the therapist's anxiety is usually good
for the patient's.

Third, and related to this, systematically asking the patient a set of
questions about his life reassures him that there is a method to the
madness of psychotherapy and gives him a sense of your competence.

Fourth, by helping us understand how and why a person has become
the way he is, the history makes us more tolerant of his foibles and
abrasiveness.

Fifth, by taking a history you are implicitly educating the patient to
the dynamic way of thinking: that his present dilemma cannot be understood in an historical vacuum, that you are expecting him to move from
talking about the present to the past and back again.

Sixth, history taking is therapeutic, though it is not intended to be.
You are evincing an interest in the course of the patient's life that he has
probably never encountered before. This consistent and empathic attention, conveyed by listening, sitting forward, looking him in the face,
nodding and grunting, remembering what he says, and asking questions, on the part of a high-status professional is reassuring. In addition,
during the initial anamnesis the patient often begins to see, for the first
time, connections between past and present and starts to entertain the
idea that there is a rhyme and reason to his distress. In optimal conditions his curiosity as a life historian is aroused and the two of you
become partners in what often has the suspense of a good detective
thriller.

Seventh, the history gives you some ability to predict the sort of
transference reactions you are likely to encounter in the course of the
subsequent psychotherapeutic work.

For example, one of my residents, a middle-aged male, was evaluating a young woman with a history of repeated sexual molestation at the hands of her grandfather. Her parents repeatedly turned their heads the other way. When the patient finally told her mother what was happening, the latter said, "You are a liar" and dropped the matter forthwith. (As it turned out, the mother herself had been molested by this man and was incapable of dealing with the memories and feelings reawakened by her daughter's communication.) With remarks like "I don't blame my parents for what my grandfather did, really, I don't. . . . but sometimes I wonder why they didn't notice," she revealed that there was tremendous unconscious hurt and resentment over her parents' refusal to protect her. Finally, she suffered from rejection by her father and a string of lovers and husbands up to the present. The resident was able to predict that her transference toward him would contain elements of these important historical themes. Indeed, she kept her distance from him at the outset, at the same time that she could barely leave the sessions. As she became more aware of her desires for intimacy with him and moved a little closer, she then began to fear that he would reject or molest her. She mistrusted him and accused him of ignoring and deprecating her communications as her mother did. Because the resident was expecting just such a transference configuration, he was better able to deal with it and he understood it was not to be taken personally. In addition, he knew to toe the line between being too aloof on the one hand (which would be perceived as rejection) and moving too close on the other (which would be perceived as seduction and molestation). Finally, he made a special effort to show her he took her communications seriously.

Your first encounter with the patient is extraordinarily important for both of you. It is significant to him because of popular misconceptions about psychiatry and for transferential reasons, the two of which are often inextricably interconnected. It is crucial to understand that, for both of these reasons, even before the patient sees you he will be convinced that he already "knows" a great deal about you. Every patient comes laden with conscious and unconscious unrealistic fears and expectations. Uncovering these and discovering whence they come occupy you both for the entire course of treatment.

As to the popular misconceptions, we all realize the aura and the stigma that surround our profession. The patient may come see you against considerable internal and external opposition. He may fear that you will read his mind and deem him crazy, incapable, or bad. He may be afraid that, if he allows himself to depend on you that he (and you) will become overwhelmed by his neediness and that he will become a mewling, puking infant in your arms. He may view you as an incompetent charlatan or an omnipotent healer who, with a few magic words, can transform his entire way of being. Or, he may view you simultaneously or alternately as both. He may expect that, like the traditional physician, you will ask a few questions and then give him a pill and tell him what to do—that, in other words, he will be the passive subject in a treatment that you control. One thing *is* certain. Because the patient experiences you as a high-status professional, your opinion of him is important even if he feigns indifference to it. Having encountered the impatience of most physicians when their authority is questioned, he may fail to speak his mind for fear of offending you. His most basic need, even if it is overlaid by a variety of defensive maneuvers, is to be liked and accepted by you. Since rejection, deprivation, and loss form the most common constellation of problems in the history and current reality of most psychiatric patients, they are particularly sensitive to *any* sign that you are not interested in them. For this reason, in the evaluation sessions, as in the psychotherapeutic ones proper, do *not* be late, repeatedly change or cancel your patient's appointment times, constantly look at your clock or watch, or answer the phone during your sessions. All of these are taken as signs that you are ambivalent about seeing him. An occasional patient, fearful of rejection, fails to come to a follow-up appointment to test your commitment to seeing him. Such patients are often rejecting you before you reject them (as a way of taking control of what they fear most) and should be called and asked why they are not following through with the evaluation or treatment and whether they wish to continue. In other words, although you cannot make a patient complete an evaluation or enter treatment who is dead set against it, you can, by your behavior, influence the *ambi*valent patient one way or the other.

As to the transferential factors, the patient approaches you with a set of attitudes and expectations derived from previous experience with designated nurturers and helpers—from his earliest interactions with parents to his recent experiences with physicians and helping professionals. After the patient sees that you are male or female, black, white, or Oriental, American or foreign, young or middle-aged, conservatively or stylishly dressed, and so forth, the initially vague and diffuse transference expectations focus down somewhat, although every therapist, no matter what his particular characteristics, is a screen upon whom are projected the patient's feelings about *all* the important early actors in his life. In the majority of cases, the patient does not openly discuss, or is not even consciously aware, of most of his attitudes. However, you can infer something about them nonetheless from the tone of his posture and voice, type and amount of eye contact, facial expressions, hesitancies and, in particular, what he tells you about the history of his experiences with significant others (especially his parents). More rare is the patient who verbally expresses the positive and, especially, negative aspects of his feelings toward you. In the case of the latter, he may demonstrate an uncanny ability to home in on your sensitive spots such as age, ethnic group, nationality, or professional experience. It is crucial that you not become defensive but that you empathically explore the reasons for his concerns about the area. If you understand his behavior as transferential, which it usually is, then it becomes more difficult to take it personally. It is also helpful to remember that the patient is coming out of acute distress more than out of any desire to prove you incompetent. He wants help desperately and, no matter how abrasive and scornful he may be on the surface, deeply hopes that you will be able to assist him. Hostile and distancing behavior is a way of dealing with *fear* of you and of those whom you unconsciously represent, in line with the adage that the best defense is a good offense. If you empathize and convey understanding, rather than meeting hostility with hostility or retreating, the cause for the patient's fear, hence his rejection, will subside. In other words, transference behavior may be defensive as much as expressive. Do not assume that a patient is nothing more than his facade. I have often seen contemptuous, scornful, and sarcastic patients break down in tears when it came time to end the session, making it clear what they had been warding off all the while.

You, the beginning evaluator, will approach the patient with your own set of attitudes, fears, and expectations, a function in part of your newness to the field and in part of your own history. As to the former, you must accept that you *will* be anxious upon meeting a new patient. Even the seasoned therapist feels mild anxiety when encountering a new patient who is, after all, a human being as yet totally unknown to him and whom he is yet unsure that he can help. A little anxiety does no harm and may even increase our attentiveness to the patient. Too much anxiety leaves us more preoccupied with treating ourselves than with listening to the patient.

Probably the most frequent cause of anxiety in the novice evaluator is his need to be liked, accepted, admired, and thought helpful and competent by the patient. In response to his own and the patient's unrealistic expectations, he may attempt too much too early or make promises on which he cannot deliver. Whenever we become caught up in pleasing and impressing the patient, we are really asking him to treat our own insecurities as a therapist, to pander to our shaky professional self-esteem. You must first hear the patient's story in intimate detail *before* you can make any meaningful therapeutic intervention. *At first all you have to do is listen.* If he presses you for direct feedback and magical interpretations, then you must explain this to him. Every patient, on some level, hopes that you will relieve him of his misery in the first session, thus making unnecessary the whole painful process of looking at oneself. I suggest that you make it a rule *not* to cure anybody in the evaluation interviews!

Finally, the psychiatric interviewer is not a distant investigator but a *"participant*-observer" (Sullivan, 1953) or, even more aptly, a "participant-*understander"* (Foudraine, 1974). Your data arise not in the patient purely, but in the field of interaction between him and yourself. You are a part of the process under investigation. You know the patient only as he impinges upon your psychic apparatus, with its complexes and considerations; similarly, your particular personality is constantly impinging upon him and influencing what you see. Consequently, you must be as aware of your own feelings and fantasies as of his.

In an earlier chapter I illustrated how your feelings can tell you not only about your own countertransference *mishegoss,* but about the patient's intentions as well. For example, if you feel "put off," it may be because it is his conscious or unconscious intention, for reasons most likely unknown to him, to distance you. If you feel sad, you may be "resonating" with his hitherto masked depression. If you feel sexually excited, it may be because the patient behaves (however subtly) seductively. If you are angry, it may be in response to the patient's (perhaps partly disguised) anger. If you feel a sense of urgency and need to rescue him, it may be because he presents himself as helpless.

Many times I have seen residents in the grip of one of these feelings and, because of their own conflicts and defenses, not conscious of it. I have observed male residents totally oblivious to the most seductive behavior in female hysterics because they were too busy (unconsciously) warding off their own anxieties. When the trainee *is* aware of his feelings toward a patient, too often he is so frantic over *what to do* about them that he mishandles the situation. One psychiatric resident told, in so many words, a female psychotic who was expressing warm and sexual feelings toward him that it was not appropriate for her to feel, much less talk about, such things. Had he *first* dealt with his own feelings about this before feeling that he had to *do* anything, he would have been able to handle it like any other patient communication—by listening and attempting to understand.

Your own history leads you to experience, consciously and unconsciously, to the degree that you are unanalyzed, your patient as the representative of a variety of figures from your past. If the patient is an age mate, you may experience him as a hateful and competitive sibling whom you must attempt to overcome and put in his place. Or you may find it particularly easy to identify with such a patient and may try to solve, vicariously, your own problems through him. Or you may have been troubled by an excessively dependent and demanding sibling and fear that your patient will be likewise. If the patient is of the opposite sex, you may feel seductive or may need to ward off your attractions to him by a variety of distancing maneuvers. The older patient may be experienced as a critical, intimidating, and patronizing parent whom you must guard against and prove your competence to. The patient may stand for various family members whom you want to "reform" in any number of ways; you may try to rewrite an improved edition of your own family history through them. If you are unaware of these issues, you might act them out or otherwise communicate them, verbally or nonverbally, to your patients, thereby influencing their behavior quite as much as will their own internal dynamics.

In the evaluation interviews you have two primary tasks: *to establish rapport* and *to gather the data* with which to construct your formulation and treatment plan. The beginner should set aside three to four 50-minute interviews to do this. The more experienced clinician can get a good baseline in an hour to an hour and a half. I favor, if at all possible, an initial 90-minute session since this allows you time to let the patient freewheel in the beginning, to do a more systematic reconnaissance in the middle, and to speak to his questions and concerns toward the end.

The simplest and most important thing is to *listen* to the patient, to pay attention to him, and to demonstrate verbally and (especially) non-verbally that you are doing so. This also happens to be one of the most therapeutic factors in psychotherapy in general. Morton Reiser (personal communication) advocates that when you see your patient you should be as "blind" to previous information about him as possible in order to be and to appear legitimately interested in his story. If you listen you will not embarrass yourself and your patient by asking for information that has already been given, which I have seen happen repeatedly in observed evaluations. If you do not hear or understand something a patient says or a phrase he uses, do not be afraid to ask him to repeat or explain it to you right then.

Unless the patient is extraordinarily anxious, psychotic, or prepsychotic, you should begin the interview with an open-ended question—e.g., "Tell me what brings you here"—and allow him the first 15 to 20 minutes to tell his story as he will, with a minimum of interference from you. This method permits you to get his associations, and to spot meaningful links between past and present, within the present and, at times, between past, present, and transference. For example, consider the following response to the opening, "Help me understand why you are here to see me today":

"Well, I've been feeling pretty low. You see, my husband left a week ago today—right after things seemed to be going a little better. Yes, I thought things were beginning to work out and—and—he just left [at this point she cries]—the way my father did when I was eight. Well, I haven't heard from Tom in a whole week. I don't know whether I will or not. Doctor— [she looks down, fidgets in her chair, and stammers] Doc—Doc—Doctor, will you be my therapist after the evaluation or will I be transferred to someone else?"

By not interrupting, by just allowing her to tell her story, the therapist learned something about the present problem, the past history, the transference, and the patient's affective state.

There are two types of data in psychiatry: the *external* (corresponding roughly to the "actual reality" of psychoanalytic theory) and the *internal* (equivalent to psychical reality and affective state). The former comprises names, dates, places, sequences, durations, happenings, and so forth. The latter corresponds to what it *feels* like to be the particular person that your patient is and how he interprets himself and his world. To perceive this latter, one must not only listen between the lines of what the patient is saying, but pay particular attention to posture, facial expression, and other nonverbal manifestations of affect. Often I have seen a trainee walk out of an observed evaluation interview able to tell me about a host of events and sequences in the patient's life without an inkling as to what they *mean* to him and without being able to describe even the most striking aspects of the patient's posture and affect. For example, one resident was able to tell me about his patient's mother's deserting him at age ten and her return four years later with a terminal illness, on a home respirator, without being able to give me the patient's reactions to either of these events! We have to speculate enough in psychiatry without having to do so on matters about which we could have simply asked the patient.

Closely allied to being perceptive to the internal data is "seeing the forest as well as the trees." Getting the external and even, to some extent, the internal data is a more active process, a *looking* or *searching*, whereas spotting the forest, the major themes, the red threads in an entire life, is more of a *seeing*, in the sense of a passive receptiveness to the patient's story and its effect on you. It takes considerable time to learn to combine active searching with passive receptivity and the broad view.

Structure is the enemy of affect, the *most important* datum you can obtain. The less structured the session, the more likely that feelings will emerge. A patient can use a tightly regimented question-and-answer format to avoid feelings. Do not ally yourself with his resistance. In the best evaluation session, with an ideal patient and interviewer, an open-ended question or facilitative comment from the latter is followed by several minutes of information from the former. Only if the patient is too fearful to proceed or plainly close to psychotic decompensation should you introduce more structure into the hours.

When you give the patient some initial time for freewheeling and structure the session as little as possible, you are more likely to perceive his characterological features, or adaptive style. Does he ramble to avoid coming to an affect-laden point? Is he uncomfortable with silences? Does he look to you to take charge of the interview and rescue him? Does he mumble or subvocalize, thus expressing ambivalence about communicating with you? Does he manifest mistrust and suspicion? Often you will perceive subtle signs of a thought disorder (e.g., loose associations or tangentiality) because you have allowed the patient a little time to himself.

Another reason to avoid being too active and controlling the sessions with a series of rapid questions is that the person is learning how to be a patient in these interviews. Being a patient means being as open and spontaneous as possible and bearing most of the responsibility for one's treatment. Consequently, while the evaluation interviews are more structured than the psychotherapy itself, there should be enough resemblance between the two that the patient does not expect to play a passive role in the treatment, with you giving him the "truth" or pulling the answers out of him. In short, I advocate an evaluation interview more structured and goal-oriented than the associative anamnesis, but less regimented than the traditional medical review of systems, the question-response type of interview.

On the other hand, there is, of course, the "difficult" patient whose silence, withdrawal, mistrust, thought disorder, personality style, or anxiety forces you to assume, from the beginning, a more active role. You should always remember that the most common causes for anxiety, withdrawal, and uncooperativeness are the patient's conscious and unconscious fears about how *you* will feel about him and react to him.

Perhaps most commonly encountered is the patient who is so anxious that he cannot relax enough to tell his story. If you remain silent he will simply become more anxious and may even get up and leave the room. With such a person you might begin by empathetically noting that he seems uncomfortable and ask him how he feels about coming to see a therapist and whether he has seen one before. If this is his first encounter with a mental health professional you should explore his preconceptions, his fears and fantasies, about psychiatry. Such questions and comments coupled with your benign, interested, and accepting attitude, will be enough to set most patients at ease and to tell you, besides, some important information about the patient. I evaluated one young woman, fresh from the movie *One Flew Over the Cuckoo's Nest*, whose anxiety disappeared when I assured her that "shock treatments" and lobotomies were not the only things psychiatrists do! If the anxious or otherwise problematic patient has had prior experience with psychiatry, find out what gives him grounds for anxiety.

The paranoid patient may manifest anxiety, withdrawal, or belligerence and an excessive need to control the session. His body language usually reveals his suspicion, mistrust, and guardedness: rigid, ramrod posture with muscles tensed for action; and hypervigilant, hostile stare, often scanning the surroundings for bugging or other devices. He may attempt to intimidate you. Do not be put off by this facade. Underneath, the paranoid is essentially *fearful* and *powerless*. He may manifest this fear with apprehensive withdrawal or he may cover it up with belligerent and domineering behavior. However, the key thing to remember is that he is fearful that you will do any number of things to him. Your consistent task is to try to minimize that fear, to show him, largely behaviorally, that he has no cause to be afraid of you. The worst response is to return the paranoid's rage and "macho" behavior. Then you *will* have a fight on your hands.

Since the paranoid's most common fear is that you will attempt to dominate him sexually, aggressively, or in a variety of ways, you must be anything but controlling in the interview. This does not mean that you withdraw, act ineffectual or doubtful, or assent or submit fearfully to everything he says, and allow him to abuse you. To remain silent simply increases the projecting that he is already engaged in and hence magnifies his anxieties; to act fearful causes him to fear that he is losing his control and perhaps lead him to that; and to withdraw is to convince him that you are malignant or indifferent. Nevertheless, you must do everything possible to allow him to feel in control of the interview: allow him to sit where he has ready access to the door and does not feel cornered, permit him to do as much of the talking as possible, and let him have some control over the frequency and duration of sessions. Some paranoids actually feel more comfortable and talk more if the door is left open and, if so, they usually indicate it to you in some fashion.

Here, more than anywhere else, a respectful and professional distance is just what the doctor ordered. A misguided friendliness might precipitate a homosexual panic or make him fear you are otherwise trying to manipulate him. Interpretive comments will be viewed as intrusions and should be avoided. Refrain from expressing observations and hunches that might aggravate any fear that you can read his mind, or otherwise violate his mental interior. If you listen to the paranoid he will, like all patients, train you to talk with him. For instance, if he complains about an earlier therapist's poking around in his childhood or asking too many questions, then do not do so yourself.

The focus should consistently be on why *he chooses* to come here, on what *he* wants out of the process, on what *he* thinks it is useful for you to know, on what *his* past experiences with psychiatrists have been, on what *he* sees as the problem. If he is there under duress, then you must empathize with his feelings about this. If frank delusions about you emerge and threaten to hinder the interview, they must be dealt with respectfully and at the patient's pace. You should neither confront them head on nor blithely acquiesce to them. While *gently* and matter of factly reasserting your professional aims and denying the patient's misattributions to you, you should explore what in his experience causes him to think that you, a professional and a total stranger, would harbor malignant intentions toward him. An empathic comment is often helpful: "Well, if you feel that my intentions are so and so, I can well see why you would have reservations about talking to me." The more consciously fearful and withdrawn paranoid can be handled by a more active approach similar to that outlined for the anxious patient, with the focus on understanding the reasons for his fear and mistrust.

With the mute and withdrawn schizophrenic or depressive you can point out your desire to be of service to him but that you cannot know anything about his life and problems unless he chooses to open up to you. If, after a few minutes, he remains silent, you can reiterate this. If this fails, you can go on to say a bit about what you already know about him, specifying the source (the doctor, the chart, and so forth). If all else fails, then you can leave it at that, informing him about your next meeting and expressing the hope that he will feel more like talking next time. Some of the great therapists of schizophrenics have sat for months with mute patients before being rewarded with a few syllables.

Or, you can—and this is more risky but I have seen it work—speculate aloud about the meaning and motives of his silence. You should limit yourself to a few ideas and they should be related to what you know about the patient from his chart or the referral source. You should spell out *what* you know about him that leads you to your speculations so that he does not feel that you are reading his mind. If you are on to something, he often indicates it by shifting his posture or, often enough, speaking to acknowledge the correctness or incorrectness of your view. In either case, at least some kind of interchange is set in motion. Or, if you know nothing whatsoever about the mute patient, you may mention what, in your experience, you have found to be common reasons for persons' reticence with a psychiatrist: fear of being judged bad or evil, of being disliked or thought incapable, or of their confidentiality being violated.

Whatever you do with the mute patient, do not view his silence as a malicious and willful attempt to foil your good intentions. His resistance is largely unconsciously motivated and for the best of historical reasons. Do not repay his withdrawal in similar coin as did one psychiatric resident I knew who would pick up magazines and thumb through them when his patients were silent!

Finally, the thought disorders of certain patients (loose associations in the schizophrenic and tangentiality in the manic) require that you structure the sessions. With certain personality styles, you must focus the discussion periodically, e.g., circumstantiality in the obsessional and global vagueness in the hysteric.

Before going on to the anatomy of the evaluation itself, I shall discuss further your style of questioning. First of all begin, as I have said, with an open-ended question and only gradually, on the basis of what you learn, narrow down and ask more specific or closed-ended questions. Avoid asking leading questions, those that suggest you are looking for something in particular. Do not ask multiple-choice questions which supply the patient with answers from which to choose. Avoid questions that can be answered with a simple "yes" or "no." The patient's resistance to elaborating on emotionally charged issues will be great enough without your assisting it. Do not ask, "Did you have a happy childhood?" lest the patient close off further discussion with an immediate "yes." Say instead, "Tell me about your childhood." Do not query, "Do you ever dream?" lest the patient respond with a rapid "no." Say, rather, "I'd like to hear about your dreams."

Avoid prefacing questions with a "*Can* you tell me . . . ?" or "*Do* you remember . . . ?" Instead, couch your questions in a way that conveys to the patient your *expectation* that he can answer them. For instance, say "Tell me . . . ," "I'd like to hear about . . . ," "What was happening when . . . ?" and so forth. If you intervene in this manner, rather than one that puts in question the patient's ability to provide the information that you seek, you will find that many more of your questions are answered. The same holds true with questions about more sensitive topics such as sex and religion. If you ask the question in a serious, neutral fashion that suggests you fully expect the patient to be able to talk about it, he usually does so.

Framing questions in a manner that can be construed as judgmental or valuational may lead the patient to suspect you are attempting to smoke out hidden problems about which he does not complain. For example, do not say, "How do you *get along with* your father?" "Who was your *favorite* parent?" "Are you *satisfied* with your marriage?" "Do you feel your mother loved you or your brother *more*?" Say, rather, "*Tell me about* your relationship with your father [mother, husband, wife, brother, sister, and so forth]." "I'd like to hear about your time with X." "What was your contact with so and so like?" Information about whether the patient felt one sibling was more favored than he by one or both parents usually comes out in the course of his conversation about the family of origin without being directly requested. Similarly, no one can talk very long about marriage or any other important relationship without consciously or unconsciously throwing out all sorts of clues about its quality.

Do not take the first "no," "I don't know," "I can't remember," "There was nothing else going on then," or pat answer ("I had a happy childhood," "I have a wonderful marriage") as the final word. In general, people with happy childhoods and wonderful marriages are not overrepresented among the patient population. "I don't know's" and facile answers usually mean "I don't want to talk about this any more." A good therapist must harbor a healthy skepticism about such comments, without at the same time being impatient, snide, or cynical. Often you can come back then, or later, and rephrase the question a bit differently and the patient will open up. For example, when the patient says, "My parents were wonderful people. That's all there is to tell," reply with, "But help me get to know them, help me get to know what you did together, what it was like growing up in your home." I wish I had a nickel for every patient who has started with "I had a wonderful childhood" and ended up telling a horror story, often within the course of a single session.

Frequently the patient wants to tell you, but feels too ashamed or guilty to come right out with it unless you first demonstrate you really want to know. In line with this, often a patient says "There is something that has been bothering me for some time, Doctor, but I don't feel I can tell you about it." If this is said in such a way that you feel the patient half wants you to coax him into talking about it, you should pursue it. Not to do so would give him the impression that you are insensitive to, or uninterested in, his communication. You approach such a statement not with "Oh come on, tell me, won't you?" but by asking the patient what makes him hesitant to talk to you about it. This is known, as we shall see in the psychotherapy section, as speaking to the resistance before the content. It is, in fact, *just as* important to know *why* the patient will not tell you as it is to know *what* he will not tell you. If you explore this you usually come up with some fear about how you would react to the communication—whether you will laugh, be judgmental, contemptuous, or hateful. Like clockwork, when you have explored the patient's motives for resisting, the hidden information emerges unbidden.

At other times you must recognize when somebody is simply not ready to face up to, much less talk about, a particular issue, and you then bide your time for a more auspicious occasion. It is far better for your evaluation summary to want for a particular piece of data than for you to sacrifice the rapport in order to obtain it. Indeed, the knowledge that a patient does not want to discuss a particular area is just as important as the information he is withholding.

Vary the wording of your questions lest you sound like a robot. Trainees observing their own videotaped interviews are often surprised by the monotonous, droning quality of their style. Vary "Tell me . . ." with "I'd like to hear . . ." with "What was____like . . ." with "How did it feel when . . . ?" with "It would be helpful if you would tell me . . . ." In addition, phrase your questions as succinctly as possible. This latter holds true especially in the psychotherapeutic sessions proper where you want your statements to be accurate and power-packed.

Avoid asking "why" questions, both in your evaluations and in your psychotherapy, since they are an invitation to intellectualize. For example, in response to a patient's account of his family's multiple moves the resident asked, "Why did your parents move you around so much?" He then received an explanation about the father's occupation. Had he asked, "What was that like?" he would have learned something more important: how it *felt* to the patient. Another patient told the resident, with no sign of affect whatsoever, about her father's suicide when she was eight. "I heard the gunshot, walked downstairs, and Mama said, 'Your father killed himself. Go back to bed'." His question, "Why did she do that?" was a pointless request for her to speculate about another's motives and ensured that her powerful feelings would remain isolated. 'Why' questions only have a place, and then but sparingly, *after* the patient has revealed his feelings and they are always used in reference to *his* motivations, not to another's. Generally much better than "Why?" are "What went into your doing so and so?" "What led you to do that?" "What was your purpose in such and such?" "What were you feeling before you said that?" If you want to know his fantasies about another person's motivations, ask him not, "Why did he do it?" but "What does it mean to you that he did it?"

Do not use emotionally loaded words like "crazy," "nervous breakdown," or "getting worse (or better)" even if your patient uses them to refer to himself. Speak instead of "problems," "difficulties," or "troubles." This may seem self-evident but I have seen trainees make this mistake.

Often, early in the first session, the patient asks "Can you help me?" "Is there hope for me?" "Am I damaged beyond repair?" "How serious are my problems, anyway?" These are questions you can never answer before you know the person and you should tell him so. In a misguided zeal to be "supportive," the novice often rushes right in with facile reassurance and ready optimism. In their heart of hearts most patients know that such reassurance, given in complete ignorance of their predicaments, is meaningless. They will think you incompetent or foolish for springing to such easy platitudes. Worse still, they may fear they are really disturbed if you must resort to such devices. First, listen to the person and get him to tell you why he fears for his state of mind. Then you can transmit something more supportive than premature reassurance: a sense of *understanding*, of genuine and accurate empathy. After a few sessions you can convey a general and realistic assessment of his problems and your recommendations (arrived at from *collaboration* with your patient). It is a rare patient to whom, following the evaluation, you cannot either offer something yourself or direct to somebody who can. *Informed* optimism and reassurance, as opposed to ignorant and premature reassurance, *are* therapeutic.

No matter how many prior psychiatric evaluations a patient has experienced, I always do my own, and generally *before* I have read any of the others'. This not only makes you more attentive, as Reiser suggests, but allows you to approach the patient with an open mind. Skill at psychiatric evaluation, formulation, and diagnosis varies greatly from clinician to clinician, and it is possible that the previous evaluator was incompetent or that he saw the patient at a markedly different point in his travels. Some patients balk at having to tell their stories again, but a brief explanation usually overcomes their reluctance and sets them talking away. A person usually finds it quite complimentary that you are as interested in his version of the story as that by "Dr. Famous" who saw him two years ago or "Dr. Wonderful" who treated him as an adolescent.[1]

We have been focusing on what *you* should ask the patient. But *he* will also be asking you questions. I have already examined his questions about prognosis and how psychotherapy works. After you have gathered preliminary information from him, he is entitled to an honest and yet general answer to both of these. Questions about diagnosis are another matter. When a patient asks you to label him, he is almost never asking you merely for a diagnosis. He is nearly always asking something else: "Is there hope for me?" "Do you think I am incompetent, evil, worthless?" "Do you like me?" "Can you give me an identity?" "Can you go ahead and tell me what's wrong with me so you can give me a prescription and we can get this whole thing over with?" Thus, you must always explore the *meaning* of this question first. After you have done this, most patients no longer press you for an answer. If they do, I usually explain briefly the difference between diagnosis in psychiatry and in medicine. I focus on how, for the most part, psychiatrists do not treat illnesses in the traditional medical sense of the word, but rather problems in living and character style, and on how the real diagnosis in psychiatry is understanding the way in which one has become the person one is today. I then explain that I shall be happy to give him my impression of the nature of his problems after we have completed the evaluation.[2]

Psychiatrically savvy patients generally know that therapists do not usually answer questions about their personal lives. Many patients do not know this, however, and may ask questions like, "Doctor, are you married?" "Do you have children?" "Where do you live?" "What's it like to be a psychiatrist?" If you know that your contact with him will be limited to the evaluation, then it does not make as much difference if you do answer them. Nevertheless, even here you should remember

---

[1] Nevertheless, I always go back later and get the old records. One can never have too much information on a patient, and you must remember the patient is telling you his life story from the perspective of one point in time. It might have sounded quite different two or five or ten years before and the old records can help you with this as well as alert you to otherwise unsuspected potential for psychotic regression or adaptive functioning. If I have already received information about the patient, I apprise him, in a general way, of its nature. This not only allows him to disabuse me of any misconceptions I may hold, but reassures him of my honesty and directness.

[2] See page 137.

that you are educating him to be a patient and if you answer his questions about your personal life, he will approach his therapist expecting him to as well. It is best to apprise the patient of the fact that a therapist does not customarily answer personal questions and to briefly explain the rationale for that. He should know it is *his* life, fantasies, fears, and so forth that you want to know about and that he has more to gain from understanding the motives of his questions than from receiving direct answers to them. That this is a bit one-sided—with him telling you all about his life, and you nothing about yours—can be acknowledged, but it should not be departed from.

There is, however, one question that you should *always* answer directly, without first exploring its meaning to the patient, and that is the request for information about your training and professional experience.[3] Such queries should be answered directly and matter of factly without defensiveness. If the patient implies that you are too young or inexperienced, treat this reaction like anything else—as something to be ventilated, explored, and understood. Questions about whether you yourself have been in therapy fall, I feel, in the same category since this is, in fact, an essential part of a therapist's education. Ideally, you can answer it with a simple "yes," because you have been. If, however, your therapy is ongoing, I would not volunteer that additional piece of information because you have then interjected a shadowy "metatherapist" into the current situation. If you equivocate about whether you have been in therapy, the patient will feel you are embarrassed by it and that will affect his attitude toward his own treatment. If he seems uncomfortable with your disclosure, then that should be explored. It may reveal more about how he feels about himself for being in therapy than about you for having been.

---

[2]With chronic schizophrenics and sufferers from uni- or bi-polar affective disorder—those with disturbances which do approximate "illnesses" in the medical sense of the term—the issue is more complex. Because of the relapses and remissions, the recurrent nature and need for treatment adherence, associated with these disorders, these patients should, at the very least, know something about the nature of their maladies and how this affects the treatment rationale. Because of the horrific popular connotations of the word "schizophrenia," one would be more chary about disclosing this diagnosis to a patient than in the corresponding case with a manic-depressive (who has often diagnosed himself anyhow). However, when a chronic schizophrenic asks directly for his diagnosis, you would need, I feel, a good reason to dissemble. He should be answered truthfully, matter of factly, without hesitation, and the nature of your educative remarks should depend upon his reaction.

[3]However, if this question does not occur until well into the psychotherapy, you should first explore what it means that the patient is bringing it up at that particular point in time. After you have thoroughly threshed this out, you should then go on to answer the question as usual.

## THE STRUCTURE OF THE EVALUATION

You should, of course, begin the interview by introducing yourself politely to the patient, following the customary social amenities. One usually shakes hands with the male patient on the first encounter, though generally not in subsequent ones and usually not in the psychotherapy itself (though this varies from culture to culture and depends upon whether the therapy is supportive or insight-oriented).

If you are a male clinician and your patient is a woman, it is generally customary to follow, as in normal social intercourse, her lead or body language in this matter. You can, incidentally, tell a good deal about a person from his handshake, as any farmer knows! Does he offer it hesitatingly out of fear of either intimacy or rejection? Is it a "macho" bone-crusher grip or a "limp fish" one? Both often reflect self-esteem problems or conflicts over aggression. Does he let go readily or reluctantly, either extreme perhaps reflecting conflicts over independence-dependency? Does he wait for you to initiate the handshake and its cessation or do it himself? Is there a seductive quality to his grasp? Is there a helpless, plaintive, "rescue me" character to it?

You should always address your patient by title and surname, unless the person is a child or early adolescent. To do otherwise is to infantilize the patient or to suggest a false intimacy where none exists. Furthermore, if you call your patient by his first name, are you prepared to allow him to call you by yours? I typically continue to address my adult patients by their title and surname throughout the course of therapy. This makes it clear that this is a collaborative relationship between two adults.[4]

Always ask the patient's permission before taking notes or utilizing recording devices. In general, I find that whatever you gain in the retrieval of "external data" by taking notes you lose in missing the aforementioned internal data. You cannot be fully attentive to your patient's verbal and nonverbal communications if you are busy with a pencil and a pad. If you practice summarizing your findings right after a session, you will train your memory such that you will not need to take notes.

Finally, you should inform the patient about the purpose of the evaluation: that your aim is to have him tell you as much as possible

---

[4]Whether you modify this in subsequent sessions depends on the patient's psychopathology and whether you are doing a more supportive or a more insight-oriented therapy. In a purely insight-oriented psychotherapy, you would *explore* the meaning of your patient's request that you "first name" him or he you. If he becomes angry about it, then you have something else to explore. At times you might honor, without first analyzing, such requests from a psychotic patient or one in supportive treatment. Nevertheless, even here you should have some idea of what it will *mean* to the patient if you do so.

about his problems, his current life, and his past history so that you *and* he can arrive at a reasonable approach to his problems.

If you are not necessarily going to be the treating as well as the evaluating clinician, as is, unfortunately, the case in many mental health centers and outpatient departments, then you should tell the patient so at the outset. He should not confide in you only to be told, at the end of several sessions, that you will not be following him. This might leave him feeling he has somehow failed you or has not been interesting enough.[5]

The standard written evaluation itself can be outlined as follows:

Identifying Data:
Chief Complaint (in the patient's own words):
Present Problem(s) (also called Present Illness):
Past History (prior history of psychiatric disorder and treatment may be described here or in a special section called Past Psychiatric History):
Past Medical History:
Family History:
Mental Status Examination:
Course of Evaluation:
Formulation:
Diagnostic Impression:
Treatment Plan:

I want to emphasize that in the evaluation interviewing, data collection (what you observe directly and what the patient reports to you) and incipient theorization at times go hand in hand, but in the write-up itself you must clearly demarcate between the data itself and your inferences and theorization about it. The narrative histories and mental status

---

[5]I am often asked how one should handle eye contact in both evaluation and therapy. This must depend largely on what seems most natural to your personality and the needs and anxieties of the particular patient. Freud himself admitted that one of the reasons for the couch was that he disliked being stared at eight or ten hours a day. Sullivan favored sitting at right angles to the patient, viewing this as less threatening to the latter and feeling his peripheral vision permitted him to pick up on major shifts in posture anyhow. I prefer sitting at a slight angle (45 degrees or less) to the patient such that he can, without physical discomfort, look directly at me or straight ahead across the room as he chooses. I generally look in his direction and nearly always maintain eye contact when either of us is talking, though in silences or if he appears particularly uncomfortable with my gaze I may look away slightly. In any event, avoid the extremes of never looking the patient in the eye or of engaging in staring contests. If he repeatedly has trouble with eye contact, then this eventually becomes grist for the mill in psychotherapy.

examination should present this data, as clean from inference as humanly possible, while the theorizing should be limited to the formulation.

In the interviews, you do not, of course, collect the information in as rigorous and mechanical a fashion as you record it. Nevertheless, you should always begin by taking an exquisitely detailed history of the present problem(s). Start, as previously mentioned, with an open-ended question and let the patient unfold his story. Pay particular attention to the first few sentences, for they often tell you a good deal about what is bothering him most and perhaps how he is defending against it. For example, one patient opened with, "I am here because of my father's heart failure, but more especially because of my fear of impotence." It soon emerged that what he stated *first* in the sentence was indeed first in order of importance, and that what he stated after was in fact a result of it. In other words, this man's fear of impotence had to do with guilt over oedipal triumph and was a graphic expression of his own powerlessness in the face of his father's progressive cardiac deterioration.

Try not to interrupt the patient in the midst of his narrative. It is easy enough to go back and request names, dates, places, and sequences. After he has painted in the broad strokes, ask him to brush in the details. First of all, find out what the patient *means* by the words with which he describes his plight. If he says he is "depressed," "nervous," "in a funk," or "down," ask him to help you understand just what he means by such words. He may reply sarcastically, "Well, Doctor, don't you know what 'depressed' means?" to which you can respond, "No two persons' depression is quite the same and I need to understand exactly what *your* depression feels like." You may come to find that what he calls "depression" is anything from the mildest and most transient "existential anxiety" to the most severe delusional psychosis.

Second, it is necessary to understand more clearly the *current context* of his disorder: both the environment in which it arose and that in which it persists. This means finding out as precisely as possible *when* the patient feels his problems began, *when* they intensified, and what was happening around him at that time. This also involves finding out *exactly when* he decided to seek your assistance, to call up and make the appointment, and *what* he was thinking about or what was happening *immediately prior* to this. The temporal contiguity between external events, the behaviors of others, and the patient's behaviors on the one hand and his internal distress on the other provides us with important clues about the meaning of his problems.

Take, for example, the following excerpt from an evaluation session with Mrs. J., a 30-year-old housewife who presented after the ingestion of half a bottle of aspirin. We were about 15 minutes into the interview. She had talked mostly about how "blue" she felt, how hard it was to do the housework, how her zest for life had gone, and how she had to drink several glasses of wine to fall asleep. Because she had told me little about the timing of her overdose and the relationship of it and her depression to her current interpersonal context, I turned to more specific questioning:

*Interviewer:* When did you decide to take the pills?

*Mrs. J:* Well, I don't know when or even why. I just know I was feeling like I didn't want to go on. [Silence]

*Interviewer:* Think back on it. Put yourself back in the situation and tell me as much as you possibly can about it.

*Mrs. J:* I don't know if I can.

*Interviewer:* I understand it's not pleasant, but I think you can.

*Mrs. J:* [Silence] Oh, O.K., I believe it was last Thursday or Friday. Yeah, come to think of it, it was Thursday. It seemed just an ordinary day like any other. I don't see that anything was that different.

*Interviewer:* It's important that you tell me what was going on when the feelings began.

*Mrs. J:* I don't remember.

*Interviewer:* Well, did you wake up feeling suicidal or did you start thinking about it later in the day?

*Mrs. J:* [Silence] Oh, I know I didn't wake up that way. It was later. [Silence] Come to think of it, it was in the afternoon, about mid-afternoon I would say.

*Interviewer:* Who was at home when you decided to take the pills?

*Mrs. J:* My husband was. [Pause] No, wait a minute, it would have been a little after 3 o'clock and he would already have left for the second shift. I guess I was alone.

*Interviewer:* What was your time with your husband like that day?

*Mrs. J:* No different from usual. He was down in his shop and I was upstairs trying to clean. Like always.

*Interviewer:* Like always?

*Mrs. J:* Yeah, we don't do too much together—at least we haven't for the last year or so. It was better before—not a whole lot better—but better. [She had previously told me she had been depressed "about a year," but had not consciously made the connection between her marital problems and the onset of her depression.] He's been away a lot lately. He gets off work at 11:30 p.m. but is often not home till 2 or 3 a.m. Says he's out drinking with the guys. I don't know.

As the interview progressed it became clear that Mrs. J. was dissatisfied with her husband. In the third interview she admitted that she was fairly certain he was having an affair, but was afraid he would leave if she confronted him with it. Like many patients, she did not *volunteer* all this information. Because it was painful she had suppressed and repressed it, but she began to open up with my gentle prodding. His *leaving* for work functioned as the precipitant for her overdose because it was symbolic of his rejection of her.

When you have obtained a well-rounded account of the present problem, your task is then to get a past history. After you have gleaned a good deal of experience doing evaluations, you will find that you can often predict with uncanny accuracy, from the account of the present problem and the patient's reactions to you, themes you will encounter in the past history. This is particularly true if you also have the patient's account of his prior psychiatric treatment in addition to that of the present problems.[6]

Thus, I advocate going from the "present problem" to the "past history of overt psychiatric problems and treatment." This helps you consider certain issues in early development that you might not otherwise: for example loss, deprivation, and rejection in the case of depressions. You will usually find a common theme or set of "precipitants"— and I use the word in an idiosyncratic fashion since the patient usually plays a role in bringing about what he is reacting to.

Any account of the patient's prior psychiatric problems should include whether he received treatment or whether and how he was "cured" by himself and his environment. If the former is true, you must find out what the treatment was like and whether he felt he benefited from it. This is particularly important, since it is not enough to know merely that a patient was in "therapy." That word is so loosely used it can mean anything from a cup of coffee and a game of checkers with one's psychiatric aide three times a week during a two-month hospitalization to years of five-times-a-week psychoanalysis. The tendency, on the part of both patient and mental health professional, is to label any interaction between the two, however brief and superficial, as "ther-

---

[6]Predicting future behavior from past behavior is another matter and much more difficult, however. An experienced therapist can predict, with uncanny accuracy, from a past history and account of the present problem, what the major transference themes will be. One can occasionally predict whether a person will engage in destructive or self-destructive behavior based on his past history. For the most part, however, we are on shaky ground in trying to predict the future. There are too many variables and factors we do not know about, chief among which is what reality will do to, or for, the patient. This is particularly true of predicting adult personality configurations or psychopathology from childhood history. We can take a child at ten and, based on his life to that point, make accurate statements about issues from his history that he will *have to deal with*, such as losses, deprivation, rejection, or abuse, but we cannot necessarily predict *how* he will deal with them. If we know enough about the sorts of coping skills available for his learning and modeling, then we are on firmer ground. However, even here, there is always the element of human creativity and the unforeseen opportunities and misfortunes provided by reality.

apy." Often, patients who say they have been in therapy for several years have *not* been at all, because of their own resistance and lack of motivation and/or the therapist's incompetence. If a patient has been in treatment, you should find out about medications, dosages, and his response to them. A caveat is in order here too. Do not infer the patient's past diagnosis from the medication he was prescribed. Trainees commonly conclude that somebody who was given a major tranquilizer must have been psychotic or someone who received an antidepressant must have been endogenously depressed. Prescribing practices vary enormously. Some psychiatrists give an antidepressant to the mildest case of the "blues," whereas others reserve it for those with severe vegetative signs and symptoms of depression and a positive family history of this disorder. Some prescribe a major tranquilizer to anybody with a little anxiety, whereas others reserve it for schizophrenia or the psychotic regressions of the borderline personality. Finally, at some point during the evaluation ask your patient to give you written permission to obtain his records from previous hospitals and therapists.

Before discussing the areas that should be covered in the past history proper, let me illustrate, again with the case of Mrs. J., how you will find that the present (and past) problems are virtually always a continuation of a lifelong theme:

*Interviewer:* Had you ever felt like overdosing before?

*Mrs. J:* Yes, just about six months ago. I almost made an appointment to see someone then. My father had died about a month before. . . . [she went on to describe this].

*Interviewer:* And before that had you ever felt that way?

*Mrs. J:* Yes, I was in a terrible down period about four years ago. We had been married about a year and I had proof positive that my husband was sleeping around with this girl at work. I let him have it one morning when he came in from work. He got so mad he just walked out and didn't come back for two weeks. If I had had any kind of pills in the house I would have taken them right then and there.

In further history-taking, it emerged that her first episode of the "blues" followed a disappointment in love her junior year of high school. The only other time she could recall any major problems was in the fifth grade when she was failing academically and staying home often with headaches. It seems that her parents had been arguing a great deal that year and almost obtained a divorce. She remembers intense relief and an improvement in her grades when their marriage improved. Even before that, however, she did not seem to receive much from her parents. Her most important nurturer, her maternal grandfather who lived in their home, died when she was six. She did not remember her reaction to this.

Thus, we see a lifelong theme of disappointment by important men. Her husband's rejection of her (symbolically expressed in the precipitant of her overdose) was only the most recent in a lifelong train of them. She habitually reacted to these rejections by feeling worthless and by turning anger against the self. This latter, her guilty feelings over her anger, and her attempt to get her husband's attention led to her suicide attempt. I shall not discuss the role she played in choosing a man like her husband and in making her marriage the way it was, although it was considerable. In other words she, like all patients, was not simply blindly, passively, mechanically *reacting* to events around her, but was acting in such a way as to help the world conform to her conscious and (mostly) unconscious interpretations and expectations of herself and it. She was reacting to a world she had in part created.

My central purpose, in presenting the sketchy scenario of Mrs. J., is to emphasize the essential understandability of human behavior (psychopathological or otherwise) when it is placed within its current and historical *interpersonal* context. This could have been demonstrated as well with a variety of cases. The contrast between the potential intelligibility of symptomatology and the patient's chaotic experience of it can be striking. The anxiety neurotic, for instance, often presents in near panic, talking in a diffuse and global way about his anxiety "attacks," perhaps attributing them to purely somatic factors (e.g., endocrine, or hypoglycemia), and bidding you explicitly or implicitly to "Do something!" If you take the bait and become ensnared in his "catastrophizing" about his symptoms, then you will be worse than useless to him. However, if you remember what you have learned from dynamic theory—that anxiety is a manifestation of people-related conflict and danger—then you will calmly but concernedly obtain sufficient interpersonal data to begin inferring the nature of the conflict and danger. In other words, you will ask him to describe his most recent episode and tell you about its circumstances (when, where, with whom; what he was doing, thinking, feeling then and before; if alone, then whom he had last been with and whom he was anticipating being with—in other words, who was in mind and in what fashion). Then you will get a history of his previous episodes, a picture of his current environment, and a skeleton past history. You will not know all the "whys" and "wherefores," but you will undoubtedly see some linkages and patterns emerge. One or two comments to this effect are often enough to give the patient some idea that there is a rhyme and reason to his distress, to diminish his "catastrophizing" somewhat, and to arouse his curiosity about himself.

Even though I have advised against "curing" the patient in the first interview, this does *not* mean that you can be blithely unconcerned with his needs and expectations. If he does not feel he is gaining anything, then he is unlikely to return. Of course, if you have been a proper interviewer, then you have conveyed your empathy and attentiveness—substantial gifts in themselves. Nevertheless, it is wise to form some idea, even in the initial session, of what the patient is looking for. Usually, it is some indication that he has been understood and accepted, and that there is hope for him after all. If he wants something that is not indicated or that you cannot deliver, then you should apprise him of this and of how you can be of assistance. When you are closing the first meeting, it is helpful to briefly recapitulate what you have gleaned so far and what you will be discussing in the next session.

In the following section is an outline of the areas that should be covered in any past history. This is a great deal and is admittedly an ideal, but it is an ideal toward which one can progressively approach with practice. The more history you become accustomed to obtaining at the outset, the less you will be content to work without it.[7] It is understood that the history is "complete" only at the end of treatment. This is to say that a history is not taken once and for all at the beginning, but that history-taking continues throughout the entire therapeutic process. Furthermore, you will return constantly to historical issues that were first raised in the evaluation, and will link them to each other, to newly uncovered historical factors, and to current and transference realities. In the course of psychotherapy, it is always helpful to review your notes periodically and to update your formulation to accord with the additional data you have obtained. This can be particularly useful in rescuing a treatment from the doldrums. Finally, lack of adequate history is one of the two most common reasons for treatment failure, the other being failure of *empathy* (which, incidentally, helps you put the italics in the right places in the history).

Although I have subdivided the data into categories, I do not mean to imply that this is the format in which you take or present your history. Emphatically it is not. You have the patient tell you his life story and you write it up in narrative fashion. Periodically, allow the patient to speak

---

[7]It is understood that it is always possible to go back later in the treatment and ask for essential information that you should have obtained initially. However, you must know that your questions will then take on additional *meaning* to the patient, depending on the context of the therapy at that time. In the beginning certain questions might stir less resistance or fewer fantasies about what you are "after" than at a later point in treatment. After six months in therapy some patients are more reluctant to discuss certain issues than they were in the beginning. Nevertheless, when you do discover that there are gaps in the past history, as you inevitably will, do not be embarrassed to ask the patient to bridge them. If you are dealing with major omissions, it is usually best to pick a quiet time in the therapy and say, for example, "I was thinking about our work together and it occurred to me that I know very little about the time from X to Z (or about when you lived at Y, or about your relationship with your sister, and so forth)."

for himself. His direct quotations can often express a point more clearly and succinctly than you can and help bring him to life for the reader. A good case history should all but read like a good novel. The history is neither taken nor presented in a choppy, categorical fashion.[8]

## THE PERSONAL HISTORY

Your patient is a person with an interesting story to tell. Approach him as one who wishes to hear and facilitate the telling of that story. Encourage him to be as graphic and concrete as possible in recounting his life. Ask him to flesh out the important relationships in which he was and is involved, to help you see the world through his eyes. Allow yourself to be receptive to themes and patterns, but suspend formulating until you have a dawning picture of the nature and evolution of his self-in-world.

Although I continually stress your investigation of the patient's inner life, I do not advocate this to the exclusion of understanding the external reality in which he moves and through which he has moved. There has been an unfortunate tendency, in some psychodynamic circles, to view the environment as but a passive screen upon which the patient projects his historically determined unconscious fears and fantasies. In fact, the self and world are in an inextricable and mutually influential interaction with one another and can be separated only for heuristic purposes; the empirical given is the *self-in-world*. The environment is not only im-pinged upon by the patient, but impinges upon him as well. It provides real possibilities and limitations with which he must come to terms. For example, it is not sufficient to spend hours discussing an individual's occupational fears and fantasies without obtaining a clear idea of the structure of his present and past work environments, of the personal-ities and institutions to whom and to which he relates and has related, and of the tasks with which he is and has been confronted. If you are too

----

[8]There is an urgent need for more rigorous research into patient nonadherence in mental health clinics. Most facilities lose as many as 50% of their clients in the transfer from evaluation to treatment, not to mention those who drop out in treatment itself. There is much speculation, and little conclusive documenta-tion, about the role of divergent therapist (evaluator)-client expectations and demographic variables. Perhaps most surprising is that the literature boasts almost no telephone follow-ups of these people to learn their side of the story! Kupers (1981, p. 54) speaks of an institutional, as well as a personal psychologi-cal, level of resistance in many lower socioeconomic class clients of public mental health clinics. "[This institutional level], containing a high concentration of feelings of powerlessness and anger, seems to have very little to do with the therapist and much to do with the setting—the public institution, the whole idea of 'seeing a shrink,' distrust of the system, and, in the case of a black client and white therapist, fears about racial configuration."

eager to view his supervisors and colleagues as nothing but parent and sibling imagoes, then you may miss important information about their personalities and the patient's interactions with them.

The following is only one of many ways of organizing the areas to be covered. Whether or not you follow my organization, you should at least have some sort of systematic outline in mind. Once more, obtain *concrete* detail about important situations, interactions, fantasies, fears, and concerns.

## I. The current picture.

A. In evaluation interviewing, I advocate that you gather this information immediately after hearing the story of the patient's present and past psychiatric problems and before taking the past history. This alerts you to the current context which is, after all, where the patient's most immediate and intense conscious concerns and feelings will be. Garner these data with an eye to empathically understanding the patient's current life structure (its components and their relative centrality) and not with a view to reducing his present relationships and preoccupations as quickly as possible to historical ones. The past must be anchored to the present, quite as much as the present to the past.
   1. Current living situation: where, what, with whom?
   2. Typical day and week.
   3. Friendships; occupation; religious, civic, and community involvement; marriage and family; recreational pursuits and hobbies; current relationships with family of origin, extended family, and in-laws.
   4. Current economic situation (it being a truism that financial problems exacerbate previously existing, often latent, interpersonal and psychological ones).
   5. Central aims, the Dream, and what the patient is striving toward; where he sees himself going; issues of adult development.

## II. Life in the family of origin.

A. *Nature and composition of the family unit into which the patient was born.*
   1. Socioeconomic status.
   2. Contemporary social, political, or historical trends that impinged upon the family.
   3. Extent of family's social network and availability of extended family; exactly *who* was living in the parental home.
   4. Ethnic group and religion, their roles in day-to-day life, and whether they constituted a minority in the patient's locale.
   5. Parents' marriage *at the time of patient's birth*, duration of marriage to that point, parents' ages, any evidence for recent stressors on marriage around this time (e.g., deaths, quarrels, illness, mother-in-law moving in, or job loss).
   6. Some inkling about whether the pregnancy was planned or unplanned: often must be inferred (e.g., if the patient was much the youngest of several siblings and born to older parents you might suspect he was unplanned).
   7. Nature and duration of the pregnancy with an eye to prematurity (a

long time in an incubator can adversely affect mother-child bonding), complications during gestation, birth, and delivery (because of the direct impact on the patient's physiological-psychological system and because a difficult gestation, birth, and delivery can adversely affect some mothers' attitudes toward their offspring).

8. Number of siblings and their ages when the patient arrived.

B. *Growing up in the parental home* (try to form a clear idea of what it was like to live in this home).

1. Bottle or breast-fed, by whom, and when weaned.
2. Thumb-sucking and other similar habits (and how the parents responded to them).
3. Developmental milestones. (If the patient can tell you little about this, it usually means his parents have told him little about it, and this in itself may tell you something about the parent-child interaction.)
4. Early childhood illnesses or operative procedures, whether they required hospitalization or prolonged bed rest and whether, and in what fashion, the parents fulfilled the patient's heightened dependency needs.
5. Earliest memories. Always get three or four of these along with their affective tone. They are particularly important as they are usually *screen memories*, condensing many typical experiences into a single graphic image. Often they are uncannily prescient of what will turn out to be life-long themes. Ask for particularly vivid or recurrent childhood dreams and nightmares.
6. Quality and quantity of interactions with the parents (prototypical for later interactions with helpers and authority figures including you):
   a. Patient's descriptions of what the parents were like.
   b. Their availability: whether he could turn to them in time of stress; whether one or both of them were emotionally or physically absent; whether the patient remembers hugging, being held, talked to, played with, and going on family outings (a virtual inability or refusal to report any memories of childhood usually means it was an overwhelmingly negative one). Watch for descriptions that suggest factors—chronic physical illness, hypochondriasis, psychosis, depression, alcoholism—in the parents which would have impaired their availability.
   c. Be alert to evidence of physical, emotional, or sexual abuse or seductive, smothering, or overprotective behavior on the part of one or both parents.
   d. Obtain a differentiated idea of the patient's interactions with each parent, whether he seemed to feel closer to one than the other (can be an ambivalent closeness), often indicated by the one he chooses to talk about *first*, and whether he felt he was the favorite child of one or the other.
   e. Know something about parental patterns of reward and punishment.
7. Physical plan of the house. This should be understood in proximity to the patient's bedroom; whether he shared a room with others; whether he had night terrors, nightmares, and other "good reasons" to try to enter the parental bedroom and, if so, how he was responded to; the closeness of his bedroom to the parental one helps determine the likelihood of primal scene perceptions; whether and where the family congregated during the day.

8. Parents' relationship with one another (crucial because the child learns how a married couple should act from them and because there is a direct relationship between the quality of the marital relationship and the patient's sense of security in the family); whether theirs was a mature love that included the children or an exclusiveness with one another that did not; whether there were yelling matches or physical fights (such that the patient came to view anger as dangerous) and how the patient reacted to them; whether the parents were emotionally distant from each other (e.g., slept in separate rooms or beds); and whether there were affairs, separations, divorce, or threats of divorce.

9. Relationship with siblings (prototypical for later interactions with peers and colleagues).
   a. Their ages in relationship to the patient's. Paying particular attention to spacing between the births and the patient's ages at births of his younger siblings (include memories of, and reactions to, these births and how they affected the parenting he received).
   b. Quality and quantity of relationships with siblings and degree of distance, affection, competitiveness, and sexuality.
   c. Whether the patient had to assume premature parenting responsibilities for a sibling such that his own needs were set aside (e.g., the "parentified child").
   d. How the patient's place in the home measures up against that of his siblings; how his achievements and parental kudos compare to theirs.

10. Traumata involving separation and loss.
    a. Deaths of family figures and the patient's ages when they occur. The most important death is that of one or both parents in childhood (people with such a history are overrepresented in the psychiatric population, particularly in the depressions). Deaths of siblings are also crucial since there are usually unconscious death wishes, in addition to love, toward them and the guilt feelings can be considerable. The death of a grandparent living within the home can have a profound impact depending upon his or her importance to the patient. How a child deals with a death, the extent of his grief work, depends largely on the *survivors'* emotional availability to him.
    b. Family moves and the ages at which they occur (a move, broadly speaking, is like a death), whether around the corner or across the country, an idea of the important persons left behind and how the patient and parents dealt with this, the degree of apprehensiveness about relocation and making new friends, and the proximity to extended family after the move.
    c. Major illness in the patient, parents, or siblings, and the impact of this on his relationship with the parents (previously referred to).
    d. Parental separation or divorce and the impact of this on the patient's subsequent relationship with each parent. Children usually feel responsible for the divorce: "If only I could have been a better child Daddy [or Mommy] wouldn't have left."
    e. Major economic reversal or natural catastrophe (bankruptcy, unemployment, flood, earthquake, and so forth).

11. Any evidence for childhood neurosis or psychopathology (obsessionality, phobias, hyperkinesis, psychosis, enuresis, encopresis, asthma or other psychosomatic conditions; night terrors; school phobia or

school problems; extreme social withdrawal; running away); to be understood within the context in which it occurred and the parental reaction to it; whether professional help was sought. Childhood psychopathology is commonly observed in the latency years.

## III. Life outside the parental home.

  A. *Social history.*
   1. Interactions outside the home.
      a. Quantity and quality: can the patient recall, for each period of his life, at least one "best friend" and close circle of friends? Were there spend-the-night parties and going home after school with friends? Was the quality mature and intimate, shallow, exploitative, all-giving or all-taking, mutually supportive, empathic, apprehensive, competitive, and so forth? Be alert for any evidence for self-defeating patterns of interaction with parents, siblings, and early childhood peers; the differentiation and nature of relationships with the same and opposite sex.
      b. Duration: were at least some of them sustained over time or is there a pattern of disappointments and severed ties?
      c. Popularity with peers: leader or follower? bullied? scapegoated? discriminated against because of ethnic, religious, or socioeconomic factors?
      d. Look especially for a sense of inferiority, shame, social incompetence and withdrawal, shyness, and so forth. If there were social fears, try to determine their nature and origin.
      e. Patient's play (age and sex appropriate?) and involvement in sports, music, and other recreational pursuits with peers.
      f. How the parents reacted to the child's socialization with peers and separation from home. Were his efforts encouraged, discouraged, or disparaged?
      g. Current social network: those with psychiatric problems tend to have smaller social networks than "normals." Continued maintenance of object relations is one of the most important indicators of the severity of the disturbance and its prognosis.
  B. *Sexual history.*
     How soon you obtain this information varies from patient to patient. Today's clinician can talk frankly to his patient about sexual issues that had to be approached more cautiously by the psychiatrist of Freud's day. The majority of individuals will be willing to discuss much of their sexual life with you by the second interview. The timing of course varies somewhat from patient to patient and depends upon the interviewing situation, e.g., whether clinician and patient are age mates of the same sex or whether they are of opposite sex and of widely differing ages. I only advocate 1) that you not raise the issue until after you have established some rapport and the patient is accustomed to talking about himself and being questioned and 2) that you broach the topic in a neutral and matter-of-fact way. In regard to this latter, if your voice and manner demonstrate that *you* are comfortable talking about sexuality, that you will not be judgmental, and that you fully *expect* the patient to be able to talk about it too (expectation again), then he *will* be able to talk about it.[9]

---

[9]See page 151.

1. Earliest years. (A reasonably complete history of the patient's earliest sexuality may take months or years to obtain since much of this is subject to repression. The following is an account of what you should look for and be wondering about, not necessarily of what you should directly question. That is, you *infer* from the patient's story whether a parent behaved seductively toward him. You do not ask this directly while still in the evaluation.)

    a. Remembrance of childhood masturbation and sex play (e.g., the "doctor game") and parents' reactions to this.

    b. Be alert for primal scene material (both in fantasy and actuality)— overseeing or overhearing the parents in intercourse (occasionally a patient shares a parental bedroom until several years of age); fantasies about what mommy and daddy do in bed.

    c. Evidence for seductiveness and overstimulation or, conversely, rejection by the parent of the opposite sex; a parent with marital difficulties at times (usually unconsciously) takes the child of opposite sex as a husband or wife surrogate.

    d. Look for evidence pointing to heterosexual or homosexual abuse at the hands of a parent, sibling, cousin, babysitter, stranger, or friend of the family, and how the parents reacted to this. (Where incest occurs, the patient often blames the parent of the same sex, as much as the seducer, for failing to protect him.)

    e. Signs of an early foundation for perversion or inversion of sexual object or aim.

    f. Latency age. Degree to which the patient's sexuality was really latent; extent of sublimation. Transient and mild episodes of homosexual play are not uncommon at this stage.

2. Adolescence and adulthood (here your questions can be much more direct and explicit).

    a. Puberty: age at onset; preparedness for by parents and peers; the patient's reactions (pride, pleasure, shame, guilt, fear, physical pain in the case of menses, and so forth); parents' attitudes toward their own puberty, sexuality, and bodies, particularly important in the case of the mother's attitude toward menstruation; parents' receptiveness to discussing sexual matters; pubertal and adolescent masturbation fantasies and practices and the patient's and parents' attitudes toward masturbation; early adolescent crushes, often on teachers and other adults outside the home (parent imagoes).

    b. Adolescent sexual experiences, ranging from dating through petting to intercourse; the quality and quantity of these and his reactions

---

[9]Occasionally, the student goes to the opposite extreme from reticence upon sexual matters and asks the patient for irrelevant detail about his sexual life. This might involve going into, without specific indications for it, intimate detail about the patient's seduction techniques, foreplay, preferred positions in intercourse, whether he and his partner talk during coitus, and so forth. This often amounts to the therapist titillating himself at the patient's expense; it might elicit in the patient an angry sense of being intruded upon or an intense erotic response. In the therapy you ask for such detail only when the context demands it and the patient does not volunteer it.

(e.g., guilt feelings, pleasure) to them; one's sense of attractiveness to the opposite sex and sense of security in one's own sexuality; and presence or absence of "steady" relationships; try to infer presence or absence of ability to fuse sensual and affectionate currents of sexuality; patterns in relationship with opposite sex; pregnancies or abortions and emotional reactions thereto; presence or absence of homosexual relationships and feelings about these.

   c. Adult pattern of relationships with the opposite sex and how this relates to one's early history; try to infer the degree to which the patient has moved toward the pinnacle of adult genitality; current sexual fantasies, practices, and masturbation; homosexuality or bi-sexuality and, if so, ego syntonic or ego dystonic; evidence for perversions like masochism, sadism, fetishism, exhibitionism, voyeurism, and the patient's feelings about his practices; try to determine the degree of sexual satisfaction in the marriage and the degree of fidelity or infidelity and his feelings about these; sexual dysfunctions such as impotence, frigidity, and fears about sexual adequacy. Be alert for subscription to self-damaging myths about sexual functioning.

C. *Marriage and family.*
  1. If unmarried or childless, his feelings about it. Try to gauge the social-familial and intrapsychic pressures to marry and raise children and the effect on self-esteem.
  2. That which first attracted the patient to his spouse; the nature and duration of the courtship; nature and residences of the early marriage. Be alert for sexual, economic, or in-law problems and difficulties of either partner in separating from the family of origin.
  3. Nature of the subsequent and current interactions between patient and spouse: quantity and quality of their time together (in particular what they talk about, degree of intimacy and emotional expressiveness, degree of mutuality in their interests and concerns); quality and quantity of the sexual experiences; the picture around home on evenings and weekends; the nature of vacation and recreational time together; the distribution of power and division of labor within and without the household and with the children; how (not whether) they argue and disagree with one another; and how the patient would characterize the spouse; separations or near divorces, infidelities, and regrets.
  4. Children: planned or unplanned; duration of the marriage at their births and impact on the marriage; nature of the patient's interactions with the children (look especially for any child with whom he identi-fies, who is made a scapegoat, or who otherwise represents an uncon-scious imago); how he feels about his parenting; and whether there is any evidence for psychopathology in the offspring.

D. *Educational history.*
  1. Early years.
    a. How the child's separation from home to preschool and/or grammar school was managed by patient and parents; any evidence for school phobia (which reflects separation anxieties on the part of both pa-tient and parents).
    b. Early experiences with peers and teachers in the classroom: How did the patient feel his academic achievement stacked up against that of his peers? Was he rewarded, punished, or ignored by the

teachers? Was he isolated for being "dumb" or "brainy" or the "teacher's pet?"

c. The patient's academic performance and how his parents reacted to it: Was his level of achievement appropriate to his intelligence? Were there any well-demarcated periods of decline in achievement, usually reflecting problems at home during the time?

d. Extracurricular activities; evidence for the ability to play.

e. Did the patient focus on academic work to the exclusion of the social tasks of childhood and adolescence?

2. Later years.

a. Performance in high school and, if he dropped out, why; academic self-esteem; major successes and disappointments in dreams of further education.

b. Involvement in college; postgraduate and professional education and feelings about his performance.

c. Current formal and informal educational pursuits.

E. *Occupational history.*

1. Preadult experiences with work.

a. Perception of, and feelings about, parents' occupational roles, including parental communications about the work world.

b. Early occupational dreams and parents' attitudes toward these. Often single successful career women feel like failures because their parents promoted marriage and family but never career.

c. Early work experiences: Did the patient have to assume premature economic responsibilities around the home such that crucial emotional and educational needs were set aside? (People who had to assume premature vocational and nurturing functions in the household are overrepresented in the depressions.)

2. Adult occupational experiences.

a. Is there an occupational dream (in the Levinsonian sense) and, if so, where does the patient feel he now stands in relationship to it? Is his work a satisfying part of his identity and does he feel successful at it or is it a trial, a bore, or merely a means of making a living? If the patient is a housewife does she regret the loss of a career? If she is a combination homemaker-career woman, be alert to the very real stresses attendant upon her and how it affects the marriage.

b. Job history: If there is frequent job-hopping, find out why (may reflect problems with authority and/or peers, even paranoia or the need to ward off latent homosexuality by fighting with peers); is there advance, stasis, or decline on the occupational-socioeconomic ladder?

c. If the patient was in the military service, find out about this and about the type of discharge.

F. *Drug and alcohol history* (for some reason a detailed accounting in this area is particularly likely to be omitted by mental health trainees).

1. Should include something about parental attitudes toward, and their use of, drugs and alcohol.

2. History of involvement with drugs and alcohol; attempt to correlate major fluctuations in usage with life events.

3. *Precise* idea of current usage and its relationship to the patient's overall adaptation and maladaptation (expect that the chronic abuser will grossly underestimate his usage); any history of drug or alcohol with-

drawal, delirium tremens, alcoholic hallucinosis, or drug-induced psychosis. (Although drug addictions and alcoholism are themselves symptomatic of underlying problems, these problems cannot usually be treated until the substance abuse is removed.)

4. It is useful to ask the patient how he acts and feels under the influence. Since alcohol is a disinhibitor, this will give you a picture of affects, fantasies, and impulses normally defended against.

G. *Religious history* (long ago surpassed sexuality as the area least likely to be investigated).

1. Whatever the patient's current affiliation (or lack of it), you should obtain a history of his early and later involvement with religion, and the parental attitudes toward it. Often someone who has consciously abandoned the religious values of his childhood nonetheless continues to be unconsciously influenced by them. The timing of major shifts in religious attitudes and practices should be noted since they often reflect major changes in interpersonal relations within or without the family.

Following the personal history are separate sections entitled "Medical History" and "Family History." The first is self-explanatory and much of this information will already have been obtained within the context of the life history. It is important to know about chronic physical conditions (e.g., diabetes or congenital heart disease) to which the patient has had to adapt, early bouts with severe infections or fractures that necessitated prolonged bed rest or withdrawal from peers, and physical conditions that may have affected the patient's self-esteem (e.g., phimosis or recurrent vaginal infections and discharge). Current medical conditions and the treatment for them should be known. Likewise, much of the "Family History" will have been obtained within the context of the patient's life story. Important information within this section includes whether there is any family history of psychiatric disorder or treatment, both because there is some evidence that severe affective disorders and schizophrenia may have a heritable, genetic component and, more importantly, because parents' psychiatric problems affect the sort of parenting a patient receives. Furthermore, it is not at all uncommon that patients identify with the psychopathology of their parents. At times, neurotic and reasonably well-adjusted individuals fear that the manic-depressive illness or schizophrenia which runs in their family is like a curse with which they will surely be smitten. If blood relatives have been treated successfully with psychotropic medications, it is important to know which ones since, if the patient has a similar problem (say a major affective disorder), he may, because of metabolic similarities, also respond to the same one(s). It is often helpful to know some history about the parents themselves. If you obtain this, as I said earlier, you will often be surprised to see patterns of faulty parenting and maladaptive behaviors being passed on from generation to generation.

In the next chapter I shall discuss the mental status examination and formulation and I shall acquaint you with a device, the life chart, that I feel is helpful in organizing the history that you have gleaned.

## SUGGESTED READINGS FOR CHAPTER 4

Readings for this chapter may be found at the end of Chapter 5.

# 5

# The Mental Status Examination and Formulation

## THE MENTAL STATUS EXAMINATION

The mental status examination is a separate section of the evaluation on paper only. You do not take the history and then say to the patient or think, "Now I will do the mental status examination." This exam starts with the first minute of the interview and ends with the last. It is of a piece with the history-taking itself. The patient is constantly telling you about his affect, his reality-testing, and his central preoccupations. You observe his physical appearance, mode of dress and hygiene, posture, mannerisms, motor activity, and style of verbal and nonverbal communication (and noncommunication). From his account of his life and problems and the way he handles your questions, you learn about his cognitive style, his recent and remote memory, and his ability to concentrate, abstract, and think logically.

Only when you suspect special sorts of problems (e.g., chronic alcoholism, schizophrenia, organic brain syndrome) should you go back and formally do certain aspects of the mental status exam. When you do you must, in a matter-of-fact way, alert the patient that you will be shifting gears somewhat. However, as MacKinnon and Michels (1971) state, if you feel the need to preface your questions with "These may sound silly but . . . ," then they usually are silly and unnecessary with that particular patient.

The written mental status examination tries to capture some of the essence of what it was like to be with the patient. This is not to say that descriptive terms should not be used in the narrative history (e.g., "he

**156**

tearfully told me . . .," "with a flushed face and quivering voice he said
. . .," "scowling, he answered . . ."), but that the mental status
section is a concentrated dose of such descriptions and that it attempts
to depict the major characteristics of the patient's presentation. Once
more, as with the narrative history, your written mental status examination should present what you see and hear and empathically "resonate"
with, as free from inference and theorizing as possible. If, for example,
you are inferring the existence of visual or auditory hallucinations from a
patient's periodic distraction, but he denies their presence, then state
plainly that this is your procedure.

In line with the rubric about staying as close as possible to what you
observe and what the patient reports, present concrete examples of the
phenomena you are describing. For instance, do not merely write "The
patient had delusions (or hallucinations or ideas of reference)" or "He
was depressed (or paranoid or manic)." The former are inferences, the
latter diagnoses. What you want are the *data* that lead you to conclude a
person is having delusions or ideas of reference or is paranoid or manic.
For example, in the case of delusions say, "Mr. K. held the firm conviction that he had discovered a mechanical process that was going to bring
global peace and that he would be appointed president of the world by a
grateful populace." In that of ideas of reference write, "Mrs. V. would
pass total strangers on the street, convinced that they were talking and
laughing about her masturbation practices." In the case of depression
you might pen something like:

> Mrs. P. walked slowly to her chair as if the effort would kill her, looked
> indecisively at me until I motioned her to sit down, and then sat wringing
> her hands and looking fixedly at the floor. Upon her face was a look of
> utter despair and resignation; her forehead was deeply furrowed. She
> admitted feeling helpless and hopeless about her situation. She hesitated
> before each question and then answered briefly and in a bland monotone.
> Not once did she initiate the conversation. Several times she asked me to
> repeat my questions and admitted to great difficulty concentrating on
> them. On three occasions she burst into tears: once when talking about the
> death of her mother six years before, once when talking about her hyster-
> ectomy four years ago, and once when talking about her son who recently
> left for college.

This example also points out how, when you mention affective eruptions, you should always specify the context in which they occurred. It is
meaningless to note that a person cried four times, laughed uncontrollably once, blew up at the examiner twice, and shifted nervously in his
chair on three occasions without knowing what he said, or what you
asked, before the display and what was being discussed during it.

In the written mental status exam, as in the narrative history, it is
often useful to have a direct quotation or two from the patient. This
illustrates or amplifies the points you are trying to make and occasional-

ly expresses them more graphically than you could yourself. It is also "kosher" to include your own affective reactions to the patient and "hunches" in the mental status exam, provided, of course, you indicate that it is *your* response that you are describing. Or, if you prefer, such information could be reserved for the "Course of Evaluation" section. If you found yourself feeling exasperated or with a headache following each session you can say so, at the same time spelling out the patient behavior to which you think it was related. If you felt fear for your safety or an urge to rescue the patient that you think was in response to his mode of presentation, then say so. If you felt the patient, while seemingly warm and open, was actually keeping his distance and withholding a good deal, then say so. If he left you feeling puzzled or a bit uneasy about him, then record this. The old-fashioned psychiatrists used to diagnose schizophrenia if they experienced a species of uncanny emotion, the "praecox feeling," with a patient. The good interviewer "resonates," like a tuning fork, with the affective "vibrations" of his patient. This is particularly important in appreciating hidden depression, anger, and anxiety.

What we call "empathy" is, by and large, a function of such resonances, which are themselves based on our transient preconscious and unconscious identifications with the patient. Relating to others by identification, rather than by object cathexis, is, you recall, the earliest mode of interaction. It persists (largely unconsciously) in all of us and is more active in some situations than in others (e.g., the well-known "emotional contagion" in groups). Most of the patient's communications about his affective state are both transmitted and received (by the therapist) subliminally through the nonverbal medium of body language and tone of voice. Much of what passes for human "intuition" is a function of this preconscious and unconscious nonverbal communication. Much of learning to be a therapist is allowing oneself to become consciously accessible to what is usually filtered out in normal social intercourse.

The following is an outline of the mental status examination though, like the history, it is presented in a smooth and narrative fashion rather than a choppy and categorical one. Although my outline comprises numerous pages, you should be able to record the significant findings of any given mental status examination in a paragraph or two. Later in the chapter I shall give an example of such a paragraph.[1]

---

[1] In psychiatry, as in general medicine, it is useful to distinguish between "signs" and "symptoms," the former being the observable manifestations of a psychical disorder, the latter its more important, internal, subjective correlates. For example, it may take the novice clinician but a few minutes to spot and record the psychomotor retardation, slumped posture, handwringing, and dejected facies of depression, while requiring many hours of skilled interviewing to flesh out the inner state that accompanies them.

## I. General appearance.

A. *Physical size, shape, and appearance:* whether the patient appears his stated age; any striking physical characteristics or handicaps.

B. *Dress:* conservative, stylish, or "mod"; staid or exhibitionistic; coordinated or clashing colors and patterns (the latter can occur in mania, schizophrenia, and certain schizoid or schizotypal characters); within the generally accepted limits or bizarre.

C. *Personal hygiene and attention to appearance:* be especially careful to note extremes in the direction of over- or under-concern.

D. *Facial expression:* tense, mournful, hostile, intensely staring, averted gaze, and so forth.

E. *Posture and mannerisms* (tell you much about a patient's character style): e.g., tense, rigid, and holding back mannerisms are often associated with issues of control and conflicts over intimacy in the obsessional and turning anger upon the self in the depressive; seductive behavior alternating with pulling away (such as the woman who continually pulls her skirt up a bit and then back down, who sits forward coquettishly and then moves back with tightly crossed arms and legs) suggests conflicts over sexuality; jerky, uncoordinated, automaton-like movements may occur in the schizophrenic; mention particularly prominent bizarre, or gender-inappropriate mannerisms.

F. *Motor activity:* motor retardation, restlessness, pacing, agitation, hand-wringing, constant looking aside, autism (e.g., rotating one's finger and looking at it intently or gazing at the light for minutes on end—refers to the private and idiosyncratic meaning of such behaviors), extrapyramidal movements, or other signs of drug-induced or spontaneous neurological disorder. (Be particularly careful to look for signs of tardive dyskinesia in the patient with a long career on antipsychotic medication.)

G. *Attitude toward the interviewer:* cooperative, overly compliant, passive-aggressive or negativistic, fearful, "macho," hostile, threatening, aloof, dependent, helpless and rescue seeking, seductive, guarded and hypervigilant, and so forth.

## II. Speech (reflects thought).

A. *Characteristics:* rapid, slow, hesitant, stuttering or stammering, slurred, lisping, effeminate, loud, raucous, or soft (subvocalization often reflects ambivalence about being heard or conflicts over assertiveness and aggression).

B. *Quantity:* taciturn or voluble.

C. *Conversation:* whether it proceeds logically and coherently; items around which it centers.

D. *Special characteristics associated with psychopathology.*
   1. Circumstantiality: the tendency to talk "all around" a topic, to avoid coming to the affect-laden point by continually sidetracking oneself with excessive detail about relatively trivial parts of the story; common in obsessional characters and in manics.

2. Tangentiality: somewhat related to circumstantiality; refers to the rapid and continual shifting of the topic of conversation, at times virtually in midsentence; most characteristic of the manic. As opposed to loose associations, a connection is generally apparent between the two lines of thought, often on the basis of a similarity in the sound of the words (clang associations such as, "Yes, I am here to see a psychiatrist for the first time—rhyme, climb, chime, mime—Doctor, what's your line?"), or a superficial similarity in content ("Yes, we were in Spain when we decided to divorce—the rain in Spain stays mainly on the plain— Doctor, the whole thing's as plain as the nose on your face"); or the lines of conversation are derailed in response to obvious stimuli from the environment.

3. Pressured speech: the patient is driven to express as much as possible in as short a time as feasible. This speech can be tangential or otherwise; it can reflect a manic process or simply a sense of crisis and a frantic desire for help as soon as possible; it can be the external manifestation of an internal and tangential *flight of ideas*—a cascading of thoughts, memories, and preoccupations pell mell one atop the other; it can also occur where one has been bottling up affects for a long time (the speech of such a patient often being anything but pressured in the second and subsequent interviews).

4. Loose associations: the patient jumps from one topic to another with absolutely no *apparent* connection between the two (e.g., "I was going to the store to buy some candy when . . . the man in the moon looked up at the sun . . . it's gray, they say, in the land of Oz . . .") This is opposed to the flight of ideas and tangentiality of the manic, where there is a discernible connection, however silly or superficial, between the trains of thought. Although you cannot discern the threads between loose associations they are there, albeit unconscious. Like all other human behaviors, the loose associations of the schizophrenic are meaningful and purposeful, if one only knows enough about the person. In most schizophrenics the loose associations are not continuous throughout the interview but occur episodically. Pay particular attention to the contexts in which the associations loosen since this will tell you something about their function, which is to defend against awareness of painful ideas, affects, and perceptions from the environment. Habitual hesitancy and pauses before answering questions may reflect a patient's frantic attempts to organize his thoughts and to prevent you from perceiving a subtle thought disorder. You can comment benignly on these pauses and ask the patient to describe what he thinks about during them.

5. Word salad: the result of a virtually continuous loosening of associations; an apparently meaningless conglomeration of words and phrases in complete violation of all rules of grammar, logic, and syntax. It is sheer primary process and is in accordance with the pleasure principle. It is often accompanied by *neologisms*—words invented by the patient and carrying a private, idiosyncratic and autistic meaning. Here again, though, if one knows enough about the patient one can arrive at some understanding of his autistic vocabulary (e.g., a young schizophrenic woman, rejected by her mother, frequently spoke of "neglection"—a compound of neglect and rejection).

6. Blocking: the patient drops off in midsentence or midthought without being able to explain why. In the neurotic it results from the threatened emergence of a repressed complex of idea and affect. In the psychotic it

may reflect intrapsychic conflict or it may occur in response to hallucinations or the intrusion of bizarre and delusional trains of thought. The schizophrenic may have the subjective sense that his thoughts are being stolen from him (*thought withdrawal*).

7. Perseveration: repetition of words, phrases, or actions without the conscious intention to do so; occurs in schizophrenia and, in particular, organic brain syndrome.

8. Echolalia (or echopraxia): parroting of the examiner's words (or behaviors); results from the schizophrenic's impaired boundaries between the representations of self and others and his vulnerability to taking on the characteristics of others. In its mildest forms it may be simply a repetition of the examiner's question before answering it (which can of course also be an attempt to buy time to organize one's answer and cover up an underlying thought disorder).

**III. Affective state** (the most important information in the psychiatric evaluation).

A. *Recognized in part* from general appearance, motor activity, posture, facial expression, tone of voice, and your empathic resonance, and *in part* from the patient's direct verbal communications (spontaneous and in response to your questions) about his affective state. The student should be able to discern (more easily said than done) subtle signs of basic affect states such as:

1. Depression (actually a final common pathway for many different affect states): the patient says he feels "sad," "blue," "down," or "in a funk"; he exhibits hand wringing, agitation, downcast gaze, furrowed brow, poverty of movement; he speaks of impatience, touchiness, ready irritability; he expresses a sense of helplessness, hopelessness, anhedonia, worthlessness, incompetence; he feels inappropriately guilty or engages in irrational self-reproach; he complains of multiple vague somatic complaints, the vegetative signs and symptoms of depression, or even somatic delusions or nihilistic ideas ("my intestines are rotting," "my brain is dead").

2. Anger: ranging from physical violence and threats to sarcasm and negativism.

3. Anxiety (like depression can be a conglomeration of many different and conflicting unconscious emotions): where there is anxiety there is fearfulness and intrapsychic conflict. It is manifested in tremulousness, sweaty palms, the tone of voice and cracking in the voice, fears of death, atypical chest pains and somatic complaints, the symptoms of hyperventilation (perioral and peripheral numbness and tingling progressing, at times, to muscle spasm, air hunger, or lightheadedness), and so forth.

4. Sensuality: varies from coy flirtatiousness and the use of words with double entendre to frank exhibitionism and sexual propositions. Patients can be conscious or unconscious of their sexual feelings and provocativeness.

5. Warmth and affection: like any other affect can be conscious or unconscious and expressed with widely varying degrees of openness, maturity, and neediness.

6. Boredom: a particularly complicated affect, which nearly always conceals more than it expresses; it is especially necessary to encourage the patient to flesh out the phenomenology and circumstances of what he

terms "boredom"; it may be a screen for anything from sexual frustration or damaged self-esteem to severe anxiety, depression, or anger.

B. *Appropriateness* of affect to thought content: a schizophrenic may laugh
uncontrollably when describing a recent death in the family or an obsessional may describe the recent dissolution of his marriage with a bland
affect (isolation of affect).

C. *Range* of affect: whether the interview is dominated by one affect; dramati-
zation or constriction of affect; lability of affect (labile affect is particularly
common in organic brain syndrome, e.g., convulsive crying followed by
uncontrollable laughter followed by petulant rage, all seemingly for "no
reason"); blunting of affect (particularly common in schizophrenia and
important to distinguish from the affect of severe retarded depression).

D. *Covering* (conscious and unconscious) of affect: it is crucial to remember,
from our theoretical chapters, that patients can use one affect (e.g., anger)
to defend against another (e.g., fear, hurt, or sexuality). Frequently depression is masked beneath an apparent cheeriness (even mania) or anxiety beneath a trumped-up composure or anger beneath an excessively
compliant, polite exterior. If you look, listen, and empathize closely, you
can often divine the suppressed or repressed affect along with the "noi-
sier" defense against it.

**IV. Perception and interpretation of self and reality.** (If they are normal and there is no evidence for delusions, hallucinations, or other gross
impairments in perception and interpretation, then this should be so
stated.)

A. *Perception and esteem of self-in-world:* obtaining this requires literally the
entire psychotherapy. The objective here is merely to gain an initial reconnaissance of this rich and complicated matter.
1. Much of the patient's perception and evaluation of himself will be
implicit in the course of conversation. To the degree that it is not, you
should specifically ask him how he views himself and his prospects;
what he particularly likes and dislikes (including enduring regrets)
about himself; how he thinks an intimate friend would characterize
him; and what a stranger would likely say about his first impression of
him. You should also glean some sense of his body image and attitude
toward the body and its functions (attractive people may have gro-
tesque images of themselves).
2. The world, the degree to which it is seen as basically rewarding and
trustworthy or as inimical and terrifying, will be inferred from his
entire presentation.

B. *Perceptual abnormalities.*
1. Hallucinations: these usually become apparent in the course of conversation if they are present; if not and the patient's history or behavior
still leads you to suspect he is hallucinating, then you should question
him tactfully and matter-of-factly. Start with an open-ended question,
such as "Have you had any experiences that seemed out of the ordinary or unexplainable or that you weren't sure were really happening
to you?" Then move to a more explicit one: "Do you ever hear voices
when no one is present or see or hear things that others don't seem to

see or hear?" Obviously neurotic and reality-oriented patients should be asked about hallucinations only if they give a history of heavy drug or alcohol abuse; otherwise, they may fear you view them as more disturbed than they actually are or they may feel insulted.

a. Visual, auditory, tactile, olfactory, or gustatory hallucinations: determine whether the patient believes in the external reality of them or understands that they are mental events. It is important to know how the patient reacts to, and feels about, his hallucinations.

b. It is crucial to ask for the content of the hallucinations: *what* he sees, *what* the "voices" say (they may be telling him to commit suicide), and so forth.

c. It is important to determine the temporal and situational variation in the presence or intensity of hallucinations (those of organic brain syndrome may intensify at night because of the diminution in orienting visual and auditory stimuli from the external world; those in schizophrenia are more likely to vary in relationship to the presence or absence of important, though problematic, individuals, situations, and affects). Auditory hallucinations are most characteristic of schizophrenia, although visual hallucinations also occur in that disorder. Hallucinations in the other sensory modalities (especially vision and touch) are more common in organic mental diseases and toxic states.

2. Illusions: erroneous perceptions, or interpretations of perceptions, of objects that actually exist in the external world, as opposed to hallucinations in which no outer object corresponds to the perception (e.g., the difference between misperceiving or misinterpreting a rustling drape as a rat or a shadow as a burglar and frankly hallucinating a rat or a burglar out of thin air). Illusions are common in excited states and in certain toxic conditions.

3. Somatic delusions (also called cenesthetic delusions or hallucinations): hallucinated organic sensations like "my brain is on fire," "my backbone has a B-B rolling up and down in it," "my uterus has turned to stone," or "my neck is swelling." It is crucial, of course, to rule out a real organic basis for complaints that border on the plausible.

4. Depersonalization, derealization: the former may range from a mild, dizzy, "floaty" feeling to the sense that "I am no longer me" or may include out-of-the-body experiences. The latter involves the feeling that objects and persons around one are not real or have somehow changed. Mild episodes of either may occur in the normal or hysteric individual, while more severe and extended occurrences are characteristic of schizophrenia. Both depersonalization and derealization are defenses against strong affects (especially anger) or conflict-laden perceptions from external reality.

5. Delusions: as with hallucinations, the presence of these usually becomes apparent in the course of the patient's conversation; if not and you suspect their presence, then question, again in a matter-of-fact way: "Have you ever felt that you possessed very unusual and special powers?" "Do you have cause to mistrust or feel persecuted by anyone in your life?" "Do you ever walk down the street and feel that strangers are talking about, or laughing at, you or that people are giving you special signals?"

a. Delusions of grandeur and special powers (including mind-reading).

    b. Delusions of persecution: often accompany delusions of grandeur and special powers.

    c. Delusions of alien control: the idea that persons or objects (e.g., "influencing machines") are controlling one's thoughts or behavior or reading one's mind.

    d. Ideas of reference: the delusion that others are closely and critically examining one's moves and perhaps sending one veiled signals, e.g., the conviction that the traffic cop, by pushing his cap back on his head while the patient drove by, is warning him to stop masturbating, or the intense feeling that one's fellow employees are continually talking and laughing about intimate details of one's private life (often involves picking up on certain key words and phrases actually uttered by one's fellows—words and phrases that touch upon one's conscious and unconscious preoccupations—and then taking them out of context and blowing them out of proportion).

6. Impairment in the ability to distinguish between fantasy and reality: the common denominator of hallucinations and delusions in general since both are in response to unconscious fears and fantasies. Nevertheless, I am referring to particular instances such as becoming "lost" in one's daydreams or reveries such that one loses the ability to distinguish where fantasy ends and actual reality begins, or being unable to distinguish when a night dream ends and waking reality begins. (Psychoses are compared to dreams from which the dreamer cannot awaken; sometimes a schizophrenic process makes its first appearance in a dream.) The patient should be questioned in a general way when circumstances warrant it.

**V. General intellectual functioning.** Like most aspects of the mental status, this is generally apparent from the patient's level of participation in the history-gathering process. Direct questions and tests designed to apprehend impaired cognitive and mnemonic functioning should be used *only if* the patient's history or behavior leads you to suspect organic mental impairment. The write-up should always include comments on the patient's cognitive functioning. In this area of testing, educational level and cultural background must of course be taken into account (e.g., a person with a second-grade education who cannot multiply or spell "world" is not necessarily organically impaired, nor is a recent immigrant who cannot give you the name of the state's governor or interpret an American proverb).

    A. *General cognitive functioning.*

        1. Alertness: general ability to *attend* to your questions and *concentrate* upon your questions and his answers. Disturbances in this area may reflect depression, mania, or schizophrenia as much as organic disturbance.

        2. Orientation to person, place, and time: impairment in the first is more ominous than in the second, and in the second more than in the third. Disturbances in orientation are usually a function of organic dysfunction, although they can be present in severe functional psychosis as well.

3. Ability to abstract: elicited by proverb interpretation (e.g., "People in glass houses shouldn't throw stones," "The watched pot never boils") and similarities (e.g., "How are a fly and tree alike?" "A lion and dog?"). When you suspect senile or presenile dementia, you can ask the patient to name objects to which you point or to point to objects that you name. Abstraction may be disturbed in schizophrenia as much as in organic mental disease.

4. Calculating ability: simple questions about addition and subtraction (e.g., "If you gave a storekeeper 50 cents for a 35-cent item, how much change would you receive?"), serial sevens, or serial threes (subtracting 7 from 100, 7 from that answer, and so on until reaching zero). This can be impaired in depression, schizophrenia, or any disorder that causes disturbances in concentration. Impaired serial subtractions can reflect deficits in recent memory as well.

5. General information: the past five presidents, the capital of France, the distance from New York to Los Angeles, and the like.

6. Reasoning and judgment (can be impaired secondary to psychopathology or "organicity"): the ability to think logically, to size up a situation, and to plan appropriate action. This is usually determined, again, from the patient's general level of participation in the interview and the history of his adaptation to the world. In problematic cases, it can be elicited by questions like: "What would you do with ten thousand dollars?" "If you were in a theater and smelled smoke what would you do?" "What would you do if you found a stamped, addressed envelope on the sidewalk?" (Such questions can also elicit psychopathy!) Where you suspect dementia, you can ask the patient to follow instructions that require him to perform several actions in sequence (a test that cuts across attention and concentration, recent memory, and general reasoning ability). For example, "When I finish speaking clap your hands, raise them to your forehead, pick up the piece of chalk, and write 'hand' backward on the blackboard."

7. Insight: basically the ability to recognize and acknowledge the presence and extent of one's psychological dysfunction; the degree to which one can offer a coherent and reasonable explanation of one's predicament and how one might extricate oneself from it. Insight can be impaired by psychopathology or organic dysfunction.

   a. Psychological mindedness: a subspecies of insight, to some extent independent of intelligence, and related to personality style and rigidity of defenses; one of the primary criteria for whether a person is a candidate for a more insight-oriented, as opposed to supportive, psychotherapeutic approach. It refers to the ability to recognize and express one's affective state and connect this to one's preoccupations and to the current environment, the ability to make connections—or respond to those made by the interviewer—between past, present, and transference, and the ability to examine one's behavior as meaningful, purposeful, and motivated.

   b. Memory: impairment can reflect organic mental disturbance or the unconsciously intentional forgetting of conflict-laden material. In "organicity" recent memory is impaired before, and more severely than, remote memory, while in hysteria or malingering it is often the reverse. The recent memory impairment secondary to conflict and repression is consistently linked to certain themes and circumstances, while that in organicity is more general and enduring. In

severe, motorically retarded depressions one may have a "pseudo-dementia" in which recent memory, among other functions, can appear grossly impaired.
1. Recent: digit span (ability to repeat forward up to 6 numbers, to reverse at least 4). Give the patient three unrelated objects to remember (e.g., cat, airplane, 43 Broadway), ask him to repeat them immediately after you (to make sure he does not have an attention deficit and is able to fix the objects in mind), and then inform him you will ask him to rename the objects in 5 or 10 minutes. Ask him whether he can tell you what he ate for breakfast. More intermediate degrees of memory are tested by his ability to recall recent current events or to give a coherent account of his present problem.
2. Remote: largely tested by his ability to give a coherent and meaningful past history and date of birth, and to recall other important instances, dates, anniversaries, and so forth.

**VI. Suicidal and Homicidal Tendencies.** When relevant, their assessment is the most difficult part of the mental status examination.

A. *Suicide:* any depressed or severely disturbed patient should *always* be questioned about this in a matter-of-fact way and without hesitation. For example, "Have things seemed so bad that you've wished you would die or thought about ending your life?" There is, in certain circles, an irrational fear that by questioning somebody about suicide you can put the idea into his head. You can assume that any depressed person has at least thought about it at one time or another. If you are in serious doubt about whether a patient is safe outside the hospital, it is better to err on the side of overcaution. If, after a thorough evaluation, you decide to let the patient remain outside, you must be decisive and unambivalent about it, communicating with your manner that it is a foregone conclusion that he will return for his next scheduled appointment and phone you in the meantime if any problems arise. Although you cannot put the idea of suicide into somebody's head, you can weaken a patient's abilities to restrain his suicidal impulses if you tell him you feel he can manage outside the hospital and *then* convey to him hesitancy, vacillation, and second thoughts about this decision as he is going out the door. This reduces his confidence in both you and his capacity for self-control. The two other ways a therapist can actively contribute to a patient's suicidal tendencies are to withdraw from him or to ignore his suicidal messages and "gestures." The former is tantamount to rejecting him (and rejection is the most common precipitant of suicide) and the latter invites him to escalate the seriousness of his attempts to get your attention, to see if you care enough to do something about them.
1. The current picture: to be evaluated first.
   a. Nature of the suicidal tendency (where it is on the continuum between fantasy and action): merely fleeting fantasies or prolonged and intense ideations? Is it merely a passive wish to die, "to go to sleep and not wake up" or "to get cancer and die," or is it an active desire to take one's life? Have the fantasies progressed to the point of planning how to do it or procuring the weapon? Are they *consciously* intended to punish people or to attract their attention rather

than to end one's life? Is the self-destructiveness not so much life-threatening or escalating as it is self-punitive or masochistic (e.g., occasionally banging one's head against the wall or scarring one's arms with superficial lacerations)? Does it have a bizarre quality such as a schizophrenic cutting himself to see if he is alive and will bleed, or suicidal tendencies in response to command hallucinations (this latter being among the most lethal sorts)? Finally, one crucial point to remember is that the patient's presence in your office or phone call to you means that he still has some will to live, that he is *ambivalent* about suicide, and hence that he can still be worked with, inside or outside a hospital.

    b. Affective accompaniments and reactions to his suicidal ideations: is the patient frightened by his suicidal ideations? Does he abhor them and wish he could stop? Does he view them as ego dystonic? If he is religious, does he view suicide as a damnable sin which he therefore would not commit? If the answer to these four questions is "yes," he is generally safer than if he appears quite comfortable with, or resigned to, the idea or shows no affect at all. You can often strengthen the ego of the frightened patient by openly exploring the nature of his ideations, pointing out to him that most depressed people have entertained the idea at one time or another and that it is not a catastrophic sign that he occasionally does too; that there is a marked difference between fantasy and action; that these thoughts do not come "out of the blue" and overtake him, but that *he* thinks them and hence has control over them; and that you are willing to work with him in controlling his behavior (e.g., by your availability by phone). With that large group of patients in the gray zone between fleeting fantasies and active planning, such a response often defuses their suicidal tendencies.

    c. Social situation: whether he lives with supportive others and maintains at least some relationships or whether he is alone or with cold, unsupportive, or actively malignant persons (individuals who may be giving him the message that they want him dead); whether he can form a relationship with the therapist, or whether he *withdraws* from him, the latter being an ominous sign.

    d. Viewpoint of his current predicament: does he still think about the future and maintain at least some hope and optimism? Does he still acknowledge his responsibilities to the living or does he feel hopeless and no longer think about the future? The latter is a worrisome sign. The preservation of a sense of humor, even gallows humor, is nearly always a positive prognostic sign. This ability is defined by Harry Stack Sullivan (1954, p. 182) as "the capacity for maintaining a sense of proportion as to [one's] place in the tapestry of life."

2. History of previous ideations and attempts: positive past history of course gives more cause for concern about subsequent attempts. (Once he has tried it, it is easier to consider suicide as an alternative "solution" and "up the ante.")

    a. Evaluate the seriousness of these attempts: e.g., potentially lethal overdose or serious injury with knife or gun.

    b. Circumstances of the attempt: alone, help at hand, or help expected to arrive upon the scene.

    c. Precipitants of the attempts: in order to determine whether the current context is similar to those in the past.

    d. How the patient feels *now* about these attempts: embarrassed and regretful; guilty; nonchalant and unconcerned, minimizing their significance and magnitude; or sorry they did not "succeed."

    e. Emotional expression: *any* expression of affect is better than none at all. Active sobbing is a preferable sign to mute and despairing withdrawal. Since suicide is largely a turning against the self, an attempt to strike out at others by smiting oneself, any direct expression of anger is welcome.

    f. Epidemiology (helpful, although you should remember that it is *individuals* suiciding who make up these statistics): the majority of completed suicides have been performed by those who have either attempted it before or at least threatened it. Often the person contemplating suicide tests his friends, family, and physicians with subtle or not-so-subtle messages—selling or giving away prized possessions, withdrawing, escalating numbers of accidents, putting one's affairs in order—to see if they care sufficiently to recognize these signs and intervene. Suicides, especially in males, increase with age. The elderly male, complaining of a variety of diffuse somatic complaints, experiencing the vegetative signs of depression without its conscious affective accompaniments, and consistently denying the existence of psychological or interpersonal problems, can surprise you by precipitously taking his life. The incidence of teenage suicides seems to be increasing; more women attempt suicide, but more men complete the attempt; divorced or single people are more at risk than married (with the elderly widower being at particularly great risk); those who have a history of important early losses overlaid by recent ones are more at risk; those with a family history of suicide (particularly that of a parent or sibling) are at greater risk; and the patient with severe and chronic medical illness is more at risk.

    g. The special case of unconscious self-destructiveness: look for a history of repeated involvement in accidents on the road, on the job, and at home. This may manifest itself in thrill-seeking, fate-tempting behaviors. Many chronic alcoholics and substance abusers engage in this. Persons with diabetes, cardiac disease, and other chronic conditions who do not comply with their treatment regimens are often unconsciously killing themselves. The first task is to get the patient to acknowledge the significance and meaning of this behavior, to talk about the feelings beneath it, and to look at the contexts in which it occurs.

    B. *Homicide:* many of the same issues are pertinent here as in suicide since each can be the reverse side of the other (suicidal and homicidal ideations occasionally alternate in the same individual). As with suicide, it is crucial to locate the patient's deliberations on the continuum from fantasy to action. Also, as with suicide, your behavior can strengthen or weaken his ego functions (his self-restraint). You can provoke him by being belligerent, moving too close physically, or manifesting excessive fearfulness. You should not try to be a hero with the patient who appears within an inch of violence and you should not sequester yourself in an office with him. His ego is strengthened by his knowing that you are in control of the situation. (See such a person in the corner of the lobby or waiting area with adequate assistance from an unobtrusive yet obviously present stand-by.) With that majority of patients whose homicidal tendencies are in the gray zone between fantasy and action and who are uncomfortable with the idea, you actually strengthen their egos by encouraging them to ventilate their fears and feelings about it, thereby indicating to them that you feel they possess enough self-control to *talk about them* without thereby *acting upon them*. As with potential suicides, when you decide to let them walk out of your office, be firm and unambivalent about it, conveying the full expectation that they will be capable of self-restraint until the next session.

1. Current picture.
   a. Where are his homicidal tendencies on the continuum from fleeting fantasy to planning to preparedness for action?
   b. Are the patient's fantasies ego syntonic and comfortable to him or is he distressed and bothered by them? Does he *want* to restrain himself? Neurotics often have such fantasies, which bother them immensely and seem quite ego alien, while virtually never acting on them.
   c. Know as much as you can about the potential victim, his current and past relationship with your patient, whom he represents unconsciously, his physical proximity to the patient, and whether he is expert at provoking the patient's violence (often a potential suicide and homicide collaborate with one another to produce a death).
   d. Does he see harming or killing a particular person as the solution to all his problems?
   e. Is the current situation similar to past ones in which the patient engaged in violence?
   f. Is he in a milieu which places no premium on the control of violence?
   g. If drugs or alcohol lower his threshold for violence, does he continue to use them?
   h. Does he control his anger in the evaluation with great difficulty and does the evaluator feel endangered?
      1. Is his homicidal tendency based on the delusion that he will be doing away with a persecutor or that he is performing the will of God (particularly ominous signs)?
      2. Can he respond to your limit-setting on the matter?
2. History: previous assault, rape, frequent brawls, and other acts of violence make it more likely that the patient will resort to them again.
   a. Seriousness of these attempts.
   b. Circumstances of these attempts: determine how actively the patient worked to "set them up" and what sorts of things "set him off."
   c. How the patient now feels about past episodes of violence: remorseful, complacent, proud, and so forth.
   d. Is the history of violence limited to physical objects or does it include persons? (Some people consistently show only the former.)
   e. A history of having been abused himself makes it more likely he will abuse others; a history of having witnessed violence between other family members makes it more likely he will resort to violence himself.
   f. Childhood history of enuresis, firesetting, and cruelty to animals is sometimes associated with adult homicidal tendencies.
3. The special case of unconscious destructiveness: as with self-destructiveness, one can be chronically and unconsciously destructive toward particular others. This can range from minor emotional abuse or neglect to life-threatening behaviors or omissions such as allowing children to

play unattended in potentially hazardous situations, continually ignoring signs of serious physical illness in a child, driving carelessly when accompanied by particular individuals, or continually making mistakes in caring for an ill and bedridden family member in the home. As with unconscious self-destructiveness, the first task is to draw the patient's attention, in a neutral and nonjudgmental way, to the pattern in his behaviors and their impact on the particular individuals involved. Your aim is to have him understand the significance and meaning of his behavior rather than to induce guilt or to mete out punishment.

The following is a sample mental status examination:

Ms. U. was a 33-year-old tall, angular brunette who appeared her stated age. She was casually dressed in green plaid pants that clashed markedly with an orange and white striped top. Her hair was a bit disheveled, her makeup askew, and she came in the office waving her arms and gesticulating wildly. "My neighbors are injecting semen into my veins while I sleep and putting it into my food while I am away. Even my parents are getting into the act now." "I don't even know if I can trust you," she said, as she arose from her chair, wide-eyed, and retreated to the door. She was frightened, angrily pounded the chair arm, and shouted loudly as she told me this story. Once or twice when she slowed down she appeared close to tears. Periodically she looked around as if fearing an assault and once or twice returned to the door and placed her ear to it as if she had heard something (although she emphatically denied, when questioned, that she heard "voices"). She was hypervigilant and watched my every move. At times she focused on the movements of my hands rather than my speech, and she was continually asking, "What do you mean?" in reference to the former. She made it plain that she felt I was hiding my true intentions and that I was giving her "double messages." She expressed the fear that I might somehow make her *want* to receive semen injections. Her associations were reasonably linear and her thought processes relatively logical whenever I could steer her away from her preoccupations with semen. Her memory was not impaired though her ability to concentrate upon my questions was disturbed. Despite a college education she interpreted proverbs concretely and self-referentially. For example, in response to "People in glass houses shouldn't throw stones" she said, "If you look at your own house you won't shatter mine. What do you think I've got in my apartment anyway?" She was oriented to person, place, and time and her fund of general information was reasonable for a college graduate. She denied homicidal preoccupations although she said, "If they do not stop this I will have to jump out of my window to end it all. I've thought about that." Her insight and judgment were psychotically impaired in that she had no awareness that she was ill. She came to the mental health center only because she could not get the police and lawyers to take her seriously. Her sole aim was to make us tell *them* to stop.

## THE PHYSICAL AND NEUROLOGICAL EXAMINATION

Because many physical illnesses can manifest themselves in disordered behavior (e.g., hypo- or hyper-thyroidism; adrenal and other endocrine problems; visceral cancers; cardiovascular, pulmonary, and renal disease; and neurological lesions), a physical examination should be an integral part of *every* psychiatric evaluation. Nevertheless, it should be performed by the attending psychiatrist only if he is *not* also the primary therapist or if his psychotherapeutic interventions are limited to brief, supportive contacts with an inpatient whom he will not follow after discharge. When the attending psychiatrist does a physical examination he should, of course, always be accompanied by an attendant, whether or not the patient is of the opposite sex. If possible, a female psychiatrist should perform the physical examination on a male paranoid since homosexual conflicts are probable in such patients. Rectal examinations on male paranoids by male physicians have precipitated homosexual panics and resulting violence. Similarly, a female physician might be indicated for hysterical women or female schizophrenics with certain sexual delusions.

The psychoanalytically informed interdict against physical examinations on one's own therapy patients has been termed anything from "theoretical hogwash" to a "violation of medical common sense." On the contrary, common sense supports the idea that one person running his eyes and hands over another's naked body will mean, consciously and unconsciously, a good deal. It might be viewed as intrusive, authoritarian, seductive, or oedipally incestuous. Of course, with the relatively unpsychologically minded candidate of a supportive and predominantly medicative approach, it might be perceived as benign and "physicianly." What is important is that one neither *knows* nor *controls* what it will mean to the patient. When you have so little control in that important a matter, it is best to avoid it altogether and ask your therapy patients to furnish you with the record of a recent physical examination or to have one performed by an internist and forwarded to you.

I performed physical examinations on two female patients when I was their inpatient psychiatric resident. Later I saw both these individuals in long-term insight-oriented psychotherapy and it became apparent from dreams, fantasies, and direct statements that the physical examination had been charged with meaning. A male colleague precipitated a transient psychotic regression in an hysterical woman with vague abdominal complaints by performing a physical examination on her.[2]

## COURSE OF EVALUATION

You should always include a few statements about the patient's manner of participation in the evaluation process. Information such as whether he attended every session, was punctual or tardy, cooperative

---

[2] The use of hypnosis, particularly by a male clinician on a female patient, can have the same effect, symbolically representing an incestuous rape.

or negativistic should be included. Tardiness and missed sessions usually reflect conscious or unconscious ambivalence about treatment and, if you suspect this, you should raise it with the patient before making any treatment recommendations. In addition to motivation, you should speak to his curiosity about himself and his "psychological mindedness." Some clinicians test these by making a tentative connection or two in the evaluation session and observing the patient's response to it. In this section, as in the mental status examination, you should include your feeling response to the patient, such as "He seemed to speak freely, but each time I felt as if he were holding me at arm's length," "I found him warm and engaging," or "After each session I felt puzzled and a little worried."

## FORMULATION

The formulation, and treatment plan that follows from it, is the capstone of your evaluation. It is your theory of how the patient has become the person he is today. Your goal is to explain, not isolated behaviors, but the patient's personality *as a whole.* Any given behavior takes on its full meaning only when placed against the backdrop of the total human being.

Whereas the previous part of your write-up functions as the data base and should be relatively free from inference and theorizing, in the formulation you can speculate and hypothesize in a controlled and sober way within the boundaries of your information. Your formulation should not be a simple restatement of the history; it should contain no more data than necessary to document and exemplify your clinical hypothesis.

The single most important activity in arriving at a formulation, in thinking dynamically, is spotting, or rather allowing yourself to be *struck* by, *parallels* throughout the patient's life course. Parallels go together to make up themes, and themes converge and interweave to form the tapestry or pattern of an entire life. From these themes and the life pattern you draw your inferences about meaning and motivation. For example, spotting parallels and themes means allowing yourself to recognize the similarities between Mr. L.'s current preoccupations with sexual *impotence,* job *performance,* and *"running out* of things to say in social situations," and the similarities between these and his childhood sense of *powerlessness* before an eminently successful father who psychologically battered him down—a father whom he was *powerless* to resuscitate following his heart attack in the family dining room when the patient was 16.

Almost as important as spotting parallels is empathically placing yourself in the patient's shoes. Using Sullivan's "one genus hypothesis" ("We are all much more simply human than otherwise"), ask yourself how you would feel, as a small child, growing up in his particular environment and how, as an adult with that history behind you, you would experience the world.

The formulation should speak to the *origins* and *purposes* of the patient's psychopathological behaviors. What function does his depression, conversion reaction, or psychosis play within the context of his historically determined view of self and world, and within the context of his current interpersonal environment? It keeps the concepts of atavism and adaptation in mind.

Since the formulation takes both historical and current factors into account in explaining any life or set of behaviors, there is no contradiction between family systems theory and psychodynamic theory. The former is concerned with the meaning and purpose of the patient's psychopathology within the context of the family and current social nexus (e.g., the role of Mr. T.'s hysterical paraplegia vis-à-vis his wife and employer) and the latter with its function within the context of the patient's history and internal world (e.g., its binding of Mr. T.'s anxiety secondary to intrapsychic conflicts with his father). There is of course no definite line between the internal interpersonal environment and the external one. The boundary between the two is fluid and we behave so as to minimize the dissonance between those two worlds and to maximize the resemblance between them. We all search out or conspire with our spouse, friends, and children to make a current outer world that corresponds to the one in which our personality developed. Our psychopathology and personality styles are then fueled from two directions, inner and outer, and by similar configurations.

Mr. Z., a 24-year-old depressed schizoid character, is a prime example of this:

His parents had lost most of their relatives during World War II. Predictably, they had intense unresolved issues around separation and loss. Because of these they were ambivalent about Mr. Z., their last child, becoming independent. Their conscious and verbal message to him was "Become a man, go off on your own, get a job, and do well in the world like your father." Their unconscious and behavioral one was "Let us do this for you because you are not capable of it; the world is a dangerous place and we must protect you from it; you can trust only us; if you form important relationships outside the family you are betraying us; if you leave us we will die." Over the years he had internalized both these messages. Each time he began to move toward independence (job, apartment, friendships) he inevitably began experiencing depressive and bizarre symptoms and sabotaged his efforts. Since he was still living with his parents, his psychopathology was as much a way of adapting to their ambivalence as it was a manifestation of his intrapsychic conflicts over independence and dependency. His psychopathology further served the purpose of 1) allowing the parents to avoid their own emotional problems and focus on his and 2) forming one of the few bridges between them.

Your formulation should enumerate the patient's repertoire of defensive maneuvers and should rank them on a scale from most to least adaptive. This is particularly helpful in those cases where you will be doing supportive psychotherapy, for you must continually decide which defenses to sap and which to shore up. You should always speak to the health-promoting forces or strengths in every patient's personality and environment and his highest level of previous functioning. (Perhaps the best prognostic indicator is the degree to which a person has been able to form and sustain relationships with others.) Your formulation should also explain any transferential reactions observed and should make some statement about transferential factors that are likely to emerge.

Although you should have a reasonably complete formulation by the end of three or four sessions, you will continue writing and rewriting the formulation until the end of treatment. It is nothing more nor less than a clinical *hypothesis*. It is not a law. Like most hypotheses, it is never totally correct or incorrect nor does it ever exhaustively explain the phenomena under consideration. You must treat your initial formulation with a curious mixture of tentativeness and conviction. Although it is not written in stone, you must be sufficiently committed to it to frame your treatment plan and early interventions in accordance with it.

You will find, from your subsequent therapeutic work with the patient, that some parts of your formulation were more "right" than others, that you initially missed some issues altogether and, especially, that you had some of the italics in the wrong places. Often you will discover that your initial formulation contained most of the building blocks of the final one, but that they were assembled incorrectly.

The final product should "feel right." It should be the most internally consistent and data-connected theory that you are able to devise, and it should have borne fruit in some degree of transformation in the patient. Finally, it should be written in clear English with a *minimum* of jargon. Too frequently students use jargon rather than spell out exactly how a patient went from point A to point E. They substitute the illusion of understanding for understanding itself. At the end of this chapter I shall include an example of the formulation process.

## DIAGNOSIS

Diagnosis will be fully discussed in the next chapter. Suffice it to say that your *formulation* of the patient's history and dynamics is the real diagnosis in dynamic psychiatry. It is from this, and not your descriptive diagnosis, that your treatment plan will follow. No two people with the same Diagnostic and Statistical Manual-III (DSM-III) label have exactly the same dynamics or hence require exactly the same approach. Your *descriptive*, as opposed to your *dynamic*, diagnosis should of course correspond to the DSM-III nomenclature and axes.

## THE TREATMENT PLAN

The treatment plan is based 1) on your formulation of the patient's account of his life and problems and speaks to the major dynamics in the patient's personality and 2) on what your patient *wants* and is *capable* of.

At the end of the evaluation you should set aside a few minutes to invite the patient to tell you how he understands his problems and what *he* wants out of treatment, how he expects to implement it, what he sees as his and your respective roles in the process, and how long he conceives it will take. This is extremely important since the patient's objectives and yours may be vastly different. Questionnaires indicate that a surprising *majority* of community mental health center patrons desire a short-term treatment with limited and specified goals. Others, on the contrary, may have unrealistically large expectations about what can be accomplished. If you have one idea about what can and should be accomplished, and your patient another, then the two of you will soon part ways in mutual dissatisfaction. It is better to help the patient to a limited success than to a monumental failure.

You *and* your patient should collaborate on the modality that seems best suited to *his* needs and capabilities: e.g., brief individual therapy, longer-term supportive or insight-oriented therapy, group therapy, family therapy, or adjunctive or primary pharmacotherapy. You must be careful not to view the mode of therapy at which you are most expert as the treatment of choice for every patient. This is particularly common for those who favor long-term insight psychotherapy. They tend to regard it as the "Cadillac" of all the therapies and feel guilty about offering a patient anything else, even though he may profit as much, or more, from another modality. It is always best, if at all possible, that the evaluating clinician also be the treating one, especially since the constellation "deprivation-rejection-loss" is one of the most common issues in the psychiatric population in general and the community mental health center in particular. Unfortunately, this is often not the case, even in some of our better outpatient treatment facilities, and it no doubt accounts for a large part of the considerable percentage who drop out between completion of the evaluation and referral to treatment.

Something may even be said for avoiding the "mental set" that everyone who comes for an evaluation needs, wants, or can profit from treatment. A patient may need treatment but not be motivated *at this time*. Such a person may be in your office primarily to please a family member or the courts or to convince you to give him a clean bill of health. In general, it is impossible to treat someone who is not in some degree of overt discomfort. There is also the occasional patient who, as a result of the catharsis and life review of the evaluation process and of what is known as the transference cure, does not feel the need for further treatment. This last factor refers to his basking in the warm glow of the positive transference to a therapist who unconsciously represents an omnipotent parent, to feeling acknowledged and accepted by such a magical figure. Merely reassuring patients that their agitation or mild depression does not mean they are going crazy and that, under similar circumstances, most people would feel a similar distress is helpful for many. (Minimizing a patient's "psychopathologizing" of his emotions is often helpful in psychotherapy. I often phrase it in terms of his "entitlement" to certain feelings given the circumstances.) I "cured" one woman after two evaluation interviews merely by letting her ventilate about her husband's recent traumatic death and by informing her that her post-traumatic dreams were not a sign of insanity but rather of the mind's attempt to work through this loss. At times patients could profit from, or will need, treatment but will not want it because of overwhelming resistance to dealing with emotionally charged issues or because admitting they need help would be too damaging to an already compromised self-esteem. Where one does not feel that somebody's life or sanity is in the balance, it is wise to respect his wishes and resistances. (Unless he is acutely suicidal or homicidal you can do nothing about it anyway.) When the patient is evenly divided on the matter and wants your opinion, you can couch it in terms of whether you think he can "*profit*" from treatment (rather than in terms of "need").

In that majority of cases in which your patient enters treatment (for our purposes, individual psychotherapy), he deserves a brief, nonintellectualized explanation of what the two of you are embarking on and, if he requests it, a "ball-park" estimate of how long the therapy will take. In any explanation the emphasis should be on the *patient's* role in the treatment, i.e., on how you will function largely as a facilitator in a process that he controls. He should know that his task is to talk about whatever is on his mind or seems significant at the time. He should also know that there will be times when, for reasons of fear and embarrassment, he will *not* want to talk about certain subjects and that it is just as important to know his motives for withholding as it is to know what he is withholding. Finally, you can tell him that the two of you are attempting to get to know his feelings and preoccupations and to identify patterns in his life—patterns of which he is not always aware and which lead to the predicaments and distress in which he so often finds himself.[3]

---

[3] In our legalistically minded age it is wise not to record anything in the patient's official chart that you would not want the patient to read (and he is legally entitled to see his record) or that you would not want read back to you in a courtroom. By the end of the treatment you should have made the average insight-oriented patient aware of your thinking about him anyway.

## THE SPECIAL CASE OF THE SUBSTANCE-ABUSING PATIENT

Patients chronically dependent on drugs or alcohol pose a different problem to the evaluator. First of all, their toxic overlay makes it difficult to know the personality characteristics and affects that lie beneath—what they are "really like" in other words. Second, since some degree of *pain*, overt emotional discomfort, is essential to successful participation in psychotherapy, their ready access to instant painkillers is a formidable foe of the therapeutic process. No therapist can compete with the immediate gratification of the pill or bottle.

Consequently, it is important to thoroughly evaluate the extent of usage. If it is relatively episodic and clearly situation-related, and the patient is able to tolerate some emotional distress, then often he can be treated psychotherapeutically just like any other patient, with fluctuations in substance abuse being dealt with like any other symptom and understood with reference to the context in which they occur and the patient's history. On the other hand, a steady, daily reliance on drugs and alcohol requires a different approach. Then it is necessary to explain to the patient that, although substance addiction is a symptom of still other problems, it becomes itself a larger problem than those which it is designed to avoid. He should be informed of the obstacles it poses to any successful psychotherapy and referred to a drug and alcohol program for evaluation and detoxification. When he has successfully completed that regimen and joined Alcoholics Anonymous or a like organization, he can return to you for psychotherapy.

The patient dependent on prescription drugs confronts you with a slightly different problem. Since his medication must be prescribed by a doctor (although he can of course buy it on the street), then you potentially have more control over it than over alcohol and "street drugs." This patient walks in and, almost before he has said "hello," asks (tells) you, "You are going to continue the Valium I've been getting from Dr. S., aren't you?" I have frequently seen residents fall into the trap of battling with the patient. For instance, one resident began to write out the prescription, then caught himself, feeling manipulated and controlled, and then changed his mind! Do not get into control battles with these patients. Remember that it takes two to engage in such battles; if you do not enter the ring with the patient, there will be no fight. You must understand that you cannot ask a highly insecure and vulnerable individual to abruptly give up something on which he has been dependent for (often) years, before he feels that you have given him something with which to replace it. The "something" to which I am referring is a relationship. You should agree to continue the patient on a safe and reasonable dosage of the medication, but apprise him that you will meanwhile be evaluating whether medication seems indicated at all and, if so, whether his is the correct one and at the right dosage. You should apprise him that you may be asking him to *collaborate* (to avoid, here again, battles over control) with you in a gradual reduction in, or discontinuance of, his medication. *After* you have established some rapport and he begins to feel he has something in the relationship, then you can begin to wean him off the medication or place him on a less addictive one and then withdraw him from that.

## THE LIFE CHART AND A SAMPLE FORMULATION

The actual composition of the psychiatric evaluation is learned only through supervised practice and cannot be conveyed through any textbook. Organizing and presenting one's findings is a painful trial-and-error process in which one learns by making mistakes and being criticized for them. Although I cannot presume to teach it in this volume, I shall present a sample organization and formulation of clinical material. My aim is to give the student some appreciation of what it is to think dynamically.

To acquaint you with an invaluable concise device for organizing history, I shall present the data in the form of a Meyerian "life chart," rather than as a narrative. The chart of necessity omits many details that would appear in the narrative. I require my students to do both the narrative and the life chart. When I feel that they have mastered the principles of organization, I then allow them to present only the narrative, though still encouraging them to construct life charts for their own use.

The life chart was invented by Adolf Meyer, the father of modern American psychiatry, who flourished from the last decade of the nineteenth century to the middle of the twentieth. More than any other man except Freud, Meyer, never himself a psychoanalyst, is responsible for the fact that every good psychiatrist takes a thorough history. The life chart correlates "age" with "event" with "reaction." "Event" corresponds to what I have referred to as the "external datum" and "reaction" to what I have called the "internal." The data for this chart are drawn from the "present problem," "past personal history," "medical history," and "family history" sections. For example, the family's moves, his parents' marital problems, his bout with rheumatic fever in childhood, and his mother's hospitalization for depression would all figure as significant events. The schematization of the life chart often makes you aware of connections between events and reactions that you might otherwise miss and alerts you to especially pivotal years.

There is only one caveat in regard to the use of this chart. To wit, the human being is not a machine which blindly and mechanically reacts to stimuli impinging upon it from the outside world. He plays an active role in the creation of that world. As often as not he helps set up the events to which he is reacting. For example, Mrs. H. in Chapter 1 dealt with her fears of rejection in a way that elicited the rebuffs that then functioned as the precipitants for her depressive reactions. Where he does not actually *arrange* the events, the problem is often his historically based neurotic *misapprehension* of them. Recall the man from Chapter 1 who unconsciously misinterpreted his father's death as a homicide and himself as the murderer. His suicide attempt was then an act of self-punishment in perfect accord with his definition of the situation. Patients continually reach out and grasp their "precipitants" in such a way that they themselves are the cause of their distress.

Table 5-1 is an example of a life chart which I shall use as the data base for a formulation.

### TABLE 5-1. Life Chart for Ms. L.

| Year | Age | Event | Reaction |
|------|-----|-------|----------|
| 1950 | 0 | Birth six weeks premature. Difficult delivery. | Brief anoxia, severe jaundice, in the hospital nursery for one month. |
| | 0-6 mo. | Lactose intolerance. | Feeding difficulties, constant crying, diarrhea and vomiting. |
| | 0-12 mo. | Has heard that mother was depressed for much of this year. | |
| 1952 | 2 yrs. | First memory: being left by her parents with a baby-sitter. | Frightened, crying, enraged. |
| 1953 | 3 yrs. | Father drafted to Korea. | Doesn't remember reaction. |
| | 3 yrs., 2 mos. | Tommy, her little brother, born. | "Mommy, throw him in the garbage can." Vomiting and diarrhea (absent since infancy) return for several weeks. |
| | 3 yrs., 6 mos. | Maternal grandfather dies. Mother goes into difficult mourning; maternal grandmother moves in. | Had seen him only a few times; "no reaction." Puzzled by mother's crying and withdrawal, patient tends to play and sit off by herself; fights with grandmother who "favored my little brother and was always trying to protect him from me." |

## TABLE 5-1. Life Chart for Ms. L., continued

| 1954 | 4 | Father returns. | "He brought me a doll and candy. I was happy." |
| | 4½ | Father joins large industrial corporation and family moves across country. | "It was hard to leave my friends but I was excited"; vomiting and diarrhea return temporarily; recalls some "shyness" and difficulty making new friends. |
| 1956 | 6 | Begins school. | "Very hard for me. My mother had to take me the whole first year. I was very shy." Many missed days in grammar school because of gastrointestinal symptoms. |
| 1956-1958 | 6-8 | Making new friends, doing well academically. | "I was coming out. Daddy was beginning to pay attention to me for my grades. Mother still spent a lot of time to herself and 'Grams' took care of little brother." |
| 1958 | 8 | Mother's first hospitalization for depression: 2 months. Father's heavy drinking begins about this time. | "We had never been that close but it was still good just knowing she was at home. It was very hard with her away. My grandmother and I fought all the time. Daddy was staying away more at nights." |
| 1959 | 9 | Family is transferred to a plant 500 miles away (in the Northwest.) | "The hardest move I ever made. Just as I was feeling part of things at school and in my neighborhood, we pick up and leave. I cried for several days and those damn stomach problems came back." |

## TABLE 5-1. Life Chart for Ms. L., continued

| | | | |
|---|---|---|---|
| 1959-1962 | 9-12 | Father's drinking increases; mother experiences two more hospitalizations for depression; fights with grandmother continue. | Difficulties making new friends, feels like an "outcast," ridiculed for her accent; grades fall at first "but then I resolved to excel at least in that and to get lost in books." |
| 1962 | 12 | Grandmother dies and mother reacts with severe depression. | "I felt like I should cry but I couldn't. Mother withdrew to her room again. I got deeper into my books." |
| 1963 | 13 | Puberty. | "Absolutely no preparation for it other than hearing my mother curse the day her periods began. I was frightened by my first flow but I kept it to myself. I felt embarrassed by my breasts. Sex was never talked about around my house and I don't think my parents had much of a relationship. I don't remember any sexual fantasies or masturbation." |
| | 13 | Another move. | "I was used to them by now. Not so hard since most of my investment was in academics anyway." |
| 1963-1968 | 13-18 | Excels in high school. Graduates as valedictorian. | "I was very proud of my performance and that was about the only attention I got from my father. Mother, as usual, was a block of wood (to everybody except my brother). Whenever I talked about what I wanted to do she made it plain I should be a housewife |

**TABLE 5-1. Life Chart for Ms. L., continued**

|  |  |  | and mother like her. I never could figure out why because *she* never seemed to enjoy *that* worth a damn." |
|---|---|---|---|
| 1968 | 18 | Begins college in the state capital, 150 miles from home. | "I had been looking forward to getting out of that cold household for years and away from my little brother, the king, but, strangely enough, I had a lot more trouble leaving than I expected. For the first time in my life I think I had some idea of what my mother had felt: down, no energy, no zest, no appetite, belly pains, and diarrhea. But I snapped out of it pretty quickly." |
|  | 18½ | The rest of the family is transferred to the Midwest. | "I elected to stay at State University although I almost packed up and went with them. I felt good about my decision." |
| 1969-1972 | 19-22 | Continues at university until graduation with an honors degree in mathematics (her father was an engineer). Other than friendship with a couple of girls, "loners like myself," her social life at college was very limited. | "It's hard to believe, but my first real depression was after graduating, after being up so high, and finding out about graduate school and all that. I moved back in with my parents for almost a year. Tommy [her brother] had just gone off to college." |
| 1973 | 23 | Begins graduate work in physics. Engages in her first dating behavior. | "I liked my work and met and dated a few boys, eggheads like myself." |
| 1975 | 25 | Meets John. | "He was totally unlike me. He was a businessman, 5 years |

## TABLE 5-1. Life Chart for Ms. L., continued

| | | | |
|---|---|---|---|
| | | | older, full of life and a party-goer. His only failing was that at times he would get a bit tipsy, but he was fun even then. He brought me out. I lost my virginity with him. I felt guilty as hell but I enjoyed it." |
| 1976 | 26½ | John leaves her and marries another woman. | "I was really depressed that summer. I moved back in with my parents and *tried* to study for my orals, but couldn't. It was the first time I sought psychiatric help and I felt terrible about it, like I was turning out just like *her* [mother]. I went home for a few weeks." |
| 1977 | 27 | She returns to graduate school, gets her orals postponed, takes and passes them at the end of the year. | "I had re-equilibrated; lost in the books again." |
| 1978 | 28 | Completes her dissertation; awarded the Ph.D. | "Felt on top of the world. *Both* my parents came to the awards this time. It was the first time I remember my mother saying anything nice to me. *Even* Tommy was there and looked proud. I moved back in with my parents until I could figure out what to do. Dated several guys. Nothing serious although a couple actually seemed interested in me!" |
| 1979 | 29 | Mother commits suicide. | "Like the bottom fell out. My father and I were out looking at apartments for me when it happened. She |

## TABLE 5-1. Life Chart for Ms. L., continued

|  |  |  | took a whole bottle of antidepressants. In a coma for a day and never came around. She fooled us. Things had looked better for some time. How could we have guessed?" It was back to the psychiatrist again for her. He gave her some Elavil and they talked 30 minutes a week for 6 months. |
| 1979-1980 | 29-30 | Takes a job with an industrial research firm in Ohio, about 200 miles from her father. | "It was a good job. I was glad to get it. But, you know, I turned down a teaching job in the same town Daddy lived in. *That* must mean something! Coming out of a depression and all, it seems I would have stayed, doesn't it? Also, since my mother's death Tommy and I have had more contact than in all the years before. It's really good. We've been able to open up to each other." |
| 1981 | 31½ | Second relationship with a man: Billy, a business executive, recently divorced, in his early forties. | "We had a good time. I sort of liked him. I don't know why but it didn't seem right any more. I just wanted to call the whole thing off. I did. Of course he was on the rebound anyway, so I don't think it was all that tough on him." |
|  | 31¾ | Promoted to a leadership position within a laboratory section which would necessitate her making | "I decide that this is it. I'm feeling down and I don't know why. I don't want to—the self-esteem thing and all—" |

## TABLE 5-1. Life Chart for Ms. L., continued

| | |
|---|---|
| a cross-country move. Visits her father a week after receiving her promotion. He is still preoccupied with her mother's death, drinking heavily, and does not seem enthusiastic about her promotion. | go back into treatment but I know I need to. So here I am." Her diarrhea returns. |

To begin with, as you skim over this life chart, you cannot fail to notice several themes, or red threads, which form the building blocks of your formulation. *Losses, moves, separations,* and *rejections* form the major one. Included in this is the patient's unsatisfactory relationship with a mother too preoccupied with her own emotional problems to give much to the patient. Issues of independence versus dependency and career success versus marriage and family are also present and intertwined with the central theme. Conflicts over sexual and emotional intimacy with men are apparent from her rejection by, and in turn rejection of, boyfriends who in some respects resemble her father (alcoholic and older). These, as well, intermingle with the theme of loss and rejection. Among other issues is competitiveness with her brother, "the king," who preempted what little attention the mother had to spare. Finally, since only two years have passed since the mother died, and since the patient's relationship with her was quite ambivalent, you can suspect there is considerable unresolved grief.

Having identified the major themes one must next assemble them into a coherent and readable construction:

The central constellation in Ms. L.'s life is that of separation, loss, and deprivation, the common denominator of which is rejection. Her first month of life was spent in the hospital nursery and one can speculate that this, along with the mother's difficult delivery, adversely affected the mother-child bonding. The mother's depression, apparently precipitated by the patient's birth, may reflect some deep-seated ambivalence on the mother's part toward her child. In any event, the depression interfered with the mother's ability to give to the patient.

Feeding difficulties secondary to a lactose intolerance further interfered with the patient's sense of being adequately filled or nurtured. Her irritability, vomiting, and diarrhea probably distanced the mother still further, and the more the latter withdrew the more the patient must have cried and somatized. A vicious circle was set in motion. Even after the discovery of the physiological basis for the gastrointestinal symptoms and the change in diet, their original association with maternal deprivation caused them to resurrect themselves at times in Ms. L.'s life when she was experiencing loss or rejection: brother's birth, beginning first grade, going off to college and, most recently, being ignored by her father.

Her first recollection, being left by her parents, is highly significant. Her life thereafter was a succession of rejections and losses, set against an ever-present backdrop of deprivation. She was exposed to three losses at age 3 (father drafted, losing what little attention she received from mother to baby brother, and grandfather's death); a move at 4½; great separation anxieties upon beginning school; mother's hospitalization at age 8; a difficult move at age 9 and the father's progressive withdrawal into alcoholism around the same time; the grandmother's death and mother's severe depression at age 12; another move at 13; leaving for college at 18, at which time she first became overtly depressed; another depression at 26½ following her rejection by John; and her mother's suicide at 29 and her own subsequent depression. Finally, her most recent episode occurred immediately after: an aborted relationship, her father's inattentiveness, and a job promotion that symbolized increasing adult independence and responsibility and that would necessitate moving a considerable distance from her father.

Markedly deficient mothering and only slightly better fathering, coupled with her mother's clear preference for her brother, left her with a diminished self-esteem. She tried to bolster this, to "overcompensate," as it were, with academic performance which got her much-needed attention from the father as well as a certain sense of triumph over the detested brother. Two coalitions resulted: a mother frustrated in her marriage joined with her son on one side and a father likewise dissatisfied joined with his daughter on the other. Her father's closeness to her, usually rather intellectualized and without much emotional demonstrativeness, was relatively short-lived, for he began drinking heavily again in just a few years.

The stimulation of Ms. L.'s oedipal fantasies by her "special" relationship with her father, and their frustration by his subsequent withdrawal, contributed to her conflicts over sexuality and to negative expectations of how men would react to her femininity. Her mother's disparaging remarks about menstruation and sexuality in general further exacerbated this, as did her parents' strict profession of fundamentalist Catholic beliefs. The strength of these conflicts is attested to by the fact that she remembers *no* adolescent sexual fantasies. She dealt with a sense of inadequacy as a woman and guilt over unconscious incestuous strivings by keeping her distance from men. She failed to work on the adolescent and early adult tasks of experimenting with intimacy with the opposite sex. Her first real dating behavior began very late—at 25—when most people have already experienced at least one relatively lasting experience with a member of the opposite sex and when many are making permanent commitments to marriage and family.

That both her significant adult relationships were with businessmen who were older and alcoholic reflects the incestuous nature of her object choices. She reacted to the first man's rejection of her by turning anger upon the self, her most frequently used maladaptive defense mechanism, with hurt and shattered self-esteem. Significantly, she ran home to her father right after this disappointment. A few years later she attempted to actively master this rejection, and pay back this man and her father, by forming a relationship with another man and then rejecting him as she had been rejected and (one presumes) *before* he could reject her. By so doing she was probably also avoiding the guilt that would be attendant upon an oedipal triumph (e.g., marrying a father imago). It may well have been guilt over the oedipal triumph represented by her mother's death that led her to turn down the previously desired teaching position at the university in her home town.

Ms. L.'s depression resulted from turning anger upon the self (or rather upon the internal representations of a number of frustrating objects), unconscious guilt over the anger, guilt over her incestuous strivings and oedipal victory over mother (who died and left her with father), and the pain of separation and rejection and the diminished self-esteem related thereto. There is a good deal of identification with the mother in her depressive symptomatology, particularly apparent in the depression which followed her mother's suicide, in which she considered taking her own life as well. She was, in other words, identifying with the lost, ambivalently loved object, rather than consciously dealing with her conflicting feelings about the loss. Her identification with father (intellectualizing and becoming a corporate scientist) was more adaptive. Even here, however, her intellectualization and academic preoccupations allowed her to avoid both her own feelings and interpersonal involvements where she might be hurt or develop conflict-laden sexual feelings. Her family history of depression and alcoholism (a maternal aunt and great aunt were also depressed and several of the father's male relatives were alcoholic or depressed) and her own vegetative signs and symptoms suggest there may be a biologically heritable component to her depression as well.

Because she was not adequately nurtured and esteemed by her parents and because her independence and sense of competence (other than academic ability) were not fostered and encouraged by them, she did not feel capable of becoming independent. This accounts for her oscillations back and forth between the university, her apartment, and the parental home and for her depressions following graduation from college and reception of a job promotion. She continued to harbor the deep-seated fantasy that she could return home, rewrite past history, and receive from her parents what she had missed out on the first time around.

She was also in the throes of the Age Thirty Transition, in which she had to reappraise an obviously deficient first adult life structure. She had failed as yet to emotionally emancipate herself from her parents and to establish her own social network on the outside. Career was about the only task on which she had worked, and even here she seemed to have "sold out" her lifelong dream of an academic career for a position in industry. Finally, she had to resolve intense conscious conflicts over career versus family, her father having given her one message (pro-career) and her mother having given her a mixed one ("be a housewife and mother but look how much I hate it").

Nevertheless, despite considerable psychopathology, the patient has coped after a fashion, has not damaged herself irreparably in any of her relationships, and has accomplished it all without becoming alcoholic like her father. There is every reason to expect that she can use her intellect adaptively (if she will allow herself to begin to know her feelings) to understand how she has arrived at this point and to make some changes in her life.

The treatment plan followed logically from this formulation and addressed the issues raised therein. Long-term insight-oriented therapy was prescribed and the possibility of instituting an antidepressant medication, if her symptoms did not improve in a reasonable length of time, was considered.

## NOTES ON SUPERVISION IN THE EVALUATION

Good supervision is crucial to the development of your evaluation interviewing skills. In order to maximize your accessibility to supervision, you must come to terms with your own self-esteem issues and castration anxiety. You must be receptive to criticism and not so concerned about pleasing the supervisor and appearing competent that you cannot be honest about your work. As a student you must also understand that no supervisor expects you to already be proficient at this work and that making mistakes is the only way you learn to be a clinician. Nevertheless, at best, you can expect to experience some anxiety in the process. Indeed, in many ways your concerns about being accepted by your supervisor will parellel your patients' concerns about being accepted by you.

Adequate supervision of the evaluation entails three processes: short-form presentation off the top of one's head, the criticism of the written report, and the observation of actual interviews. It is helpful when one's fellow trainees participate in this process since it desensitizes them to their anxieties about evaluating each other's work and being evaluated themselves and helps them to actively master, to take ownership of, the principles the supervisor is trying to teach.

The presentation "off the top of your head" forces you to spontaneously organize the material and to see the forest as well as the trees. It forces you to present your own feeling-toned reaction to the patient and to make him come alive in a few graphic sentences for the supervisor and your colleagues. Many times you will become aware of aspects about the patient which you did not realize you knew or you will get a better sense of where the italics lie and of his character style.

The written presentation is, of course, the bread and butter of evaluation supervision. It is helpful, again, if some of this supervision can occur in a case conference format, where one's fellow trainees have read the protocol and can join in the supervision process. It takes many months to learn to do an adequate evaluation write-up and formulation.

Slips or parapraxes that occur in your verbal or written presentation often tell you as much about the patient as about you, though you must have a thorough knowledge of yourself to know when a slip results more from your own psychopathology or character style than in response to the patient's. For example, in one evaluation summary the resident wrote, "Mrs. B. said 'If my husband were transferred to New York I would *not* quit my job and go with him.' " She actually said, "I *would* quit my job and go with him." However, from the context of the rest of her history and personal presentation it was clear that she was considerably more committed to her business career than to her marriage and family. The resident's "slip" therefore told us something about the patient rather than about him. This is only one example of the general rule that the resident "knows" more about his patient than he thinks he does. Often he dismisses his slips, hunches, and vague feelings about a patient as meaningless when they are not at all.

The observed interview, through the one-way mirror, and videotapes in which you can observe yourself afterwards are invaluable for honing one's actual interviewing skills. Good supervision of this sort can make you aware of habitual mismoves that it would take years to discover, if at all, on your own. Here you can flesh out the general principles of interviewing and make them come alive. You can also learn about your own professional and personal style in this process. You may find that you consistently barge in whenever a patient is feeling sad or angry, that you obtain the external data to the exclusion of the internal, that you become impatient with people who cannot tell you outright what their problem is, or that you behave condescendingly. You may discover that you tend to nod your head up and down, smile, say "uhm-uhm" when you are anxious—often conveying unintended messages at inappropriate times, that you keep your distance too much, that you are too mechanical, that you do too much of the patient's work for him, that you are too active, that you consistently ask leading or closed-ended questions, that you continually begin questions with a "Can you. . . .," that you stumble and stammer whenever you ask for sexual history, that you seem to rush each patient out the door at the end of the interview, that you look at your watch whenever a patient is talking about warmth and emotional intimacy, and so forth. It is often helpful, as long as you do not feel you must become a carbon copy of him, to coerce your supervisor into modeling an interview or two for you as well. It is as reassuring to see what he does wrong as it is informative to see what he does right!

## SUGGESTED READINGS FOR CHAPTERS 4 AND 5

Mac Kinnon, R. and Michels, R.: *The Psychiatric Interview in Clinical Practice.* Philadelphia, W. B. Saunders Co., 1971. A good exposition of evaluation interviewing with nice tips on adapting one's style to different character and psychopathological types.

Sullivan, H. S.: *The Psychiatric Interview.* New York, W. W. Norton & Co., Inc., 1954. One of the first systematic treatments of the subjects by a dean of American psychiatry and still worth reading.

Tarachow, S.: *An Introduction to Psychotherapy.* New York, International Universities Press, 1963. See Chapters 13 and 14 for a superb example of how a dynamic psychiatrist thinks.

# 6
# Diagnosis

I shall begin this chapter with the riddle with which I open any discussion of psychiatric diagnosis with my students: "If there are two million schizophrenics in this country, how many ways of becoming schizophrenic are there in America?" The answer—"two million"— makes an important point about the role of diagnosis in psychiatry, which will become clear in this chapter.

Diagnosis is the central element in mainstream medicine, where it refers to the identification of *disease entities*—well-delineated disorders in bodily function with demonstrable etiologies, pathopnysiologies, and reasonably predictable courses of illness. When one speaks of a "good" internist, one is usually referring to his diagnostic acumen. Arriving at a diagnosis is crucial to such a physician because a relatively specific treatment plan follows as a matter of course.

Of course I am referring to the ideal. In actual practice it is often not that simple, even in internal medicine. A certain number of the internist's diagnoses are syndromes (collections of signs and symptoms whose pathophysiologies remain obscure). Even here, however, medicine's history of one brilliant elucidation of etiology after another gives the internist reason for optimism that eventually these syndromes too will be subdivided into the disease entities that constitute them. The same could be said of his attitude toward those disorders for which inadequate therapeutic interventions exist at this time.

Nevertheless, the internist is so accustomed to speaking of "diseases" that he usually forgets that nosology is not merely a description of what is "out there," in concrete reality, but is partly the mind's way of

190

ordering its otherwise chaotic experience. Each disease involves, to some degree, the entire human organism and its psyche as well. Consequently, it is a violation of reality to wall off a pathogenic process in an organ or organ system from the host and environment in which it is embedded. Thus, disease entities are cognitive constructions that correspond only more or less accurately to the realities to which they refer.

Furthermore, even in those cases of relatively well understood and discrete illness (e.g., peptic ulcer disease, diabetes mellitus, atherosclerotic cardiovascular disease), the interaction of psyche, soma, heredity, and environment is so complex that one hardly "explains" the patient or knows his treatment once one has labeled him. As Warren Garrison, emergency medicine specialist and psychiatrist, told me, on any given day he sees the same bacterial pneumonia present in several different ways, with several different histories, and necessitating several different treatments.

Finally, the general physician is liable to forget that what counts as an illness is, to some extent, culturally determined. For example, malaria was once so endemic to our Mississippi Valley that it was not considered a disease at all! Rather, it was accepted by the inhabitants as an unavoidable part of the human condition. The same is true today for yaws in parts of Africa.

If diagnosis, seemingly simple and straightforward, is actually this complicated in a "hard" clinical discipline like internal medicine, then how much more difficult is it in a "soft" one like psychiatry? There are at least five crucial differences between diagnosis in psychiatry and in the rest of medicine.

1. The majority of what the psychiatrist treats cannot be construed as manifestations of "illness" or "disease" in the sense that the internist understands it. Rather, the psychiatrist deals with *historically based distortions in one's view of self-in-world which lead to chronically maladaptive behavior patterns*—i.e., "problems in living."

Unlike the internist or surgeon, we encounter, not discrete dysfunctions in single organs, organ systems, or even groups of organ systems, but rather the disordered behavior of a thinking and feeling total-human-being-in-a-society. That is, the substrate of psychiatric *disorder* (a term I favor, after Meyer, to "illness") is not merely the biological human organism (in particular, its central nervous system), but its inextricable interaction with society as well. Even conditions such as schizophrenia and the major affective disorders (unipolar and bipolar manic-depressive illness), many cases of which doubtless have a genetically heritable or biological component, cannot qualify as disease entities in the medical sense of the term. Instead, they are "syndromes," final common pathways for what in some individuals approximate problems in living and in others genuine illnesses.

2. "Disorder" in psychiatry is even more obviously a response of the total human being than "disease" in medicine. For example, so-called "endogenous" depression or schizophrenia is not a discrete pathological process that insinuates itself into an otherwise intact psychological organism. Rather, it is such an idiosyncratic response of the whole person that it is perhaps preferable to speak of the "psychiatrically disordered" rather than of their "disorders," and of the "depressed" and "schizophrenic" rather than of "depression" and "schizophrenia." Mark Vonnegut puts it poetically in his Preface to *Eden Express,* that fine book describing his own psychotic breaks:

> Most diseases can be separated from one's self and seen as foreign intruding entities. Schizophrenia is very poorly behaved in this respect. Colds, ulcers, flu, and cancer are things we get. Schizophrenic is something we are. It affects the things we most identify with as making us what we are . . . [It is] always weaving itself inextricably into what we call ourselves.*

3. Whereas most medical diagnoses are at the same time descriptive *and* etiological, most psychiatric ones are not. They are usually either descriptive *or* etiological, but not both. The DSM-III (Diagnostic and Statistical Manual-III) nosological categories are, by and large, descriptive. By contrast, diagnosis in dynamic psychiatry is etiological. It refers to the elucidation of the dynamics of the maladaptive behavior.

4. Since psychiatric disturbances are disorders in psychosocial adaptation, what is considered psychopathology must inevitably vary from society to society and even in subgroups within the same society. Psychiatric diagnoses are infinitely more culture-bound than those in general medicine. Psychiatrists' styles in diagnosing change over time and from nation to nation, only in part, one suspects, because of differing incidence rates and patterns of psychopathology. British psychiatrists are more likely to diagnose manic-depressive illness; their American counterparts, schizophrenia.

5. There is not currently (and never will be, despite all the mandates of the federal government) the same degree of specificity between diagnosis and treatment in psychiatry that exists in the rest of medicine. The major affective disorders and schizophrenias are closest to being treatment-specific diagnoses, and even these have infinite variations. Some schizophrenics respond well to medication alone, although finding the right one(s) is often an exciting and hazardous odyssey. Others require a more concerted approach involving pharmacology, environmental manipulation, relearning, and various forms of supportive psychotherapy. Still others require medication and what approximates to long-term

---

*From Vonnegut, M.: *Eden Express.* New York, Bantam Books, Inc., 1976.

insight-oriented psychotherapy. Some respond best to the latter alone. When one "prescribes" psychotherapy, one should know that it is somewhat different for each patient. Psychotherapy, unlike medications, cannot be standardized.

To return to our riddle, my point of course is that it is far more helpful to know the current picture and history of the human individual to whom the label "schizophrenia" has been appended than to know that he meets the DSM-III criteria for that disorder. You must know not merely that he "has it," but what his schizophrenia feels like, how it came about, and to what it was, and is, a miscarried attempt to adapt. This is even truer of those DSM-III categories like "dysthymic disorder" and the neurotic and characterological reaction types, in which there is no evidence for concomitant biological dysfunction. What does it profit you to know that a person is possessed by a demon known as "dysthymic disorder," without knowing the history, dynamics, and self-world view of the neurotically depressed individual? No two "dysthymics" mean the same thing when they refer to their "depression."

It is insulting to a human being to try to subsume his entire history and way of being under a single label as if that sufficiently explained him.

In short, we are more interested in the dynamic, than in the descriptive, diagnosis, and a DSM that took account of all these would have as many entries as there are psychiatrically disturbed people in the world! People can manifest the identical observable unit of behavior for totally different underlying reasons, in which case it is not even accurate to speak of it as the same. Schizophrenia, for example, is a descriptive diagnosis in which the relative weight of biological and psychosocial factors varies from patient to patient and where the history and dynamics are in no two the same. Although the descriptive label, "schizophrenic," alerts you to the potential usefulness of medication, the overall approach to the patient is dictated by his particular dynamics *whether or not* you are doing insight-oriented psychotherapy with him. For example, you approach a schizophrenic who withdraws out of strong conflicts over latent homosexuality quite differently from one who isolates himself because he fears his dependent longings will devour his objects. In psychosis, as in neurosis, it is the dynamic, rather than the descriptive, diagnosis upon which one builds one's treatment plan.

Thus, in dynamic psychiatry the *formulation* is the real diagnosis. As set forth in Chapter 5, the diagnosis entails 1) the identification of important themes and maladaptive behavior patterns and their history and dynamics—what they "mean," and their "purpose"; 2) the assessment of ego functioning, including the identification of preferred sublimations and defensive maneuvers (and their hierarchical ordering as to adaptiveness), the highest previous level of functioning, and the evaluation of reality testing; 3) the assessment of past and current object relations; 4) the prognostication of transference and countertransference situations likely to arise, given the patient's history and your own sex, race, age, and history; and 5) the consideration of any apparently biological factors in the patient's disorder. The mode of treatment the patient can best profit from and participate in will follow from this diagnosis.

A complete presentation of psychiatric nosology would require a volume in itself. DSM-III is readily available, and I refer the student to Freedman, Kaplan, and Sadock's textbook. In this chapter I shall only provide a rough outline as a preliminary guide.

At the minimum, you should be able to recognize the five major categories of disordered human behavior: organic brain syndrome, schizophrenia, affective disorders (the depressions and mania), symptom and character neuroses, and the personality or character disorders.

## ORGANIC BRAIN SYNDROME

*Organic brain syndrome* refers to a constellation of signs and symptoms that manifest a variety of etiologies. It and depression are the most commonly encountered psychiatric disorders in the patient population of the nonpsychiatric physican. The syndrome is characterized by disturbance in *consciousness* and *attention, orientation, intellectual functioning, memory, affect, personality, motor activity,* and the *perception* and *interpretation of reality.* The hallmark of all these signs and symptoms is their *fluctuating intensity* within the same patient and in the course of a single day.

For example, the patient who is disoriented at 7:00 AM may be oriented at noon, the one who cannot tell you the names of his children in the morning may tell you their names and birth dates in the afternoon, the one who is confused at lunch may be lucid at dinner, and the one who is reality-oriented at 6:00 PM may be hallucinating at 9:00. This lability is particularly apparent in the case of affect. In the patient whose affect is not blunted, he may alternate between tears and laughter, and between depression and euphoria, in an explosive manner. More specific manifestations of, and tests for, organic mental dysfunction have been discussed in Chapter 5 and are not repeated here (e.g., hallucinations predominantly visual or tactile and worsening at night, recent memory affected more than remote, and so forth).

The organic brain syndromes are excellent illustrations of how, even in these most biological of psychiatric disorders, a dynamic approach cannot be dispensed with. This is because the total picture of any patient with organic mental disease results from a combination of biological and psychosocial factors. No two people react to the same organic mental affliction in the same way. Declining mental function is a crisis that strains the person's remaining adaptive capacities to the utmost. Prior adaptive styles (i.e., personality patterns) frequently become exaggerated in the patient's frantic attempt to both deny and cope with his organic dysfunction. Thus, a person who was mildly obsessive-compulsive may develop a florid obsessive-compulsive symptom neurosis and a person who was always a bit suspicious may become flagrantly paranoid. Therefore, one should suspect organic mental disorder in any patient who presents with a first episode of apparent neurosis or psychosis in middle or late adulthood—most functional disorders initially manifesting themselves in the first half of life.

Likewise, the patient's delusions, hallucinations, and bizarre speech and behaviors are not explicable without reference to his psychodynamics. Organic mental dysfunction affects the biological substrate of ego and superego functioning in such a way that there is a general diminution in defensive processes, a disinhibition of previously repressed fantasies and affects. This accounts for the coarse expressions of sexuality and aggression that often occur in hitherto prim and proper victims of organicity. The hallucinations, illusions, and delusions are likewise the manifestation of these. In other words, although the organic dysfunction accounts for the *process* of formation of delusions and hallucinations, it does not explain their *content*. The content—whether one is hallucinating a dead parent or a snake, whether he has delusions that he is a sinner or a saint, whether he is persecuted by a neighbor or his spouse—depends on his history and dynamics. In addition, we have all seen an elderly friend or relative "use" (unconsciously) his organic impairment to forget what he does not wish to remember and to inattend to that which he wants to avoid.

Social factors can affect the content of hallucinations and delusions and the situation in which they occur. It is not uncommon that organic mental patients are more disordered in some settings than in others, such as in stressful home environments or in new and unfamiliar places.

Organic mental disorders are divided into two broad categories: acute and chronic. The former is synonymous with "reversible" and has a more rapid and noisy onset, whereas the latter is synonymous with "irreversible" and has a more quiet, insidious mode of presentation. Untreated, the former may become the latter. Acute organic brain syndrome is often termed "delirium" and chronic is often termed "dementia." Acute organicity is more likely to result from physiological lesions and extracranial processes and chronic from structural and intracranial processes. The former is often associated with infectious or toxic processes, the latter with vascular and neoplastic disease.

The following are the etiological categories of organic brain syndrome: infectious (central nervous system or systemic), vascular (cerebral hemorrhage or atherosclerosis), neoplastic (malignant or nonmalignant, primary intracranial or metastatic systemic), primary degenerative (e.g., Alzheimer's disease and other neurological processes), metabolic-endo-crine (e.g., uremia, hyper- or hypoglycemia, or thyroid, adrenal, or nutritional deficiencies), toxic (e.g., alcohol, drugs, anesthetics, heavy metals, carbon monoxide), traumatic (e.g., epidural or subdural hemato-ma), and systemic (e.g., congestive heart failure, chronic obstructive pulmonary disease).

The treatment is both etiological and symptomatic. The former varies of course with the causative agent, while the latter depends upon the presentation. Hallucinations and delusions can be treated with support-ive psychotherapy and *low doses* of antipsychotic medication, particular-ly the high-potency phenothiazines and butyrophenones like trifluoper-azine (Stelazine) and haloperidol (Haldol). Agitation can be treated with talking therapy and, again, with *low doses* of antipsychotics or tranquiliz-ers such as hydroxyzine hydrochloride (Atarax) or hydroxyzine pamoate (Vistaril). Often, *no* medication is the treatment of choice. Mental status frequently improves merely by the removal, rather than the addition, of a psychotropic or other medication, especially in the elderly patient. Since hallucinations, delusions, and confusion are exacerbated by senso-ry deprivation, one should resort to leaving on a night light, leaving the patient's door open a crack, and discouraging excessive withdrawal. (Too much sensory stimulation, by contrast, is just as bad as too little.) Calendars and watches, a nursing staff that reminds the patient of time, place, and their names and functions, and friends and family who visit regularly all minimize disorientation. Finally, like all patients, those with organic brain syndrome function more adaptively in the presence of concerned and caring personnel than in that of hostile or indifferent ones. The whole area of psychotherapy with the chronically "organic" patient is—and will, unfortunately, probably remain—an untouched one.

## SCHIZOPHRENIA

*Schizophrenia* has doubtless received more attention than any other disorder in psychiatry. It is the closest thing to hell on earth. Although recognizable descriptions of schizophrenia occur in medical writings from ancient times, the syndrome itself was not codified until relatively recently. Morel, over a hundred years ago, termed it "dementia prae-cox" and Kraepelin and Bleuler, at the turn of our century, conceptual-ized it basically as we do today.

Schizophrenia is the most severe of the psychiatric dysfunctions and manifests itself in disturbances in affect, cognition, object relatedness, identity, perception, psychomotor behavior and, in particular, the reali-ty-orienting and defensive functions of the ego. Its incidence through-out time and space appears to be fairly constant, with the primary variations occurring in the content of the hallucinations and delusions rather than in the broad strokes of the syndrome itself. For example, in New Guinea demons are "in" and flying saucers and x rays are "out," while in the contemporary United States radiation and the Mafia are "in" and spirits are "out."

The "schiz" in schizophrenia refers to the fragmenting of the representations of self and reality in this disorder. In other words, there is not an integration of the various representations of self and those of objects into a consistent and coherent picture of self and world. There is, furthermore, a blurring of the boundaries between representations of self and those of world such that a schizophrenic may attribute his toothache to a window or may perceive the breaking of that window as the shattering of his soul. He may regard his rage as yours rather than as his own, or be convinced that you can read his mind or are inserting thoughts into it. The "integration" that occurs during the recovery process refers to the remelding together of the disparate pictures of self and others into unified images of self and world. This is accompanied by the repression of unintegratable, ego dystonic images of self and world that were previously all too conscious. The schizophrenic's exquisite sensitivity to loss, his object hunger, results from a paucity of representations of integrated objects and from an inability to fix an object in mind for any length of time. His withdrawal is a way of dealing with his most profound fear—that of fusion with his objects, the loss of self.

Many of the signs and symptoms of schizophrenia were discussed in the section on the mental status exam and are merely briefly repeated here. Bleuler, the great Swiss psychiatrist, hinged the diagnosis upon the identification of four *primary* signs (the 4 A's): *autism*—bizarrely private, idiosyncratic, fantasies and behaviors which the patient finds virtually impossible to explain to the examiner; *affect* that is flattened or inappropriate—a poverty of affect, a stonelike facies and demeanor, or affect grossly incongruous to the topic of conversation; loosening of *associations*—a derailing of one's train of thought; and *ambivalence*—intense love and hatred toward the same object. *Secondary* signs for Bleuler included delusions and hallucinations.

Over the years, psychiatrists have grown disillusioned with the utility of Bleuler's criteria. Although autism (also called "dereism") and loose associations are undoubtedly characteristic of many schizophrenics, blunted affect and ambivalence are less clearly associated with the disorder. Although you will certainly see some schizophrenics with both of these signs, they do not seem to be a primary feature of the disorder—in particular, ambivalence, which occurs to some degree in most psychiatric patients, as in most normal individuals. The extreme withdrawal and listlessness of severe depression is sometimes misinterpreted as blunted affect. Currently most psychiatrists favor Schneider's criteria. His *first rank* symptoms include two of Bleuler's secondary signs (delusions and hallucinations) and one of his primary signs (loose associations).

DSM-III cleaves closely to the Schneiderian scheme. Its criteria are: bizarre, paranoid, and somatic delusions; auditory hallucinations; loosening of associations and poverty of speech (if the latter is associated with blunted or inappropriate affect, delusions or hallucinations, or catatonic or other grossly disorganized behavior); deterioration of previous level of functioning; continuous signs of the illness for *at least six months* during some point in the patient's life with *active signs at present;* a prodromal and residual phase (including such things as social isolation, hypochondriacal complaints and bizarre somatic preoccupations, impaired occupational functioning, peculiar behavior, impaired hygiene); onset of prodromal or active phase of the disorder before age 45; and absence of organic brain disease or mental retardation.

The schizophrenic disorders are further subdivided into the "disorganized" (formerly called "hebephrenic"), "catatonic" (withdrawn or excited), "paranoid," "undifferentiated," and "residual." "Schizoaffective disorder," formerly classified as a form of schizophrenia with predominantly depressive or euphoric and excited features, is currently considered in a separate category. The new criteria for this last emphasize major affective disturbance in which a *mood-incongruent* hallucination, delusion, or other psychotic feature is present. By contrast, the symptoms of the other schizophrenic subtypes tend to be ego syntonic.

Many dysfunctions that would formerly have been classified as schizophrenic are now termed *schizophreniform,* primarily because their duration is less than six months and because there is a more prominent reactive component. It is important to distinguish this last from drug-induced psychoses. A schizophreniform disorder must have persisted for at least two weeks. Drugs can either cause psychosis directly or else unmask a previously latent psychosis.

The schizophrenic disorders proper are closer to what Langfeldt termed "process" schizophrenia, whereas the schizophreniform dysfunctions are closer to what he called "reactive." The classical process schizophrenic is one who exhibited a childhood history of introversion, shyness, and withdrawal and whose disorder has an insidious onset with a first outbreak in the late teens to early twenties. This type is often considered to have a heavier genetic loading. The prognosis of the process type is considered more guarded than that of the reactive. Although external precipitants are usually considered to be absent or minimal compared to the reactive type, I have never encountered an episode of schizophrenia where precipitants were not to be found if one only looked. Common stressors include losses, rejections, and separations—a death, disappointment in love, or leaving home for the first time for college, occupation, or military service. Major or minor physical illnesses commonly precipitate a first episode,[1] in part, perhaps, because they raise the issues of dependency which are so prominent in the "oral" preoccupations of the schizophrenic. By contrast, the reactive schizophrenic is less likely to exhibit a schizoid premorbid personality, has often reached a somewhat higher level of adaptation, and is assaulted by more obvious stressors from his environment.

It would require a volume in itself to recount the theories of schizophrenia. They range from the purely biological to the purely social to the purely psychological to those which take account of all three. Adoption and other studies do suggest that there is a biologically heritable metabolic component in many cases, although the statistics are far from unequivocal (see Lidz, 1981). Faris and Dunham and others have pointed to the association of schizophrenia with urban crowding and lower socioeconomic status. Jackson (1960) and Lidz, et al. (1965) have focused on the family, with emphasis upon how the patient's family both teaches schizophrenic behavior and makes it adaptive. Psychoanalytic writers have focused on the early mother-child interaction and disturbances in the oral period. Behaviorists look at the reinforcement value and the conditioning and modeling of isolated schizophrenic behaviors.

My primary intention, however, is not to discuss the descriptive diagnosis of schizophrenia or the various theories of its etiology. The reader can refer to DSM-III and Freedman, Kaplan, and Sadock's (1980) textbook. My aim is to impress upon the student that, whatever their biological components, schizophrenic behaviors are *meaningful* within the context of the patient's current and historical interpersonal environments. People who believe that schizophrenia is all genes and dopamine will not take the time or ask the questions to discover the meaningfulness of the patient's "word salad" or bizarre behavior. There is nothing more heartening than to see the student, previously convinced that schizophrenia is all chemistry, take sufficient history to understand what is ostensibly the most "senseless" behavior.

Granted, there seems to be a talent for schizophrenic behaviors of which not everyone is possessed.[2] This talent is probably the gift of both biological and social inheritance, with the weight of each varying from individual to individual. (Biology helps us understand the biological

---

[1] By contrast, physical illness or injury in a chronic schizophrenic may induce a temporary remission in symptoms.

[2] Or rather, a talent of which not everyone is possessed to the same *degree*. In early childhood we were all capable of schizophrenic-like experience and behavior, and in dreams we continue to be. The closest approximations to schizophrenia in waking normal adults are occasions such as awakening from a particularly vivid dream and being momentarily unaware of its unreality and the experience of hypnagogic or hypnapompic hallucinations or disorientation.

substrate of schizophrenic symptoms, but it will never explain their content and the circumstances in which they occur.) However, once the capability for such behavior is given, it then becomes a response to *intrapsychic conflict* like any other. Schizophrenic behaviors are, by and large, defensive maneuvers—ways of avoiding the anxiety attendant upon conflict-laden perceptions from the external environment and upon conflictual drives from within. Like neurotic symptoms, they generally express some of what they are defending against.

I shall illustrate the meaningfulness of schizophrenic symptomatology with a patient, Mr. M:

> Mr. M. was a 40-year-old man with an alcoholic, philandering father and a psychotic mother, toward whom he was much closer than to the father. During his mother's frequent hospitalizations he was left at home to virtually fend for himself. When Mr. M. was 12 years old, his mother was diagnosed as having a brain tumor. Surgery was performed and she spent her remaining days in a state mental hospital. Mr. M. was placed in an orphanage at the time. He religiously visited his mother, who could hardly recognize him. He saw his father very little after this time. A particularly traumatic event occurred at age 19 when his mother delivered a child in the hospital. His first psychotic break occurred within a few weeks of that time and involved the delusional fear that people were after him to cut off his arms, visual hallucinations of people being butchered, and "voices" telling him he was a rapist and deserved death. His second break occurred shortly after his father's death in an auto accident and involved similar delusions and hallucinations. His third break followed the discovery of cancer in, and subsequent radical mastectomy of, the aunt (mother's sister) to whom he was closest. Again, he was preoccupied with delusional fears of mutilation. The fourth and current episode followed his discovery that his wife was having extramarital affairs. He entered a bar "to get drunk" immediately after learning of this. While walking to the pay phone, after a few drinks, to call his wife and "have it out with her," he began hallucinating "men and women being butchered" by "green-eyed monsters" with huge meat cleavers. He ran in fear from the bar and was committed shortly thereafter.

Each of the four psychotic breaks followed the loss of, disappointment in, or illness of a loved one. Themes of destruction, mutilation, and recrimination were prominent. I understood his hallucinations and delusions as frantic attempts to defend against the onslaught of previously unconscious sexual and, especially, aggressive fantasies. The mother's delivery of a child destroyed any images of her purity and simultaneously stirred up and frustrated his oedipal desires. He reacted to the former by producing self-condemnatory voices calling him a "rapist" and to the latter with rage, which he projected in the form of hallucinations and delusions. This rage was in part "oral," as well, since the mother, with her repeated absences, had frustrated her son's dependent strivings. The content of his delusions, the preoccupation with mutilation, was in part a function of his fear that he would be surgically manipulated as was his mother—a castration equivalent (arm equals penis). His second psychotic episode followed the death of the father, toward whom he was ambivalent. Again, his symptoms consisted of projected rage and fear of punishment for what in this case amounted to an oedipal triumph. The operation on the aunt, to whom he was close but who had often turned him away, stimulated the same complex of sexual and aggressive feelings and fears. Finally, the wife's affair must have awakened memories of his mother's extramarital affair and pregnancy in addition to being a major event in its own right. Once more, projected rage was predominant. One might predict with reasonable assurance that, however fortunate this man's future might be, he probably will experience at least one more psychotic break following the death of his mother.

If historical determinism and psychic causality were manifest in his delusions and hallucinations, they were also in his thought disorder and affective disturbance. Loose associations and blocking, like his inappropriate laughter, were not continuous but occurred, like clockwork, whenever his wife, mother, aunt, or old girl friends were mentioned. When asked to describe his parents' relationship, he laughed uncontrollably, then became angry, and said "You already know all about it. Don't ask for answers you already have." In other words, these symptoms were serving a defensive function by taking his mind away from conflict-laden material.

This man also illustrates an important point for the interviewer of the schizophrenic. Such patients suffer from a failure of the usual neurotic defenses and the consequent need to erect psychotic ones against the imminent consciousness of forbidden desires. This, coupled with their loss of self-other boundaries, makes them particularly fearful that people will read their minds. You must avoid giving them any impression that this is in fact the case. Residents' intentions to impress both patient and supervisor with precipitous "deep" interpretations have often proved disastrous. One resident's questioning about the patient's mother, right after asking him about his girl friend, precipitated a rage and the delusion (! ?) that she was reading his mind. She had obviously intruded on a precariously repressed Oedipus complex. In a neurotic, where such material would have been more repressed, her procedure would probably have elicited little or no observable response.

Schizophrenics are treated with a variety of measures: from drugs and electroconvulsive therapy to psychotherapy. A host of unusual treatments from vitamins to hemodialysis have been tried as well. The tremendous optimism in the wake of the discovery of the antipsychotic medications has waned somewhat now that we understand they offer a largely symptomatic, rather than etiological, treatment and now that we are aware of long-term side-effects such as tardive dyskinesia. Nevertheless, the drugs are highly beneficial and, used judiciously, account for an untold reduction in suffering. With medication, many acute episodes can now be treated outside the hospital. However, overmedication can make a patient less, not more, amenable to psychotherapy and can stifle symptomatology that seems to be in part, as Freud (1924) and Boisen (1939) have suggested, the schizophrenic's attempt to restore self-integration and resume object relations. Resocialization and educational therapies, both on and off the hospital ward, are invaluable. Supportive and, in cases, insight-oriented psychotherapies remain indispensable modalities, both in conjunction with medications and by themselves. The early nineteenth-century "moral treatment" of schizophrenics, which offered only milieu and supportive therapies, showed impressive results. Anyone who still doubts that the schizophrenic's behavior is meaningful and that he can be successfully treated by psychotherapy should read the beautiful case histories of Harold Searles (1965).

The student should remember that all that is psychotic is not necessarily schizophrenic. To its everlasting credit, DSM-III has refined and sharpened the diagnostic criteria for schizophrenia—a syndrome that was previously overdiagnosed. Because of the social and vocational stigma attached to a diagnosis of "schizophrenia" and because of the unfortunate and erroneous mental set that such a label evokes in many psychiatrists subsequently encountering the patient (e.g., he only needs drugs, he will not respond to psychotherapy, and he will not progress or will inevitably deteriorate), you are not helping the patient by precipitously diagnosing him "schizophrenic."

It is possible for those with a history of lifelong adaptation to become transiently psychotic under the right stress. A mother became disorganized and hallucinated for several days following the death of her infant. A physically active 40-year-old man became transiently psychotic a few days after immobilization in a body cast (in part because of relative sensory deprivation and in part because his preferred outlet for discharge of aggression was removed). If such behavior lasts no more than two weeks, it is termed a "brief psychotic reaction." The aforementioned "schizophreniform disorder" refers to similar behavior which lasts for two weeks to six months and in which there is a less clearly demonstrable psychosocial stressor. As in the brief reactive psychosis, there is usually no evidence for a positive family history of schizophrenia. Certain personality disorders—in particular, the borderline, schizotypal, and histrionic—may exhibit transient psychotic symptomatology. This can be particularly colorful in the so-called "hysterical psychosis" (see Freud and Breuer's *Studies on Hysteria* for fine examples).

There is an unfortunate tendency to misdiagnose mania as schizophrenia. Similarly, all paranoids do not suffer from paranoid schizophrenia. Paranoia vera ("true paranoia"), now termed "paranoid disorder," is characterized by a fixed and well-delineated delusional system in an otherwise intact and well-organized personality. I treated a young physicist who functioned well socially and occupationally and whose thinking was linear and logical, as long as one did not impinge upon his delusion that there was a "crime-queer syndicate" headquartered at Hiltons all across the nation.

The mere presence of hallucinations is insufficient for a diagnosis of schizophrenia. My impression is that occasional hallucinations are more common in the nonpsychiatric general population than most people suspect. People can hallucinate in response to sensory deprivation or loneliness. Several well-functioning and drug-free truck drivers have told me about auditory hallucinations that "kept them company" and were quite pleasurable. One of Canada's greatest prime ministers, McKenzie King, apparently talked with his dead mother for years and years (Stanley Jackson, personal communication). Freud hallucinated his fiancée's voice on several lonely occasions in Paris in 1885. A variety of drug-induced and toxic states can of course present as psychosis. The confusion of amphetamine intoxication with paranoid schizophrenia is a classic example, as is the psychosis of "PCP." Finally, a number of culture-bound psychoses correspond only approximately to our diagnostic categories. All behavior that appears eccentric or peculiar to that dictated by our cultural norms cannot be called "schizophrenic." Behavior appropriate to a foreign culture's definition of reality may not be so to ours, e.g., belief in voodoo, bewitchment, and spirit possession.

## AFFECTIVE DISORDERS

DSM-III divides these into the major affective disorders (formerly called manic-depressive illness) and the more neurotic or characterological depressions (e.g., dysthymic, cyclothymic, and atypical affective disorders). These disturbances have plagued man for years, and the medical and nonmedical literature throughout the ages is replete with accounts of them. They are characterized, as the name suggests, by a constellation of signs and symptoms at the center of which is a euphoric or, more commonly, dysphoric disturbance of affect. They are quite common; DSM-III estimates that 18 to 23% of women and 8 to 11% of men have experienced at least one major depressive episode.

The word "depressed" is so loosely used today that it is necessary for the patient to be explicit about what he means by it. Likewise, your psychiatric reporting must spell out whether you are referring to a simple case of the "existential blahs" or the syndrome of clinical depression. I shall first discuss depression and then mania and hypomania.

Most people have experienced the "blues," or have been in a "funk," or "down in the dumps." In "normals" such feelings are mild, transient, and clearly situation-related. Some people, however, such as the neurotic depressives (dysthymics) are more subject to such moods and find it harder to shake them. Neurotic depressions are more intense and prolonged versions of the downs that most of us experience occasionally. They are also referred to as the exogenous or reactive depressions, since the external precipitants are usually more obvious than in their so-called endogenous counterparts (major affective disorders), which are thought to have a genetically heritable biological component.[3]

The *neurotically depressed individual* experiences a variety of disturbances in mood, behavior, and outlook on life. He is melancholy, tearful, and performs previously pleasurable activities without zest or gusto. In contrast, however, to the more endogenously depressed individual, his depressive mood is generally not continuous. Rather, it is *mercurial.* He may be depressed for several hours and then feel all right for a while. If there is a diurnal variation in mood, he is more likely to feel better in the morning and "neuroticize" himself progressively into depression as the day goes on. Furthermore, in contrast to the individual with the sustained anhedonia of endogenous depression, he is often capable of experiencing some pleasure from time to time. He often has a diminished self-esteem and sense of inadequacy. He may feel guilty and self-reproachful out of proportion to any real misdeeds. He frequently feels chronically tired, and experiences decreased efficiency at work and home and impaired concentration secondary to conscious and unconscious preoccupations. It is more difficult to make and implement decisions. He is impatient, irritable, and often anxious as well. He is less likely to have the vegetative signs and symptoms that accompany the endogenous depressions. He may, however, have vague and diffuse somatic complaints such as headaches. If he is insomniac, he is more likely to have difficulty falling asleep (here again, because of his neuroticizing) than the early morning awakening that is more characteristic of the endogenous depressions. A positive family history of depression is less often obtained with the neurotic than with the sufferer from major affective disorder.

---

[3]It is important to distinguish between the affect depression and the clinical syndrome of depression. It is the latter with which we are concerned here. The affect depression is not limited to the neurotic and major affective disorders but may accompany any psychiatric disorder, from schizophrenia to obsessive-compulsive neurosis. Nor do affects such as anxiety and depression exist in pure culture, but rather in varying degrees of admixture with one another. Brenner (1976) has a useful way of differentiating between anxiety and depression. He defines the former as the experience of "unpleasure" associated with an image of impending calamity, the latter as the experience of "unpleasure" associated with a calamity that has already transpired. In this regard, he speaks of defenses against the "unpleasure" of depression, quite as much as against the "unpleasure" of anxiety.

Those with *major affective disorders* experience many of the same symptoms as those with neurotic depression but more intensely. Whereas the latter describes his mood as "blue," the former may say, "I feel as if a black veil has been drawn over my life, as if I am in a dark and deep valley." He may sob continuously or he may be in an apathetic heap, too despairing to even cry. Whereas the neurotic's depression is mercurial, the melancholia and anhedonia of endogenous depression is steady and unrelenting. If there is any diurnal variation in mood, he tends to feel worse in the morning and a little better as the day wears on. Whereas the neurotic may be indecisive and sluggish, the endogenously depressed person can be virtually paralyzed in total anergia; he may even come to resemble the catatonic. Whereas the neurotic is subject to bouts of pessimism and occasional thoughts of death or suicide, the endogenous may feel utterly hopeless and be obsessed with death and suicide. In extreme circumstances he may feel that he is already dead or is rotting away inside. Other delusions, and even hallucinations, consistent with themes of personal inadequacy, nihilism, guilt, and deserved punishment may be present. The diminished self-esteem and sense of inadequacy of the neurotic become a conviction in one's total worthlessness and helplessness in the endogenous depressive. His social withdrawal can be profound. He is more likely to experience the vegetative signs and symptoms of depression: insomnia (especially early morning awakening) or hypersomnia, hypophagia and weight loss or hyperphagia and weight gain, decreased libido, and constipation. He is more likely than the neurotic to have had prior, relatively well demarcated, episodes of depression lasting weeks or months, with remissions in between. (Neurotics, by contrast, often have a virtually lifelong lowgrade, mercurial depression). He gives a positive family history of depression (often of depression in female relatives and alcoholism in males) more frequently than the neurotic.

A special class of patients presents with the anergia, vegetative signs, and diffuse somatic complaints or even somatic delusions of endogenous depression, but without the subjective emotional sensation of depression. Frequently these are elderly patients who are often somewhat agitated as well. With their somaticizing ("depressive equivalents") and defenses against depressive affect, they are difficult to treat and particularly prone to surprise you with precipitous completed suicide.

Pertinent to our discussion is differentiation between normal grief and pathological mourning. The latter is essentially a manifestation of major affective or severe dysthymic disorders. Many in the throes of an acute grief reaction have been mistakenly "psychopathologized" and given medications which actually interfered with, rather than assisted, their grief work. Table 6-1 compares and contrasts normal grief with pathological mourning.

**TABLE 6-1. Reaction of the Survivor: Comparison and Contrast of Normal Mourning and Pathological Grief\*†**

| Normal Mourning<br>(In general, as common sense would suggest, the younger the deceased, the more difficult and prolonged the mourning.) | Pathological Grief<br>(An ambivalent or extremely dependent relationship toward the deceased usually predisposes to this.) |
|---|---|
| 1. *Sad and dejected affect;* temporary loss of zest for life. | 1. *Absence of any affect* for a prolonged period following the death (affect may appear much later and in response to a seemingly inappropriate event). |
| 2. *Preoccupation with the image of the deceased.* | 2. *Overactive without a sense of loss;* perhaps even euphoric. |
| 3. *Hostility toward the deceased* for deserting us (may exist outside of our awareness and be displaced onto doctor or hospital). | 3. *Marked identification* with the deceased: developing his somatic symptoms or attempting to take on his occupation or character style (Freud understood this as an attempt to become like the lost object rather than to acknowledge the loss). |
| 4. *Guilt feelings* over real or imagined acts of commission or omission toward the deceased (these guilt feelings may be projected onto the hospital or doctor). We may also feel guilt in response to our hostility toward the dead and in response to our (often unconscious) pleasure at surviving him ("survivor guilt"). | 4. *Prolonged alteration in relationships to friends and relatives* (prolonged social isolation or irritability). |
| 5. *Somatic complaints* often present. | 5. *In general, the extreme exaggeration or prolongation of signs of normal mourning* (e.g., extreme and unremitting hostility toward doctor or hospital, crying to the point of inability to function for a long period, refusal to give up the image of the deceased). |
| 6. *Some loss or disorganization of habitual patterns of conduct.* | 6. *Guilt feelings and self-recrimination often severe.* Guilt is often over death wishes toward the deceased |

*Continued on next page*

**TABLE 6-1. Reaction of the Survivor: Comparison and Contrast of Normal Mourning and Pathological Grief\*† (Continued)**

| Normal Mourning (In general, as common sense would suggest, the younger the deceased, the more difficult and prolonged the mourning.) | Pathological Grief (An ambivalent or extremely dependent relationship toward the deceased usually predisposes to this.) |
|---|---|
| 6. Continued | (based on "omnipotence of thoughts"—the magical idea that "wishing makes it so"). Self-accusations are (as in depression) often disguised accusations against the deceased for his shortcomings. Consciously or unconsciously (e.g., sudden bout of accident proneness) self-punitive behavior may result. |
| 7. *Possibly some mild identification with the deceased,* may shade over into pathological mourning. | 7. *Anniversary reactions* often occur in cases of missed mourning. (Recall the patient who fell and injured herself on a rock in a river where her loved one drowned—on the first anniversary of his death). |
| 8. *Self-esteem is usually maintained* (Freud believed this is the primary distinction between mourning and melancholia). | 8. *Any of the signs and symptoms of clinical depression* (agitated or retarded type). |
| 9. More intense phase subsides in 6 weeks to 3 months; often some residual mourning for up to one or two years. | 9. *Persistent denial* of the loved one's death which may take the form of hallucinations or alcoholism. |
| 10. Often some temporary decrease in interest in friends and loved ones. | 10. *Medical illness* (Lindemann noted that 33 of 41 patients with ulcerative colitis developed their disease in close temporal relationship to the loss of an important person; it is well known that mortality among widowers greatly increases in the period immediately following the loss). |

\*Lindemann's classical 1944 article on grief was useful in preparing this table.
†Compare and contrast columns as wholes; individually numbered items do not correspond with one another.

Manic and hypomanic syndromes are the reverse side of the depressive. They are essentially "defenses" against underlying dysphoric affect. Frequently the same individual experiences both manic and depressive episodes (bipolar affective disorder or, as it was formerly called, manic-depressive illness, circular type). Often, you can sense the depression underneath the facade of frenzied cheeriness. If you can get a manic to slow down, he often admits this himself. Manic episodes include periods of hyperactivity lasting a week to months and a sensation of boundless energy, decreased need for sleep, pressured speech, flight of ideas, grandiosity, elation, and easy distractibility. The manic may dress bizarrely, go on buying sprees, invest money foolishly, and engage in a host of reckless behaviors reflecting grossly impaired judgment. If he feels thwarted or hindered in any way, the manic may become angry and aggressive. Delusions or hallucinations congruent with the elated mood and sense of inordinate self-worth and power may occur. "Hypomania" refers to a constellation of behaviors similar to those of the manic, only less intense and more reality oriented. A variety of actions known as "counterdepressive behaviors" function as hypomanic equivalents. These can include thrill-seeking, dare-devil activities, workaholism, alcoholism, and some cases of pathological gambling and lying.

Generally, theories of the etiology of depression may be divided according to whether they view the major affective (endogenous depressive) and dysthymic (neurotic depressive) disorders as on a continuum or as two discrete entities. The evidence is equivocal at present. I shall present my own view, containing elements from both theories, although the reader must form his own opinion.

The central issues in the endogenous depressions tend to be "oral" ones, though other preoccupations are certainly present as well. We postulate that the disturbances in the mother-child relationship are neither so early nor so severe as in the schizophrenic. Nevertheless, deprivation, rejection, and abuse are sufficient to leave the infant deeply unfulfilled and with pessimistic expectations of his environment. *He reacts to this frustration with hurt, rage, and a diminished sense of self-worth.* Since any tantrums often serve to distance the parents still further or evoke punitive responses, he soon learns to internalize his anger, to turn it against the self, or rather against the representation of the object within the self. This primal constellation of hurt, internalized rage, and diminished self-esteem goes to make up what is experienced and manifested as depression. It is important that you understand this: the affect that the sufferer describes as "depression" is a wastebasket filled with a host of more discrete affects. As a depressed patient begins to improve in psychotherapy, the vague and pervasive affect of depression is replaced by "purer" expressions of the hurt, sadness, disappointment, anger, and guilt feelings that lie beneath it.

Upon this foundation of early deprivation or abuse is laid subsequent experience with rejection and loss. A variety of events, such as family moves, parental withdrawal, divorce, or deaths, count as the losses which are essentially perceived as rejections. Epidemiology shows that depressives are more likely than "normals" to have experienced major losses in the first 12 years of life, particularly the deaths of important individuals like parents, siblings, and live-in grandparents or other relatives. The death of a parent is essentially experienced as a rejection, as a desertion, and arouses not only hurt and disappointment, but a good deal of rage as well (which is internalized in conformity with rules about speaking ill of the dead). The more dependent or ambivalent the relationship with the deceased, the more problematic the mourning because of guilt over one's anger at him for leaving in the first case and because of this and guilt over one's sense of triumph and relief at his death in the second. The degree of emotional scarring depends largely on how available the survivors are to help the child with his grief work. All too frequently the remaining parent discourages, rather than encourages, the abreaction and recollection that is essential to a healthy mourning.[4] The death of a sibling is almost as problematic as the death of a parent, but for different reasons. Each child harbors conscious and unconscious murderous fantasies about his sibling. When a sibling dies this is perceived, on one level, as a triumph over him. The child, in his magical thinking, reacts as if his wishing somehow made it so and is likely to harbor a residue of fratricidal guilt all his life.

In addition to having an early history of deprivation, many depressives had to assume adult responsibilities prematurely. Often I have seen the woman, who functioned as a surrogate parent for her siblings from eight or ten, married or entered the work world prematurely, and who developed a lifelong pattern of giving rather than receiving, suddenly collapse in middle age. Her despair and self-reproach conceal a good deal of reproach for those historical and current others who have failed her and are in part a bid for the attention which she so desires.

Compared to its endogenous counterpart, neurotic depression is a

---

[4]Freud explained the normal mourning process as a hypercathexis of the image of the deceased in the service of an eventual decathexis of it—this latter the prerequisite for redirecting one's mental energies toward the living and the tasks of current life. This phase of hypercathexis is recognized and institutionalized in most cultures. This is less so, unfortunately, in our own where one is likely to be enjoined, as was one of my patients who had lost his best friend, not to dwell upon the dead. This teenager was chided by his mother for spending hours in his room listening to records cut by his deceased older friend—chided, in other words, for doing exactly what he was supposed to do. Another man recalled the difficult grieving for his father whom he lost at the age of ten. "He was on my mind for weeks. I was failing in school. Finally, one day I decided I would have to go on living and the daydreams stopped."

more descriptive than etiological diagnosis. That is, a wider variety of dynamics is likely to participate in producing the clinical syndrome of neurotic depression than the predominantly oral ones in major affective disorders. The neurotic depressive is more apt to have important oedipal issues intertwined with the preoedipal ones (recall Mrs. A. from Chapter 1). Damage to self-esteem, a sense of having violated one's ideals, frustrated longings, and countless other issues can precipitate neurotic depressions.

In addition to the psychodynamic factors, the evidence for genetically heritable biological ones in the major affective disorders is overwhelming. Certain defects in the metabolism of catecholamines seem to exist in these patients. They tend to present with a positive family history of depression (or alcoholism and depression as previously outlined). By contrast, there is little or no evidence for biological factors in most cases of neurotic depression (dysthymic disorders). Nevertheless, it is important to remember that there is no hard-and-fast line between genetic and psychodynamic factors in the endogenous depressive. His parents bequeath much more to him than their genes. These same genes raise him. His depression is as much the heritage of their depressively impaired childrearing and of identification with them as of their chromosomes.

In short, neurotic and endogenous depressions often share similar dynamics and are set in motion by precipitants which these patients, in atavistic fashion, have played a role in creating. They differ most in that the affective reaction set off by the precipitant somehow mobilizes a biological mechanism in the latter which then becomes autonomous and takes on a life of its own.[5]

I want to emphasize again that one cannot understand the endogenously depressed person without knowing his dynamics and the precipitants of his disorder. It is a myth that a prime differentiating characteristic between neurotic and endogenous depression is the absence of a precipitant in the latter. It may be harder to identify in the sufferer from the major depressions, but I have never encountered a patient where one or several could not be identified. The same is true of manic episodes. The most common stressors are a loss (including loss of self-esteem) or perceived rejection, which function both as events in their own right and as aggravants of unresolved feelings about similar episodes in the past.

There are treatment implications here. First of all, in the neurotic depressive, insight-oriented psychotherapy is the treatment of choice. Although antidepressant medications may be helpful for the more se-

---

[5]I am resorting to the mind-body split (as in the discussion on organic brain syndrome) but for purely heuristic purposes and not because I disbelieve in the fundamental unity of the psychobiological human organism.

verely depressed and agitated neurotics, in general they are not indicated. If the patient does respond it is often to the placebo effect ("transference cure," e.g., symbolically being fed by you). By contrast, in the endogenous depressive the relative autonomy of the biology set in motion makes antidepressants mandatory. Nevertheless, if this is *all* you do you may succeed in alleviating his current depression, but you will do nothing to help him understand the maladaptive behavior patterns that create the situations that precipitate the affective response that precipitates his biological dysfunction.

For example, I treated a bipolar manic-depressive patient, with an overwhelming family history of this disorder and a history of early loss and deprivation, whose manic and depressive episodes were precipitated by disappointments in love. Certain enduring behavior patterns, devised to deal with a pathological home environment, ensured that he would arrange a rejection from every woman with whom he became involved. I treated the biological component of his disorder with lithium carbonate and the psychodynamic with a modified insight-oriented psychotherapy.

Table 6-2 compares and contrasts neurotic and endogenous depression.

### TABLE 6-2. Depression

| Exogenous (Neurotic or Dysthymic) | Endogenous (Major Affective Disorder) |
| --- | --- |
| 1. Mood characterized by "feeling blue," "down in the dumps," often with associated anxiety and irritability. | 1. Melancholic affect is much deeper and more severe and the person is more likely to exhibit psychomotor retardation than anxiety (though the latter may occur). |
| 2. Depressive affect is mercurial. | 2. Affective disturbance is unrelenting. |
| 3. Can usually derive some pleasure from the right situations. | 3. Persistent anhedonia. |
| 4. If there is a marked diurnal variation in mood, the patient is most likely to feel better in the morning and worse toward evening. | 4. If there is diurnal variation, he is more likely to feel worse in the morning and better as the day wears on. |
| 5. May be intensely pessimistic or despairing, but usually retains some optimism about the future. | 5. Often a deep sense of hopelessness, of despair. |
| 6. Feels inadequate but rarely a sense of total helplessness. | 6. A sense of utter helplessness. |

*Continued on next page*

## TABLE 6-2. Depression (Continued)

| Exogenous (Neurotic or Dysthymic) | Endogenous (Major Affective Disorder) |
|---|---|
| 7. Self-reproach and decreased self-esteem. | 7. Impairment in self-esteem and sense of guilt can become delusional, e.g., an intelligent or wealthy patient may insist he is retarded and indigent. |
| 8. Diffuse somatic complaints. | 8. Diffuse somatic complaints and, at times, frank somatic delusions. |
| 9. Reality testing intact. | 9. May experience mood-congruent hallucinations or delusions. |
| 10. May engage in self-destructive behavior. | 10. May engage in self-destructive behavior, particularly surprising in the improving depressive who suddenly recovers enough energy to enact what he has been considering all along. |
| 11. Experiences tiredness and increased difficulty getting things done, but can usually manage. | 11. May have a profound anergia. |
| 12. Disturbances in concentration and melancholy ruminations. | 12. Both are usually more severe. |
| 13. Less likely to have insomnia and the vegetative signs. If the former is present, it is usually difficulty in falling asleep. | 13. Vegetative signs usually present. Sleeping disturbances characterized by early-morning awakening or hypersomnia. |
| 14. External precipitants more obvious. | 14. External precipitants *always* present but often less obvious. |
| 15. Past history is usually one of a chronic, mild, and mercurial depression with occasional exacerbations. | 15. Past history of discrete episodes (weeks to months) of depression or mania with pain-free intervals (months to years). |
| 16. Family history of depression is variable. More likely to elicit a family history of neurotic and characterological disorders. | 16. Strongly positive family history of depression and alcoholism. |
| 17. Usually no demonstrable laboratory abnormalities associated with the depression. | 17. Often demonstrable blood and urine abnormalities in catecholamine metabolites. |
| 18. Insight-oriented psychotherapy is the treatment of choice. Antidepressants seldom indicated (occasional agitated neurotic depressives respond to amitriptyline or doxepin). | 18. Antidepressant medication (and/or lithium carbonate in the unipolar or bipolar manic) and a modified insight-oriented psychotherapy are the treatment of choice. Those with psychomotor retardation seem to respond better to imipramine and those with agitation to amitriptyline or doxepin. |

## SYMPTOM AND CHARACTER NEUROSES

The dynamics of neurotic behaviors were intensively discussed and exemplified in Chapter 3; therefore, I shall only resketch the broad outline here. Then I shall briefly acquaint the reader with the subclassifications of neurosis.

The neuroses are maladaptive ways of dealing with the anxiety secondary to unconscious intrapsychic conflict. They are characterized either by discrete ego dystonic and unpleasurable behaviors known as symptoms or by atavistic behavioral patterns that no longer protect their owner from anxiety and which themselves begin to be perceived as ego alien and painful. Most neurotics today present with the latter, with perhaps a few discrete symptoms embedded in a maladaptive character style. Both a neurotic character and a neurotic symptom are to be viewed as unsuccessful defensive maneuvers, or *compromises,* in that they invariably express a bit of what they ward off. They are only partially successful at binding the anxiety of conflict. The neurotic character continually imposes his historically determined viewpoint and expectations upon those in his environment, thus ensuring that the traumata of childhood remain the traumata of adult life.

The neurotic is the most sought-after insight-oriented psychotherapy candidate since he is both hurting (hence motivated, unlike the character disorder) and reality oriented (hence able to exercise some observing ego, unlike the psychotic). His ego and defenses are sufficiently intact that he can tolerate the relative deprivation of an exploratory and interpretive psychotherapy.

In this section I shall discuss: the obsessive-compulsive neurosis, or "disorder," as it is now called; the conversion hysterias and the hypochondriacal neurosis, or "somatoform disorders," as DSM-III now terms them; the "anxiety disorders" (phobic and anxiety neuroses); and dissociative hysteria, now called the "dissociative disorders." It is important to remember that these are merely labels to which the patients themselves recalcitrantly refuse to be tied. There are no pure cultures of hysteria, obsessionality, phobia, and so forth. The behavioral repertoire of most people includes mechanisms characteristic of a variety of syndromes.

### Obsessive-Compulsive Disorders

The classical symptomatic neuroses of Freud's day were the *obsessive-compulsive* and *hysterical.* The Rat Man and the hysterical paraplegic, both described in Chapter 3, are excellent examples of them and, rather than repeat that discussion here, I shall simply refer the reader back to it. It is, however, important to note that the premorbid personality of the obsessive-compulsive neurotic is virtually always obsessional, whereas the premorbid personality of the hysterical neurotic is not always hysterical or histrionic.

As previously mentioned, today's clinician is more likely to encounter an obsessional or hysterical character neurosis than the corresponding symptom neurosis. Again, in Chapter 3 I discussed the concept of character neurosis and illustrated it with an *obsessive-compulsive character neurosis* (or *"compulsive personality disorder"* as it is called in DSM-III). These "living machines," as Reich (1945) has called them, are engaged in a host of intellectual and ritualistic maneuvers designed to keep *affect* (sadness, anger, sensuality, and especially warmth) *at bay*. They are "long" on thinking and "short" on feeling. They frequently "know," in an intellectualized fashion, a great deal about themselves, although the italics are almost invariably in the wrong places and the affect is split off. The clinician's task is to get them to *feel*, and he often has to inject a little affect into his comments and questions to do so. They have a perfection-ism that leads to a preoccupation with the trees to the exclusion of the forest. They have definite ways of doing things, can be stubborn when opposed, and are frugal to the point of stinginess. They tend to be immersed in work to the detriment of enjoyment and interpersonal relationships. Their obsessive ruminations often lead to indecisiveness and procrastination. They doubt everything, from their own abilities, to whether their family and friends love them, to whether they turned off the coffee percolator in the morning.

With such individuals it is often easy to discern the childhood neuro-sis that lies behind every adult one. You invariably find that they resorted, as children, to a variety of ritualized ways of repressing or undoing unacceptable impulses. For example, one man's preoccupation with even numbers—avoiding odd-numbered hotel rooms, retouching objects he accidentally brushed against once, being careful to pause in his reading on an even numbered page—began at age five to six when he was preoccupied with the number six. As it turned out, this preoccu-pation was precipitated by his father's long hospitalization for a serious illness. There were six members in his family and this was his way of undoing his, partly conscious, wish that one (his father) or more (his siblings) of them would die.

## Somatoform Disorders

The *hysterical character neurosis* is an ego-dystonic variation on the hysterical, or histrionic, personality style characterized by self-dramati-zation, an inordinate need to be the center of attention, vanity and egocentrism, affective storms, overreactions to minor incidents, dependency and demanding behavior, and a tendency to diffuse and global thinking and affectively tinged judgments. Their language is laced with superlatives and interjections. The hysterical character neu-rotic, in contrast to the obsessional, feels intensely, if mercurially, and yet knows little about the ideas and events to which these feelings are related. Furthermore, the hysteric's conscious feelings are frequently defenses against other, more troublesome unconscious ones. Since the hysteric is "long" on feelings and "short" on thinking, your aim is to help him organize and think more precisely about his experiences, to show him his feelings are connected to specific persons and issues, and to help him understand the more significant feelings that lie beneath.[6]

*Hypochondriacal disorder* is now classified with hysteria, although developmentally and dynamically the two bear little relationship to one another. Hypochrondria represents a more regressive stance than hysteria (where the conflicts tend to be oedipal). Object relations are more disturbed in hypochondria, with the patient withdrawing his cathexes from persons and redirecting them onto representations of his bodily organs. He then has a heightened awareness of even the most minor bodily sensations, which then become misinterpreted as abnormal. These bodily preoccupations ward off awareness of conflict-laden or painful affects and ideas. They can be a response to loss, e.g., of bodily function (menopause) or of important persons (spouse), an unconscious bid for attention or a way of expressing anger, a disguised sexual gratification, and any number of other things. I have seen hypochondriasis first arise following the death of a hypochondriacal parent, with whom the patient then identified. Their unshakable belief in an organic basis for their symptoms, despite all medical evidence to the contrary, lends an almost delusional cast to the picture. It is important to differentiate hypochondriasis from the somatic delusions of schizophrenia and from depressive equivalents.

Most hypochondriacs have had frustrating and angering encounters with physicians who, after a thorough physical and laboratory workup, tell them they have no problems, which is of course not the case. Nevertheless, many of these patients are probably best handled by a patient and psychologically minded general physician rather than a psychiatrist. The doctor must be willing to listen to them seriously and sympathetically and see them regularly, only gradually reducing the frequency of appointments. While focusing on their bodily sensations and disabilities, one looks for doors to gingerly open onto affective and interpersonal issues.

---

[6]Shapiro (1965) suggests that we come into the world with the biologically based potential to favor certain perceptual-cognitive styles. The hysteric, in choosing repression, dissociation, and other such defenses, presumably is utilizing the vague, diffuse, and global cognitive style that was already at his disposal. Similarly, the rigid, isolating, intellectualizing obsessional is simply resorting to his natural mode of cognition for defensive purposes.

## Anxiety Disorders

The phobic and anxiety neuroses are now classified under the "anxiety disorders." The *phobic* displaces the scene of his unconscious intrapsychic conflict from the persons and situations to whom and to which it was originally related onto objects or situations that bear some unconscious, associative, symbolic connection with them. If the object of the phobia is then encountered, the unconscious fantasy is stimulated, threatens to rise into conscious awareness, and anxiety is experienced. This may progress to a *panic attack,* which is characterized by a sense of impending doom, depersonalization or derealization, and a host of somatic symptoms including dyspnea, palpitations, chest pain, vertigo, paresthesias, hot and cold flashes, sweating, faintness, and tremulousness.

If the object of the phobia can be avoided, the repression is maintained and the person is relatively calm. Freud's "Little Hans" is an excellent example of a phobic neurosis. He also illustrates the three mental mechanisms of this disorder: symbolization, displacement, and projection. Little Hans displaced and projected his oedipal rage onto the horse, which unconsciously symbolized his father, and henceforth both feared and hated that formerly beloved animal. Many agoraphobics are avoiding situations where they might be tempted to "step out" on their spouses. A phobia of driving may be a way of dealing with unconscious desires to run someone over.

*Anxiety neurosis* is similar to phobic disorder except that the sufferer is not as adept at limiting the anxiety to discrete objects and situations. Because of this absence of specific symptoms, the anxiety in this disorder is often called "free floating." It is more continuous and generalized. Nevertheless, it is always worse in some *situations* and with some *persons* than with others, and this is a clue to the nature of the underlying conflicts (sexual, aggressive, and so forth).

## Dissociative Disorders

The dissociative disorders were formerly classified under hysterical neurosis. Minor and transient episodes of dissociation are not necessarily pathological and may even be culturally rewarded (e.g., certain trance states and group cultic phenomena). *Psychogenic amnesia* results from the repression of a whole, conflict-laden segment of the patient's history. *Psychogenic fugue* is a sudden flight from home with the repression of one's previous identity. I encountered a young woman (previously mentioned) who, having repressed her former identity, "came to" in the backseat of a car, with a strange man, hundreds of miles away from home. The precipitant of her amnesia and fugue was a seduction attempt by her elderly father a few days after her mother's death. She dealt with her overwhelming disillusionment, rage, sexual feelings, and oedipal guilt by simply repressing all memory of the incident, her mother's death, and of virtually her entire life history as well. Her fugue personality, which landed her in the arms of a strange man, was different from her normally straitlaced demeanor. She was essentially both defending against the oedipal fantasies stimulated by her father (by fleeing from him) and expressing them (by acting them out with the stranger).

*Multiple personality* is the most famous of these disorders. Cases were first described over a century ago and hardly a year has gone by without new reports, some purportedly involving virtually dozens of "personalities." Some of these "personalities" are aware of the existence of the others and some not. I have no doubt that cases of spontaneous multiple personality actually occur. However, the recent practice of hypnotizing these individuals, to "bring them out," can result in an iatrogenic proliferation of "personalities." I observed the hospital course of a patient treated in this manner. She went from an initial vague statement ("Sometimes I feel like a different person") to several "personalities" in just a few days. She was not only, like all hysterics, notoriously suggestible, but was receiving considerable attention from her male psychiatrist, the ward staff, and the audiovisual crew for her "personalities" which, finally, could be brought out merely by pushing imaginary, hypnotically induced "buttons" on her forehead! When one has what appears to be a legitimate multiple personality, it is important to treat the patient consistently as *one* individual, rather than as a crowd of persons. Talking to him in terms of different "personalities," rather than in terms of the disavowed feelings and fantasies of a single human individual, does not promote the integration you are striving to attain.

The last of the dissociative group is *depersonalization neurosis*, or *"disorder."* As the name suggests, this is a condition in which depersonalization, in the absence of schizophrenia or any other psychiatric disorder, dominates the picture. Depersonalization refers to a loss of, or change in, the sensation of one's reality. It may include a sense of being in a dream, in a mechanical state, out of one's body, in unreal surroundings (derealization), and a sense of paralysis and dizziness. Depersonalization is ego dystonic and reality testing is intact. Brief episodes of depersonalization, not grossly interfering with social or occupational functioning, are common in adolescents and young adults. Depersonalization is essentially a defensive maneuver, a means of withdrawing from something or someone and one's feelings about it or him, and particular attention should be paid to where and when it occurs. Commonly it is a defense against overwhelming anger. One patient experienced it briefly before public speaking engagements, in which case it turned out to be related to conflicts over exhibitionism. Many of these patients (like those with panic attacks) fear that their experiences are a sign of impending insanity, and a simple matter-of-fact statement about the symptom's prevalence, function, and lack of progression is sufficient to set them at ease about that.

## CHARACTER OR PERSONALITY DISORDERS

In Chapter 3 I defined and exemplified the general concept of the character disorders. They are maladaptive behavior patterns which, in contrast to the neuroses, are ego syntonic and generally experienced as painful only when they bring one into conflict with the environment. Reality testing is preserved. The character disorders are not without unconscious intrapsychic conflict, but they tend to *act it out* rather than to experience it as symptoms or dysphoria. Recall the example of the psychopath who acted out his unconscious oedipal conflicts by mugging men and raping women rather than by becoming impotent or developing an anxiety disorder.

In this section I shall describe the antisocial, narcissistic, borderline, dependent, passive-aggressive, paranoid, schizotypal, and schizoid personality disorders. The "histrionic" and "compulsive" character disorders were described under the "hysterical" and "obsessive-compulsive" character neuroses. There is considerable overlap among them. For example, the antisocial personality often demonstrates borderline and narcissistic traits, the paranoid displays narcissism, the obsessive-compulsive exhibits paranoid features, and the borderline displays characteristics of the dependent personality. My earlier warning about the dangers of reifying diagnoses is a particularly relevant caveat here. These labels are useful primarily as shorthand communication devices and do not replace an understanding of the idiosyncratic individual. In reality, there are as many personality types and exaggerations thereof ("disorders") as there are individuals.

### Antisocial Personality Disorder

The antisocial personality (formerly called the "sociopathic" or "psychopathic" character) exhibits a chronic history of violation of the rights of others with little or no remorse, inability to sustain employment, impaired parenting abilities, promiscuity and difficulty maintaining enduring attachments to the opposite sex, aggressiveness, failure to honor financial and other obligations, impulsivity and general inability to postpone present gratification or endure present pain for future gain, lying, and recklessness.

The prototypes of these behaviors begin in childhood with delinquency, school problems, precocious sexual behavior, drug and alcohol abuse, and the like. The antisocial individual tends to have an early history of deprivation and abuse and harbors a lifelong residue of frustration and rage about this. Less frequent is a history of "overindulgence" from parents who did not enjoin frustration tolerance, postponement of gratification, and a sense of personal responsibility. Insofar as his parents were sufficiently present to identify with, they often functioned as models for psychopathic behavior. Parental withdrawal and psychopathy are responsible for the antisocial personality's "Swiss cheese" and socially deviant superego. Indeed at times he has an ego ideal that positively awards his predatory behavior. Depending upon his skill and place in society, he may end up anywhere from prison to positions of prestige and authority.

Upon initial contact, he can appear as anything but a criminal, manipulator, or confidence man. He may be likable and fluent, but if you experience him over any length of time you will see glaring inconsistencies in his story and will sense the shallow and instrumental quality of his relationship with you.

It is difficult to effectively treat these patients once they reach early adulthood. The treatment of choice is resocialization and entails months or years in a highly organized and consistent milieu. Working with these individuals forms one exception to the rule that the psychiatrist keeps his own values in the background. Here he must firmly and explicitly, though not punitively, represent the values of society to the patient. In order to minimize our antipathy toward (and jealousy of) these individuals who casually indulge what we work hard and long to suppress and repress in ourselves, we must keep constantly before us the historical reasons for their behavior.

### Narcissistic Personality Disorder

Owing to the work of Kernberg (1976) and Kohut (1971), the *narcissistic* and *borderline personalities* are today's most talked-about psychiatric diagnoses. Thought to be on the rise, such characters may well reflect the decreasing stability of the American family, society's generally increased preoccupation with self, and the current premium on self-expression to the detriment of old-fashioned notions of self-restraint. Both personality types are characterized by predominantly oral pathology, although oedipal issues are invariably present as well.

Freud (1914) distinguished between narcissistic and object libido. The former invests representations of self and its symbolic extensions (productions and possessions). The latter cathects the representations of one's fellows. Freud coined the term "primary narcissism" to denote the infant's sense of omnipotence at the mother's breast.

Failing to appreciate that the mother is an object apart from himself, the infant is posited to see "himself" (i.e., the undifferentiated infant-mother matrix) as magically possessing or controlling—indeed, as being one with—the source of his physical and emotional sustenance. Within a few months, as a result of the maturation of his perceptual-cognitive apparatus and in response to the inevitable frustrations at the hands of his mother, he begins to be painfully aware of his separateness from her (recall Chapter 2).

His infantile omnipotence is destroyed forever, with subsequent triumphs and happinesses in life being pale beside it. If this trauma is sufficiently severe, then the small child may attempt to compensate for it by fashioning an internal representation of an omni-benevolent, omnipotent parent, which he then merges with representations of himself. He replaces the lost mother-child paradise with an internal ersatz of it. If this "secondary narcissism" is sufficiently powerful, it forms the basis for the so-called "grandiose self" (the fusion of representations of self and parent).

Narcissistic and borderline configurations are similar in many respects. The former is thought to represent a more mature and integrated level of functioning than the latter. Narcissism, in the sense of some degree of love of and concern with the self, is ubiquitous. Indeed, life could not go on without it. Certain neurotic personality types such as the hysterical and obsessive-compulsive are overly narcissistic. In some schizophrenics this can reach a pitch of virtually total absorption in the self and its processes. Many consider the antisocial personality as a subspecies of the narcissistic one.

In the narcissistic personality disorder a grandiose sense of his importance and ability alternates with a feeling of total worthlessness and incapability. The latter can be precipitated by the slightest criticism or failure to receive anticipated praise and is accompanied by mild depression or "narcissistic rage" (i.e., anger secondary to injuries to self-esteem). In other words, his self-esteem is towering, but shaky, and requires continual bracing from those below. The slightest ill wind can topple it. Often he denies his underlying sense of inadequacy by the continual disparagement of his fellows.

To support his fantasies of limitless success, wealth, beauty, power, and brilliance—goals that he often does not make the concrete efforts to realize—he must rope in kudos from those around him. His exhibitionism, in contrast to that of the hysteric, is often described as having a "cold" quality. When middle age approaches and his powers and attractiveness wane, he is particularly vulnerable to severe depression and a sense of inner poverty and shallowness.

Disturbances in interpersonal relationships include a sense of entitlement to special dispensations without concomitant responsibilities and a sense that the rules do not apply to him (the "psychology of the exception"), interpersonal exploitation, lack of empathy, and relationships that alternate between idealization and devaluation. He frequently relates to others, not as real persons, but as part objects or as unconscious representations of his grandiose self-image and aspirations. When called to task for any minor delinquencies, he is more likely to experience shame than guilt. When he loves he does so narcissistically, loving the other's love for him rather than the person himself. Like the borderline, the narcissist has experienced such early frustration and disappointment that he is afraid to become close to others lest his monumental rage be evoked by his unconscious expectation that they too will frustrate and disappoint his intense needs and unrealistic expectations of them.

The narcissist's preoccupation with self and with others' opinions of him frequently leads to mild ideas of reference, or the sense that others are scrutinizing him. Under severe stress he may regress transiently to psychotic, especially paranoid, levels of functioning.

In order to counteract any antipathy to the narcissist's arrogance and self-centeredness, the therapist must recognize that he has not chosen to be this way, that he is suffering, and that his most fundamental dynamic is a sense of worthlessness and internal poverty, to which the grandiose self-image is simply a garishly misleading and fragile facade.

## Borderline Personality Disorder

The term "borderline" has become, unfortunately, a wastebasket diagnosis into which are tossed a variety of highly dependent, infantile, rageful, and impulse-ridden characters. Often the term is used to mean only that the therapist experiences the patient as a demanding, hostile nuisance or that he does not understand him. Some diagnose it purely descriptively, whereas others, such as Kernberg, insist that the criteria must be dynamic ones. This disparity accounts for some of the confusion surrounding the term.

The term was originally coined to refer to conditions that look like a hybrid between neurosis and schizophrenia, that appear to be on the borderland between the two. Such patients do exhibit some characteristics of each. At one time it was thought that the borderline syndrome was simply a way station for an individual on the road from neurosis to psychosis. Today we view the syndrome as a "stable instability," an enduring personality organization that does not deteriorate into schizophrenia.

Descriptively, the borderline demonstrates impulsivity and unpredictability, often engaging in physically or socially self-destructive behaviors: gambling, substance abuse, sexual promiscuity, self-mutilation, and suicide gestures and attempts. There is a pattern of intense yet chaotic interpersonal relationships characterized by alternating idealization and devaluation (splitting) of the same object and by manipulativeness. Affective storms, particularly temper trantrums, and rapidly changing moods are characteristic. There are chronic complaints of emptiness and boredom, and little tolerance for being left alone or for dysphoric affect. Identity disturbances around gender, career, values, self-image, and so forth at times of stress may resemble the self-object boundary problems of schizophrenics and schizotypal personalities. Boundary problems and primary process thinking are often elicited by relatively unstructured psychological tests such as the Rorshach and TAT. At times of stress the borderline may transiently regress to psychotic functioning in other areas as well, but such episodes are short-lived and he quickly reintegrates to his prior level of functioning. For example, during our termination session a hospitalized borderline painted her face like a clown, with a big smile on it, and huddled in a corner moving her hands bizarrely. In response to an interpretation about her rage, sadness, and disillusionment about my leaving, she came out of the corner and raged and cried for the rest of the session. Her psychosis had lasted perhaps 15 to 20 minutes and she was reality-oriented by the end of the session.

Kernberg has most extensively elucidated the dynamics of the borderline personality, and each student should read his books.

Such personalities are characterized by an excessive use of projective identification, primitive idealization and, especially, splitting. Splitting manifests itself in the treatment in the patient's alternate *idealization* and *devaluation* of the therapist. It is an activation of alternating ego states, each of which is comprised by a representation of the self, of the object, and an affective charge. The aforementioned young lady had periods of days or weeks when she would react to me as if I were the nicest, most benevolent father and lover in the world and she, by implication, the most deserving daughter and girl friend. On other days I was seen as a cruel and depriving "bastard," and her behavior was correspondingly "witchy" to me. It must be stressed that this was not some sort of multiple personality phenomenon. She retained perfect memories for the times in which she felt differently toward me, but could not affectively connect with them. This same curious compartmentalization exists at times in the borderline's impulsive behaviors, where a customarily prudish individual can talk about her episodic promiscuity, cognitively aware that it is she who has engaged in such behaviors but, for all the affect she shows about it, acting as if it were somebody else. When one attemps to integrate the split attitudes, considerable anxiety results. Related to splitting is the tendency to view situations and people in an all-or-none fashion: either you totally care about them, as a lover or parent, in a way that no therapist can pretend to care about a patient, or else you hate or are indifferent to them.

The borderline's pathological maneuvers, like splitting, arise to deal with the residue of *overwhelming rage, hurt,* and *disillusionment* attendant upon an upbringing that included physical and/or emotional deprivation and abuse. By keeping apart the representations of malignant parent-bad child interactions, the borderline attempts to preserve that paucity of representations of nurturing parent-good child interactions from destruction. One of my patients expressed this in response to my premature attempt to have her recognize her rage toward her parents: "Don't you see? I *have* to protect these people. They're all I've got. If I start hating them and spewing that anger out, I'm afraid there won't be anything left in me. I *have* to believe I've forgiven them."

The borderline is among the most difficult patients to treat in psychotherapy and yet, paradoxically, this therapy is often his only hope. There is no magic pill for this patient. He is treated with a modification of insight-oriented psychotherapy, which includes support, limit setting, and the lending of ego. He often presents with a vapid look, complaining he feels nothing and is empty inside. You soon discover that this apparent affectlessness is actually a barricade against a legion of powerful feelings and against the fear that you, too, will hate, deprive, and reject him. In comparison with neurotics, the transference unfolds more quickly. At times the patient loses his observing ego and experiences a *transference psychosis*, not merely feeling and acting toward you as if you were his father, mother, or other historically significant figure, but at times actually believing it and *acting out*, rather than talking about, his feelings (e.g., by throwing your ashtray or becoming physically threatening, undressing in your office, "shadowing" you, and intruding into your private life). When interpretation fails to control such behavior, you must resort to immediate and consistent limit-setting. Failure to do so will result in a gratification of the patient's unrealistic desires and an escalation of the level of acting out such that a talking therapy may become unworkable and you must then discharge or transfer him.

His central issues, like those of the dependent personality and those of the formerly termed infantile characters and the "primitive" (or oral) hysterics, concern dependency. Paradoxically, this excessive "dependency" reflects, as Kernberg (1975, p. 202) remarks, an inability to trust others sufficiently to depend on them. For example, one patient's repeated phone calls to me were a function of his fear that I would completely forget about him (and he about me) unless he repeatedly reminded me of his continued existence between the sessions.

Borderlines frequently exhibit the aforementioned psychology of the exception. Feeling that they have already been deprived and have suffered enough, they now feel entitled to sit back, be fed, and allowed to rage with impunity. Oedipal issues are present but are intertwined with more intense oral ones. Often what passes for oedipal behavior is a vehicle for simultaneously expressing and covering up what are predominantly oral issues.

They are filled with warm, dependent longings and rage secondary to past deprivation. You will be the target now of one of these, then of the other. Not occasionally, the same behavior expresses both their neediness and their rage: late-night phone calls, showing up between the sessions, and suicide gestures and attempts. They are geniuses at evoking countertransference responses in you similar to those of their parents. Although I am always painfully aware of the role these latter played in their problems, I also come to understand how the parents can at times want to throttle their offspring.

The most therapeutic course you can follow with these patients is to demonstrate, by sticking with them, that you are not a carbon copy of their parents and that you view them as worthwhile human beings. At the same time you must convey that you will not allow yourself to be abused and manipulated and that you have limits beyond which they cannot go. Whatever immediate gratification they receive from abusing you will be more than offset in the long run by their guilt feelings and loss of respect for you. Finally, as an antidote to the rageful and judgmental feelings that can be elicited by their often ill-mannered behavior, you must constantly bear in mind that they have good historical reasons for their behavior. Often, in their more tranquil and reflective moments they are embarrassed by their aggressive and boisterous antics. One young woman interspersed stormy episodes of the most obstreperous disregard for my rights as a person with impassioned love letters in which she apologized for her behavior, asserted that she did not like being that way, and expressed her appreciation for what I was trying to do.

### Dependent Personality Disorder

DSM-III's *dependent personality disorder* contains some elements of both the borderline and the passive-aggressive personalities. These are individuals who have a profound sense of incapability and allow others to do for them what adults would ordinarily be expected to do for themselves. They tend to see others as being the source of, and the potential solution to, their problems. Such a personality configuration usually stems from a childhood involving either excessive deprivation or excessive gratification with no encouragement of, or even with active punishment for, independent strivings. Often there is inappropriate gratification in some areas, such as food and material goods, and deprivation in others, such as emotional nurturance. The parents frequently have unresolved issues around separation and loss which make it impossible for them to foster the child's independence. They often paint a picture of the world as a cold and dangerous place. At times they lead the child to feel that his separation from them would constitute a betrayal that might precipitate their deaths. Such patients are absolved from the demands of an independent adult life and from the traumata of separation, but at a fearful price—their individual autonomy and self-expression. They tend to repress their anger or express it in a passive-aggressive manner rather than risk losing the object of their dependency.

## Passive-Aggressive Personality Disorder

The *passive-aggressive personality* is characterized by persistent resistance to the normal demands of his occupational, familial, and social roles. He expresses anger indirectly through procrastination, forgetfulness, stubbornness, dawdling, and unconsciously intentional inefficiency. All of us are capable of such behavior from time to time. The resident who is continually behind on his paperwork may be acting out authority conflicts with his supervisor. The physician who keeps forgetting to sign his patient's insurance forms may be unconsciously expressing his dislike for him. Passive aggression is the mode of discharging anger of one who feels like an underdog and who fears retaliation or rejection from the object of his aggression.

## Paranoid Personality Disorder

The *paranoid personality* is guarded, hypervigilant, concerned with ferreting out hidden motives and special meanings, mistrustful, and uncomfortable relying on others. He tends to shift the blame for his own problems onto them. He may be pathologically jealous of his spouse, feels easily slighted, and positively abhors warm and tender feelings—anything that might lead him to feel dependent upon, hence vulnerable to, others. The paranoid ideations of this personality type do not reach the delusional intensity of those in paranoia or paranoid schizophrenia. Nor are there the other bizarre signs and symptoms of schizophrenia. What is striking here is not so much any symptomatic content, but a pervasive personality style characterized by projection. They flock to organizations like the Ku Klux Klan, the Nazi party, and other extremist paramilitary groups where they mutually reinforce one another's projections. Obsessive-compulsive characters frequently exhibit characteristics of the paranoid personality and vice versa. Indeed, when obsessionals decompensate, they often begin to look increasingly paranoid.

Paranoid personalities have an uncanny knack of inducing others to conform their behaviors to their projections. Mrs. S., a prim and proper 65-year-old woman, is an excellent example:

Both her brief marriages ended in divorce because of her sexual frigidity and her husbands' alcoholic and philandering behavior. She was possessed by extraordinarily strong unconscious conflicts over sexuality and aggression. Seven years before entering treatment she moved into a large old house at the edge of a turbulent lower socioeconomic neighborhood. She missed no opportunity to lash out at the local youths for their "idle and shiftless" behavior, drinking, sexual promiscuity, marijuana smoking, and littering. She was scrupulously careful to keep her blinds closed and on several occasions accused them of voyeurism. Needless to say, she was waving a red flag before a bull. Within a few months the boys were openly ridiculing her, dumping garbage into her yard, trespassing, smoking "pot" under her window, shouting obscenities—delivering tenfold on her expectations. Her rash reactions only escalated their behavior. Soon she was the butt of ridicule of the entire neighborhood and the local police as well. Now people *were* talking about and looking at her, as she feared.

## Schizotypal and Schizoid Personality Disorders

*Schizoid* and *schizotypal* personalities are often compared and contrasted with one another. Like schizophrenia, the major affective disorders, and the narcissistic, borderline, and dependent characters, disturbances in very early childhood (the oral period) are thought to loom disproportionately large in their genesis. The essential disturbances in the schizoid personality are related to affect and interpersonal relations. Such an individual is cold and aloof, frequently responding to your questions about feelings as if you are speaking a foreign vocabulary. Often they can only describe feelings in terms of their bodily concomitants rather than their subjective emotional states. For example, one man only knew he was anxious if he felt his pulse to be racing. The closest another could come to feeling and expressing warm feelings was describing a certain physical sensation in her stomach. These individuals tend to maintain significant relationships with only one or two persons. Both schizoid and schizotypal personalities may have a rich and bizarre fantasy life, in stark contrast to the poverty of their actual reality. Usually they jealously guard this inner world from the scrutiny of others since their reality-testing is sufficiently intact to know that it would be viewed as "weird," "bad," or "nutty."

The schizotypal personality exhibits the aforementioned traits, but differs from the schizoid in that perceptual and cognitive distortions of reality and bizarre and eccentric behavioral characteristics may also be present. The former may include magical thinking, such as preoccupations with the occult and paranormal, ideas of reference, illusions, depersonalization and derealization not associated with panic attacks, and paranoid ideation. Under extreme stress there may be transient regression to frank psychosis. Chronic schizophrenia seems to be more common in the families of schizotypal characters than in those of "normals" or of schizoids. Many of these individuals would formerly be diagnosed as "simple schizophrenics." Many "residual schizophrenics" may have a picture resembling this one.

## PSYCHOPHYSIOLOGIC, OR PSYCHOSOMATIC, DISORDERS

I shall mention these but briefly since our present understanding of them is so incomplete. You can refer to DSM-III for their nosology. The classical seven are: asthma, peptic ulcer disease, ulcerative colitis, rheumatoid arthritis, hyperthyroidism, hypertension, and the neurodermatoses. Freedman, Kaplan, and Sadock's (1980) textbook provides a good discussion of the historical and current thinking on these matters.

At one time each type of psychophysiologic disorder was thought to be the symbolic expression of a specific underlying dynamic. Asthma, for example, was seen as invariably linked to separation anxieties, rheumatoid arthritis to repressed rage, ulcerative colitis to depression, and so forth. Most physicians continue to believe that psychological factors play a role, along with biologic ones, in the genesis, exacerbations, and remissions of these disorders, though they no longer cleave to the specificity hypotheses. Rather, they tend to view the various psychophysiologic reactions as nonspecific manifestations of psychological stress, mediated through the autonomic nervous system.

Every psychiatrist has experienced the waxing and waning of patients' psychophysiologic symptoms in the course of therapy. Such symptoms are not usually addressed directly. Instead, one strives to identify the interpersonal and temporal contexts in which they occur and takes these as clues to the nature of the stress that precipitates them. For example, an asthmatic patient would wheeze toward the end of virtually every session. This, coupled with the fact that her childhood asthma began during her mother's hospitalization for depression, alerted me that separation was a major unaddressed problem for her. Her asthma did indeed respond to my interpretations along these lines (seeming to bear out the specificity hypothesis).

The relationship between body and mind is far from elucidated. Most psychiatrists believe they are two different facets of a common reality and that hence all disorders, psychical or physical, should be conceptualized as unitary disturbances of the total human being. There is no somatic illness without psychological concomitants and no psychological disorder without somatic correlates.

SECTION

# III

# TREATMENT

# 7

# Dynamic Psychotherapy: General and Philosophical Considerations

This third and last section is the capstone of the book. The theory and evaluation are important only insofar as they form the foundation for treatment. We turn to this at present. I shall begin by discussing some general and philosophical considerations about dynamically based psychotherapy.

There then follow three chapters on insight-oriented treatment, one on supportive psychotherapy, and one on dynamically based hospital psychiatry. This entire section is intended only as an introduction and orientation. If it is the capstone of the volume, it is but a stepping-stone to the fascinating world of dynamic psychotherapy. At the end of these chapters I list several fine elementary, intermediate, and advanced works which devote themselves exclusively to the practice of dynamic psychotherapy. I also include a list of books dealing with more specialized forms of treatment: brief therapy, work with schizophrenics, with borderline, narcissistic, and character-disordered individuals, and with adolescents. Psychotherapy with children is a separate area altogether and is not discussed at all in this book.

In these chapters I am as concerned with fostering a set of *attitudes* as with disseminating a body of knowledge and procedures. The former is the matrix in which the latter must occur if it is to be effective.

Although psychotherapy, broadly speaking, is the oldest medical procedure, the psychotherapist, as we think of him today, is a surprisingly recent phenomenon. Until the dawn of the nineteenth century

**231**

those in emotional distress were most likely to be handled by family, friends, or clergy. The patient's disordered behavior was commonly interpreted, by both his neighbors and himself, as a manifestation of alienation from his community and its ideals. In line with this, the cure consisted of the sufferer's confession of waywardness and recommitment to the social network and its religious, philosophical, or political creed.

The modern centuries have of course been the scene of a progressive breakdown of these small and cohesive communities and their larger ideals. Dynamic psychotherapy, as Rieff (1966) has taught us, arose in response to the Western individual's need for a therapy that would no longer depend for its effect upon his actual and symbolic return to such a community and its belief system. As Freud (1926, p. 256) himself said, "We do not seek to bring him relief by receiving him into the Catholic, Protestant, or socialist community. We seek rather to enrich him from his own internal sources." The psychotherapist is hence the last recourse for many of those suffering in today's atomistic and kaleidoscopically changing world.

As therapists we are the champions of our patients' *psychosocial adaptation*. By this I mean the optimum fit between the individual and his environment: his working with, upon, and at times even against his environment to maximize the development of his potential for pleasure and productivity and to minimize the actualization of his potential for harmfulness to self and others. The therapist is not interested in the patient's acquiring affective and cognitive self-knowledge for its own sake, as a kind of *summum bonum*, but because he has found that such awareness makes possible major and long-lasting adaptive changes. The therapist implicitly (in insight-oriented treatment) and explicitly (in supportive treatment) supports that which promotes adaptation, while giving the patient the *opportunity* to remove, as a result of his new insights, the obstacles to pleasurably and productively being in the world. I choose the phrase "giving him the *opportunity*" because that is the most we can do. We cannot, nor should we think ourselves brilliant enough to, nor should we desire to, force any particular program for living upon our patients. We are in the business of increasing options, and nothing more.

The therapist has been praised and condemned, depending upon one's point of view, now as the agent of society, now as that of the individual. Since he is the advocate for the patient's psychosocial adaptation, he is actually the champion of both. Optimum adaptation requires that the needs of *both* the individual and society be taken into account. Neither the patient nor his community stands to profit from his psychopathology.

## WHAT IS DYNAMIC PSYCHOTHERAPY AND HOW DOES IT WORK?

First of all, the term refers to any form of verbal treatment which bases its understanding of, and interventions with, the patient on psychodynamic theory. Freud once said, when asked to define psychoanalysis, that it is any therapy which takes account of the unconscious, resistance, and transference. Broadly speaking, dynamic psychotherapy is divided into psychoanalysis, insight-oriented psychotherapy, and supportive treatment.

The one attitude common to the practitioners of all three is the consistent attempt to *understand* what their patients are telling them, and in the fullest possible context. At every point in treatment the dynamic therapist is asking himself, "What does it mean that this *particular patient*, with his *particular history and current preoccupations*, is doing or saying (or not doing or not saying) this *particular thing* at this *particular time* with *me?* What are his conscious and unconscious purposes in so behaving? What are the affect-laden fantasies and/or fears behind it?" *All* one's interventions either are designed to get the patient to answer such questions or are based upon answers he has already (wittingly or unwittingly) given you.

The three forms of dynamic treatment are differentiated from one another by the degree to which the treatment is carried by the *analysis* of the transference and resistances (by which I mean the attempt to elucidate the unconscious, historically based fears and fantasies beneath them) and the extent to which it is carried by the conscious and deliberate attempt to shore up, rather than to dissect, defenses and by the use of the positive transference as a suggestive lever.

Psychoanalysis places the highest premium on affective and cognitive understanding and on the therapist's remaining as neutral and verbally inactive as possible lest he contaminate the transference with his own issues and considerations. The overwhelming burden of the treatment is carried by the patient, or "analysand," with the therapist limiting his comments to questions and facilitating remarks and to the much rarer clarifications, confrontations, and interpretations. There is virtually nothing in the way of direction, advice, exhortations, reward or punishment, and buttressing of defenses. It places the maximum possible emphasis on the patient's willingness and ability to tolerate emotional pain and deprivation (of the succors of a "real" relationship) at the hands of the analyst. He must be able to recover, at the end of each session, from what is often profound regression and go out into the world and contain powerful affects and fantasies until the next hour.

Insight-oriented psychotherapy cleaves as closely to the interpretive model of psychoanalysis as the aptitudes and desires of both patient and therapist will allow. The bulk of this treatment is still carried by the analysis of the resistance and transference, with the important difference that the therapist keeps a higher profile than in psychoanalysis—indeed, quite literally, since he sits in plain view of the patient rather than behind the couch. He is thus more of a real person, and his presence has more influence on the patient's productions than that of the psychoanalyst. It is more likely that the therapist's facial expressions and nonverbal reactions will act as subliminal cues, rewards, and punishments for the patient's conversation and behavior. The therapist must decide which defenses to analyze and which to leave alone or even, at times, to strengthen. Because he sees his patient less frequently and over a shorter duration than the psychoanalyst, he must be more active in focusing the patient's attention on problematic areas and central conflicts.

In supportive psychotherapy, insight formation and analysis of the transference and resistance also play a role, but a less important one than in psychoanalysis and insight-oriented treatment. You use your dynamic understanding of the patient's history and current environment to make conscious decisions about which defenses to sap and which to support. You use the patient's transference to you as a means of reinforcement for desired behaviors. You permit yourself, at opportune times, to be more of a real person to him, which means leaving certain aspects of the doctor-patient relationship unanalyzed. Whereas in analysis and insight therapy you are concerned with fostering internal (*autoplastic*) changes, which will then allow the individual to act more effectively upon his environment, in supportive treatment you may resort to active environmental manipulation (*alloplastic* change). This subject is discussed in Chapter 11.

How, then, does dynamically based psychotherapy work? Answering this question involves taking account of factors specific to it and to those characteristic of the "talking therapies" in general.

To begin with, incredible as it may seem, some people do not believe that psychotherapy works at all. Some of these are actually psychiatrists! Anyone who has ever been in emotional pain, some sort of quandary, or even worse, and then felt the healing balm that words from a concerned friend can be has experienced the power of human communication, which is what psychotherapy is based upon. If human social intercourse can be efficacious at all—and I believe that most of the world's population would agree that it can—then it stands to reason that, like other human endeavors, the general principles underlying it can be elucidated and their application refined. This is what psychotherapy is all about: making the potentially and naturally therapeutic potency in human verbal and nonverbal interaction explicit and systematic. The prime motive of clinicians who cleave to the absurd notion that psychotherapy does not work is the wish to absolve themselves of any responsibility to come to know their patients as troubled human individuals.

## Therapeutic Factors in Psychotherapy

I shall first examine the nonspecific factors, those common to successful psychotherapy whether it be performed by family physicians, witch doctors, clergymen, psychiatrists, social workers, clinical psychologists, nurses, or whomever. By "nonspecific" I do not mean that these factors are irreducible entities, that they cannot be explained psychodynamically. I mean only that their operation is not peculiar to psychodynamic psychotherapy. You will notice that the positive transference is the engine for many of these vehicles.

The *relationship* is the most important of the nonspecific factors, whatever the school. The psychoanalyst Alexander considered the atmosphere of good will and acceptance in which the treatment transpires to be as important as the complicated theoretical and technical superstructure of dynamic psychiatry. The power of the relationship is carried, quite apart from your technical expertness, by the positive transference, the charisma accruing to your status as a trained and socially designated healer and, above all, by your personal characteristics.

The most therapeutic aspect of relationship is *presence.* "Presence" is so experiential a concept that it is difficult to explicate in words. It entails being with the patient with as much of oneself as possible, listening attentively, communicating honestly and sensitively, and attempting to grasp him in the immediacy and totality of his existence. It means *knowing* him as a fellow human being, rather than merely *knowing about* him as an *object* of scientific scrutiny. Indeed, since a person is always more than the sum total of the data that we can garner about him, viewing him purely "technically" or "scientifically" is actually less scientific than appreciating him as a living whole. This grasp of his totality of being must be the matrix in which we obtain, and to which we relate, the historical and dynamic data.

Because of our human finitude, the level of our presence fluctuates from time to time and patient to patient and with the vicissitudes of our personal lives. There will be occasions when our minds may be on the golf course, on our vacation next month, on a paper we wish to write, on a committee meeting we do not want to attend, or on last night's argument with our spouse. Much of the therapist's task is recognizing when one's presence is impaired and identifying the factors in oneself (and at times the patient) that are responsible for it. Viewing the client in a purely "technical" or "scientific" mode, as merely a bundle of historical data, symptoms, mechanisms, and dynamisms, as simply grist for the formulation mill, is one of the most potent and insidious ways of destroying presence, of distancing ourselves from him.

In an optimum therapeutic relationship the clinician is genuine, receptive, accurately empathic, nonpossessively warm, concerned, and interested. He permits the patient to tell his story in an atmosphere of acceptance rather than the one of warp and rejection to which he is likely to have been exposed. Many patients never have experienced the consistent caring and interest of another human being, particularly one as socially valued and respected as a health care professional. Feeling liked and approved of by the real person and parent imago that you are is occasionally enough to launch a patient onto a precipitous flight into health—the so-called transference cure.

Restoring *hope* is another of the nonspecific factors. It operates not only in mental healing, but in physical as well, it being well known that medical patients can die from want of hope. As I said in Chapter 4, however, the hope that we convey must be genuine and based on a knowledge of the facts of the case. It must be *informed* hope. The correct stance does not minimize the magnitude of the patient's problems or the struggle that lies ahead, but conveys that it is humanly possible, with a helping professional at one's side, to recover from emotional distress, even from profound emotional distress. As with many of the therapist's communications, hopefulness is conveyed largely nonverbally, in one's tone of voice, attitude, facial expressions, and the calm and confident expectation that the patient can recover if he will work with you. Because of our social and transference charge, we are more effective conductors of hope than the patient's grandmother, best friend, next-door neighbor, or an acquaintance on the bus.

In your attempt to restore hope the patient often meets you more than halfway. Although he may appear pessimistic, he is actually frantically seeking grounds for optimism, however slight. He is likely to have, as Jerome Frank (1974) says, an "expectation of benefit" from the outset. It has been documented that this can be so powerful that the patient begins feeling better from the time he phones for the appointment! As long as these expectations are positive, and yet not too extravagant and unrealistic, they will work in favor of the therapy. Insofar as they are a function of your position as a socially respected healer, mundane things like displaying diplomas and professional books, being housed in a university or clinic, having a well-appointed office, and dressing like a professional also play a role in fostering the curative potency with which a patient endows you. Both restoration of hope and expectation of benefit are in some respects a function of your persuasive, or suggestive, power, which I shall treat subsequently.

Jerome Frank (1974) has also written about the therapeutic importance of the *"sense of mastery."* Many of your patients will feel like helpless failures. Successfully giving you a history and finding they can participate in talking therapy, keep you interested, and arrive at insights about themselves and others provide them with much-needed success experiences. Part of the curative effect of occupational and recreational therapies doubtless rests on strengthening this sense of mastery.

Fuller Torrey (1972) has examined the common ingredients in successful psychotherapy from culture to culture. Among these are catharsis, confession, and what he calls the "Rumpelstiltskin principle." The beneficent effect of *catharsis* has been recognized for centuries. It is the basis of the old adage, "Get It off your chest." The discharge of potent, pent-up affect in a therapeutic setting can provide tremendous relief. Usually one time is not enough. Repeated emotional discharge, accompanied by some understanding of the source of affect, is likely to be necessary. Catharsis is especially healing to those who have failed to mourn a loss or who feel guilty about something.

This last brings us to *confession*. The Catholic Church of course still acknowledges its curative power, and Chinese group psychotherapy makes use of it as well. Talking about real or imagined guilt to a benign and nonjudgmental listener, who personifies, in dynamic terms, the parental introjection in one's superego, can be therapeutic. Most patients feel guilty about something: fantasies, impulses, as well as real commissions and omissions of all sorts.

Often the therapist combines a bit of *education* (another of the nonspecific factors) with his function as confessor. Many people who harbor sexual, aggressive, and other impulses, often toward close friends and family members, do not know that such feelings and fantasies are ubiquitous to humankind. Learning this helps them feel less cut off from humanity, and anything that reconnects us to the human community is, as I shall elaborate upon, therapeutic. Many also need reminding that there is a marathon distance between a wish and a deed. If, on the other hand, a patient feels legitimately guilty about something, such as abusing or neglecting a child or spouse, misusing a friend, or engaging in dangerous and illicit activities, then he is helped by understanding the motives of his behavior and appreciating its impact on others.

Related to, and in some ways subsuming, confession and education is the *symbolic reconnection* of the patient to the rest of humanity. I am not referring to reintegration into those cohesive communities with gripping belief systems that are now so hard to come by. I simply mean decreasing the terrible distance he feels his psychopathology puts between him and his fellows. In the previous paragraph I mentioned the role that education can play in this reaffiliation. However, a far more important factor is the patient's *feeling understood* by you. If you can empathize with, and understand, him, then the two of you must speak the same language after all. You become the first link in his symbolic and actual reconnection to humankind.

The *"Rumpelstiltskin principle"* is a poetic way of referring to what is more prosaically called the *"principle of attribution."* That troublesome gnome, Rumpelstiltskin, was banished when the princess discovered his name. Similarly, there is ample evidence that simply labeling a behavior or assigning a cause to a reaction, symptom, or feeling can reduce one's anxiety and at times even alleviate the maladaptive behavior altogether. One young woman was virtually cured when I informed her that her jitters, palpitations, symptoms of hyperventilation, and sense of impending catastrophe did not mean, as she feared, that she was going crazy, but that they were manifestations of the garden variety of anxiety attack.

Even when one's interpretations or attributions are not completely accurate they may still have a therapeutic effect, in part because of the magical transference potency with which the patient endows your statements. (In addition, if you can uncover a sufficient reason for his psychopathological behavior then, by implication, he has acquired sufficient grounds or permission for changing them.) However, this does not mean that you can facilely throw out attributions in complete disregard of the patient's history and life circumstances. Interpretations, which we shall discuss in Chapter 9, should be consistent with one another and tied closely to the data.

One of the most potent nonspecific therapeutic factors of all is *persuasion* or *suggestion*. Frank (1974) points out that most psychiatric patients are anxious and in a heightened state of dependency, both of which have been experimentally shown to raise one's susceptibility to suggestion. The therapist's power of persuasion derives from the positive transference and the aura attached to his profession. In supportive psychotherapy, as we shall see, it is often used quite consciously and explicitly. In insight-oriented psychotherapy it is generally not capitalized on directly, but is more of a fringe benefit of the relationship and of one's interpretive and educative work. An example of this last is the aforementioned case of the woman with the post-traumatic dreams and depression, secondary to the drowning of her husband (see Chapter 5). By attributing them to her unresolved feelings about her spouse and his death, I contributed to a remarkably rapid recovery. Was what I did suggestion or was it a correct attribution and the encouragement of catharsis? I think it was all three. My statement to her (that if she could discuss the trauma and do her grief work then the dreams would diminish and her depression would improve) was based on empirical and theoretical conviction. I never say something to a patient that I do not consider justified by my experience and the facts of the case. However, at the same time I am willing to accept that, phrased in the right manner, my interventions carry considerable suggestive power as well. Similarly, your quiet but consistent optimism and your faith in the patient function, in effect, as a powerful suggestion that he can both do and profit from this work.

In every treatment—insight-oriented or otherwise—you are to some extent taken into the patient's psychic apparatus. This is the species of symbolic immortality vouchsafed to the psychotherapist. With your consistently benign and attentive attitude, you are immortalized in internal representations within the patient's ego ideal and superego. There you come to crowd out the portraits of hostile and unrealistically demanding individuals from his past. You also become brick for the patient's ego, implicitly educating him, in your interactions, to new perspectives and modes of problem solving.

Finally, certain mechanisms elucidated by behaviorists also operate in dynamic, as in other, forms of treatment. Responding to the patient's fears and anxiety-laden fantasies with a serene acceptance constitutes a variation on systematic desensitization. Modeling is a complementary explanation for what I alluded to in the previous paragraph. The therapist's witting and unwitting reinforcement of desired behaviors (or withholding of rewards for undesired ones) unquestionably occurs.[1]

## Therapeutic Factors of Insight-Oriented Therapy

Now I shall turn from the therapeutic factors common to all forms of psychotherapy, including supportive and insight-oriented treatment, to those peculiar to *insight-oriented therapy* itself.

"How does this stuff work, anyway?" several impertinent trainees have asked me. Every student is entitled to a straight answer to this question. Indeed, he should have such a clear idea of the therapeutic rationale for his work that he could explain it understandably, if asked, to his afternoon bus driver. *Dynamically based insight-oriented treatment attempts to make the patient affectively and cognitively aware of maladaptive patterns of behavior and the historically based conflicts and distortions in view of self and world from which they result, to the end of broadening his options in reality.* This is achieved by educating the patient about his defensive maneuvers, by elucidating the unconscious fantasies, feelings, and danger situations which they arise to treat, and by interpreting the historical roots of the patient's current and transference behaviors.

---

[1] It is important to note that dynamic concepts contribute as much or more to the elucidation of behaviorist principles and practices as the latter do to the former. For example, object relations theory, with its consideration of identification and introjection and the dimensions of history and meaning, considerably enriches the more diffuse and mechanistic notion of modeling. Similarly, systematic desensitization, however standardized a procedure it may appear to be, occurs in the presence of a therapist who represents many different things and individuals to the patient. Its efficacy is, in part, a function of transference and of your introjection into the ego and superego. Similarly, that to which you are desensitizing the patient has a history and unconscious meanings, *whether or not* you choose to examine them.

The therapist's neutrality, lack of self-disclosure, and verbal "inactivity" are all designed to allow for the maximum possible historical, intrapsychic determination of the associations, inhibitions in associating, feelings, fantasies, slips, remembering, forgetting, silences, reporting of dreams, and other behaviors that are the stuff of therapy. By influencing the nature of the patient's fears and fantasies as little as possible with your own interventions, you allow him not merely to recollect, but to act out a truer picture of his past in the present. He transfers, in other words, his neurosis from the past and present outside world to your office. In this current edition of his conflicts the patient, as De Wald (1971, p. 207) explains, has a more fully developed ego, the benefits of subsequent life experience, and wider opportunities for developing solutions to his conflicts than in the original edition.

The more you are simply a benign and understanding listener, the greater is the contrast between the patient's historically grounded expectations of you and their lack of justification by any of your own actions. Being struck by this contrast, the patient slowly becomes aware that he is living atavistically, in the past not the present. This living awareness that his fears and fantasies are more appropriate to a child of three, five, or ten than to an adult of 30, 40, or 50 is the most transformative aspect of insight-oriented psychotherapy. It is the patient's *experience* of this transference and your *analysis* of it, rather than your jointly making intellectualized connections between past and current outside reality, that bypass his relationship with you, that make this process more than an exercise in academic history. Any treatment that bypasses the transference is two-dimensional.

In sum, the hallmark of dynamically based insight therapy, that which differentiates it from all others, is its concern with the expansion of consciousness and the range of operation of the ego, not merely by making conscious that which was deeply unconscious, but by enriching the context of what one has always known about himself, and helping him to know it in a more affective way.

You may be struck that my discussion of the nonspecific factors in insight-oriented psychotherapy is far lengthier than that of the specific ones. It may even be, as some have argued, that the former play a greater role in the healing process than the latter. The latter, however, make the crucial difference between a temporary alleviation of distress and the restructuring of a personality such that one stops becoming the cause of that distress. I shall spend the next three chapters unpacking the previous three paragraphs.

If insight-oriented therapy expands one's awareness of one's motives, how, then, is this necessarily transformative? It is commonly misconceived that therapy functions as a classroom, in which a patient learns about himself and then goes out and wisely chooses to apply the knowledge that his brilliant and kindly therapist has helped him attain, or else foolishly and recalcitrantly refrains from it. This would be as if the therapist, like the lecturer, said, "Now, there you have the theory, the truth about yourself. My job is finished. It is up to you to go down the hall to the lab and put it into practice."

A person does not first discover some fixed and static truth about himself and then consciously decide to change or remain the same, having coolly weighed the benefits and deficits accruing to each. If the balance of forces within a mind has truly shifted, if his neurotically distorted view of self and world have truly been altered, then the patient will change his behavior as a *matter of course*, without any prodding or exhortation on your part. He will change simply because he *no longer needs* his old, unsatisfactory ways of seeking and avoiding (often simultaneously) gratification. This is because *the old dangers are no longer there* now that he is no longer living in the same reality. In other words, since all behaviors (psychopathological ones included) exist for some adaptive advantage (either within the context of the internal or the external worlds, or of both), then when the intrapsychic and current realities to which they are adaptive change, the behaviors will too. In other words, when Mrs. H., from Chapter 1, realized that the danger she feared from intimacy with men was an historical, currently unrealistic one, then her aloof and rejecting behavior was no longer adaptive within the context of psychic reality. She no longer *had* to withdraw from men, but had increased her conscious options tremendously. When she began exercising these options, her behavior no longer induced men to act toward her as she feared. Since men started relating to her differently, her old, neurotic pattern was no longer adaptive within the context of external reality as well. Her changed view of self and world resulted in changed behaviors which resulted in different reactions to her; these reactions in turn made it easier for her to change still further. A beneficent circle was set in motion. Her growth and development did not cease with the end of psychotherapy; rather, they were only just beginning.

Transformation is the true test of dynamic understanding. If an individual's patterns of behavior do not change, then he has not come to a full affective and cognitive awareness, permeating past, present, and transference, of the unconscious purposes of his behavior. You and he remove the dangers and the behavior *will* change. You cannot predict the final content of his choices, but only that choices will be made.

If, however, transformation fails to occur, it does not necessarily—though it may—mean that you have been remiss. The defenses of some individuals are so strong, so cursedly effective, that Sigmund Freud himself could not budge them or provide the incentive for change. The unconscious dangers some fear are so powerful that no amount of therapy will lead to much change. The sadistic, masochistic, and dependent gratifications of certain neurotic behaviors are so great that reality's pale possibilities are deemed (unconsciously) not worth the risk.

In the case of others the intrapsychic dynamics have indeed been altered, but the environment to which the neurotic behaviors have been adaptive has not. In this case the old behaviors may persist or the patient may be faced with the conscious decision to accept an unsatisfactory reality or to take steps to find and create a new one. This is what Mrs. A. was confronted with vis-à-vis her husband. When it became apparent he had no motivation to change and to adapt to her changes, she decided to leave him. When another patient, Mr. Z., realized that his socially self-destructive, "crazy" behavior was in large measure a way of getting back at his parents and me (as their transferential representative) for past emotional deprivation, abuse, and tyranny, and that he needed to express his anger and seek his nurturance in this fashion lest he lose his fragile, perennially depressed parents, he began to experiment with more direct expressions of his feelings and needs. Nevertheless, the real behavioral changes did not occur, despite his insights, until he moved out of the home where his self-repression and ambivalence over independence *were* adaptive.

Before addressing some characteristics of the ideal psychotherapist, I want to discuss a beautiful paradox in the curative nature of insight therapy. To wit, the dynamic therapist concerns himself largely with fantasy, and yet his discipline is the most severe education to reality known to man. Helping people become more realistic about the possibilities, dangers, and limitations of life, and one's responsibility in the matter, is the ultimate goal of dynamic psychotherapy. The therapist's realism about what can and cannot be accomplished in any therapeutic interchange is an important lever. A personality is built up over many years and is never totally reconstructed. Nor does such refashioning as occurs happen overnight, dynamic psychotherapy being a hard education to patience as well. It is difficult to overestimate how much reducing unrealistic expectations out of life—such as the romantic view that the omnipotent, omni-benevolent parent is coming at any minute to make life blissful—frees us to take our pleasures and make our contributions in a world that, at best, will never be without its measure of pain and sorrow.

In short, making people happy is not our business. Our work ends with helping the patient to become more realistic and to increase his options. We may in fact assist him in removing inhibitions that keep him from adding aspects to his life—interesting and productive work, satisfying relationships, new modes of playful regeneration, or commitment to the furtherance of religious, social, philosophical, or political ideals—that may eventually lead to happiness. However, we shall not share the credit for what he has taken hold of, only for that of which he has let go.

If happiness occurs, so much the better, but we shall accept it graciously, as the product of an unforeseeable conspiracy between the patient and his world. Otherwise, we remind our patients, as Freud (1895, p. 351) did his, that "much will be gained if we succeed in transforming your hysterical misery into common unhappiness."

## THE THERAPIST

You have chosen to do the hardest work in the world. Although psychotherapy has its rewards—or who would practice it?—you are, as Sullivan said, simply immature if you think it should be enjoyable. Psychotherapy, like giving birth, is carried through in pain, with the difference that the psychic obstetrician, unlike the ordinary one, is in there with the suffering himself. *No* amount of your own therapy will spare you the task of reimmersing yourself, day in and day out, in sheer human misery. The temptation to retreat from soul-to-soul contact with patients into full-time teaching, writing, administration, or medication dispensation is strong and ever-present. If you are an individual who has a "constitutional" inability to brook the suffering of self and others, who wants to still these waters or dam them as soon as possible, then this is emphatically not your line of endeavor.[2]

Dynamic psychotherapy has been called by some an art, and by others a science. I believe that it is neither an art, although it emphasizes intuition, feeling, fantasy, form, and pattern, nor a science, although it operates out of a systematic body of theory and observation and has rigorous canons of evidence. It straddles the fence between the two. It is a *craft*, in other words, being more systematic, less personally innovative than art, and less rigorous and exact, more artistically creative than science.

Like all crafts, and unlike certain forms of artistic expression, dynamic psychotherapy is teachable. In contrast to many endeavors, however, it does require from the would-be knower and practitioner certain qualities of *temperament*, or *"character"* (in the old-fashioned sense of the word)—and not merely of intellect—unequally distributed among the population at large. Because of the extraordinary power over the patient with which his transference and self-disclosure and your status endow you, you must possess an integrity the like of no other professional. We exploit our patients enough through learning, income, teaching, and professional writing without using them to gratify unmet desires for sex

---

[2]Indeed, if you do not experience, at least once in the course of a working week, the overpowering desire to become something like a used-car salesman, then you are either holding back from your patients or treating people who probably do not need a psychiatrist anyway. Read Lawrence Kubie's (1970) "The Retreat from Patients" on this score.

and affection, our longings to know more about their special areas of expertise (e.g., gardening, the stock market), and any inclinations to entertain our cocktail friends with their cherished secrets.[3]

You must possess a basic curiosity about human nature, defenses against dysphoria sufficiently unsuccessful to prompt your introspection and "patienthood," courage, a respect for the interior life (human fantasies and feelings), a conviction in the intrinsic worth of the human being and the ever-present possibility of his melioration, the willingness to set aside your own needs in the best interests of the patient, and a talent, previously alluded to as "psychological mindedness," which embodies the ability to spot thematic patterns and parallels and to make connections between circumstances and feelings, fantasies and feelings, between all of these and behaviors, and between past, present, and transference. Given a modicum of these aptitudes you can, through reading and, more particularly, apprenticeship to senior craftsmen, practice and feel your way into this difficult trade that none of us ever truly masters.

The ideal therapist is best considered in terms of a number of paradoxes, or seeming contradictions. Synthesizing these antitheses, navigating between the Scylla and Charybdis of these dilemmas, is what becoming a therapist is all about. The most important of these polarities, and the one that overarches all the others, is that between *theory-technique* and *humanness*.

More than to anything else, this book is dedicated to convincing you of the eminent utility of thinking dynamically. You must be well schooled in metapsychology, the gathering and formulating of history, and the general principles of translating your theoretically based understandings into an idiom intelligible to the patient. You must, in the midst of this process, retain something of the neutrality and observational detachment of the good scientist. Yet, at the same time, you have to recognize that at no point are you confronted with "mechanisms," an "ego," "id," "superego," and so forth, but rather with complex, warm and breathing, hurting and hoping, more or less whole human beings much like yourself. In other words you must be human as well. Thinking dynamically is thinking with soul. Freud, Sullivan, Fromm-Reichmann, the masters of our craft, were not merely great intellects, but great human beings as well.

---

[3]Something too seldom discussed is the burden that the secrecy of this work imposes upon the psychiatrist. We function daily as the repository of that which the patient would sooner be rid. The necessity to keep this to ourselves can be wearing. The need to unload a bit of it onto the shoulders of students and colleagues, as much as any desire to teach and learn, is probably a prime reason for case conferences, lectures, impromptu clinical discussions, case reporting, textbook writing, and so forth.

This humanness consists basically of the possession of *empathy*. Empathy does not come from your knowledge of any particular theory, but rather from your own experience as a human being. It means being able to put yourself in another's shoes, to feel your way into his psyche in an uncritical, unpitying, nonsuperior, and nonpossessive way. It is relating, in Buber's terms, to the patient as "thou" rather than "it." It is a talent which virtually all of us possess to some degree, and which can be honed wonderfully with practice. If it is present, your patient will know it and be the better for it. If it is not, than he will know that too and, though you spin the most brilliant clinical hypotheses, you will be "as sounding brass, or a tinkling cymbal," and the treatment will come to naught.

You must possess a combination of patience, forbearance, kindness, and the loving charity that Christians call *agape* and Carl Rogers calls "unconditional positive regard," and yet at the same time be able to set limits when they are indicated and to refuse to let yourself be abused beyond a certain point and in any fashion but verbally. You must be as committed to your client as a good trial lawyer is to his, and yet you must love the truth and recognize that you are not engaged in the placement of blame or ultimate responsibility for the patient's predicament. Indeed, the practice of psychotherapy fosters strenuously, as Schafer (1976) and others have argued, a *tragic* view of the human condition: that people are the products of the worst errors, perpetrated (by themselves and others) out of what are often the best conscious intentions and for no other reason than that the actor, with his particular history and circumstances, could do no otherwise. You must be tactful and sensitive to your patient's resistances and sore spots at the same time that you are not too "nice" to deal with his maladaptive behavior patterns, to divest him, when appropriate, of his cherished defenses against emotional pain, and to withhold yourself sufficiently so that you do not gratify, rather than analyze, his acting out or warp the unfolding transference.

You must desire, above all, to be useful to the patient and yet realize that he is, like all human beings, fully entitled to fail. He has all the trumps and it is he, and not you, who decides the outcome of the game. At no time should you engage in the pretense that you are willing or able to assume responsibility for the maintenance and direction of his life between the sessions. You prove helpful to him by empathizing and consistently attempting to understand him, not by becoming frantic or maudlin. Too much solicitude on your part will eventually prove insufferable to both of you. Some patients, especially borderlines, will use your solicitude self-destructively, as a weapon against you; others will be infantilized or thrown into a superheated dependent-erotic-rageful transference toward you.

If your professional self-esteem or sense of personal well-being is riding on the patient's recovery, then you will not be useful to him. Fromm-Reichmann (1950) wrote of the young man who began to recover only when he learned that she would be neither made nor broken by his success or failure and that his responsibility was only to himself and not to her self-regard. Freud advised Jung, when the latter was becoming emotionally embroiled with a difficult patient, to "First, leave off wanting to cure." You have only to be there with your patient, attempt to understand him, and serenely and diligently pursue your craft. In short, you are, paradoxically, more likely to hit your target if you do not aim directly at it.

You must retain some of the capacity to react, internally, to the patient as would his parent, spouse, friend, or the man on the street. Yet, you must not *act* upon these feelings and judgments, but should treat them as important information about the patient's unconscious intentions toward you and those whom you represent. You must know enough about yourself to know when these feelings issue more from your own *mishegoss* than in reaction to the patient's.

You must maintain a certain ingenuousness toward your patient, accepting his statements as consciously honest intentions to tell the truth at the same time that you recognize they will invariably conceal as much as they reveal. They are, in other words, compromises that are simultaneously expressive and defensive. You accept the husk that is offered you at the same time that you attempt to get to the kernel beneath. Naive and suspicious, "wise as a serpent, gentle as a dove," is how the therapist must be.

You must allow your patient to become attached to and dependent upon you, but always in the service of his eventual independence and separation. You do him no favor by *giving* him "truths," making decisions for him, providing "guidance," and otherwise fostering the illusion that he has at last found the omnipotent parent after which we all unconsciously seek.

You must remember your formulation of his particular case and what dynamic theory has taught you about psychopathology and human nature in general at the same time that you permit yourself to be surprised by the patient. You must possess sufficient confidence in your clinical hypotheses to follow them up and test them in the treatment, while you also recognize that you will never, even in the most "complete" analyses, understand all the historical and current factors in any given behavior, symptom, or dream, much less in the patient's personality as a whole. Nor will you, in most cases, know beyond a reasonable level of assurance, that your particular line of explanation is necessarily the only, or even the most cogent, one. The dynamic psychiatrist, like the scientist, is doomed never to possess certainty or the absolute truth, only progressive approximations of it. You are in the business of *providing explanations,* not of uncovering some absolute truth that is waiting to be discovered. It is enough if your hypothesis fits the data, conforms with what we have learned about human nature, feels right to you and your patient and, above all, bears fruit in some degree of transformation in his life.

As a therapist you must be confident in the worth of your chosen profession and your competence in it at the same time that you recognize you cannot practice your trade without your patient. He provides you with the experiences with which you grow professionally, the information with which you work, and the income that is your livelihood. Therapy is a true *collaboration* between two individuals, each with the expertise appropriate to his role.

Indeed, you must be humble enough to recognize that the patient has much to teach you. Not only does he furnish you with his history and signal you when you are overlooking important issues or proceeding in such a way as to offend his sensibilities, but he has much to teach you about yourself. For example, my patients have taught me that I have at one time or another tended: to try to rush them impatiently into insight formation and behavioral change rather than permitting them to relinquish their resistances at their own pace; to do too much of their work for them rather than allowing them to make their own connections and arrive at their own insights, thus unwittingly fostering dependency and adversely affecting their self-esteems; to behave in such a way as to defuse and circumvent their anger at me; to be uncomfortable with their overt manifestations of dependency and warmth; and to want to quash or flee from intensely sorrowful affect.

As a psychotherapist you are your own instrument in a more complete way than is any other healing practitioner. You bring all of yourself and your experience in the business of living into your consulting room. Not only your theoretical knowledge and ratiocination, but your eyes and ears, empathic resonance, intuitive responses, associations, fantasies, and visual imagery are all called upon. Because your data are filtered through your own psychic apparatus, you must take pains to have it as clear and clean as possible. Areas of unresolved unconscious conflict function as blind spots, i.e., you are so busy maintaining your own repressions, defending against your anxiety, that you cannot attend to communications that impinge upon your complexes. Where distortions in this lens cannot be polished away, they must as least be recognized. You need not be a psychological saint. In other words, it is permissible to have unresolved conflicts and sensitive spots so long as you are aware of them! If you are consciously aware of your countertransferences to the patient, there is less chance that you will act inappropriately on them.

For these and six other related reasons I strongly advocate personal therapy for the would-be therapist.

1. If you have not experienced the difference that increased self-awareness can make in your own life, then you will never be more than superficially or intellectually convinced of the efficacy of psychotherapy. The person who has experienced the therapeutically induced transformation of his own life will not be concerned with all the attempts to statistically prove or disprove the contention that psychotherapy works.[4]

2. You will never fully taste the unconscious until you have experienced its operation in yourself. How well I remember how struck I was to discover that many of my most enduring behaviors had purposes and motivations of which I was *totally* unaware and that many of my fears, feelings, and fantasies were displaced from their original objects to others who unconsciously stood for them in the present. Trying to translate the feeling accompanying such insights must be somewhat like a Zen practitioner's trying to explain *satori* to an outsider.

3. There is a certain immorality and hypocrisy in exacting from your patient what you have been unwilling to exact from yourself. How can you ask him to painfully peel away his defenses, layer by layer, to look at himself with Nietzsche's "fearless Oedipus eyes" and unstopped "Ulysses ears, " if you have not had the courage to do the same?

4. Your own treatment will make you more sensitive to what the patient experiences vis-à-vis the therapist. If you have never laid on the couch or sat opposite your therapist and felt your mind go blank midway through a train of thought, or sweated out whether to disclose some silly, hostile, or embarrassing idea to someone who, after all, you have every "good" rational and financial reason to be honest with and unafraid of, then you will not appreciate that the patient's conscious and unconscious resistances are not merely malicious attempts to foil your good intentions. Finding yourself with intense and "inappropriate" feelings for, and fantasies about, your therapist gives you a three-dimensional understanding of what a patient goes through in transference. In particular, you come to understand the supercharged nature of transference time, of how the therapist's every move is laden with significance to his patient. Only through your own "patienthood" can

---

[4]As a patient, you will not, however, necessarily be more able than patients in general to articulate most of the factors that led to the changes you experience. In other words, you will not be able to link, in mechanical and linear fashion, piece of work "A" to transformation "B"! You will, of course, learn a great deal about hitherto unconscious conflicts and danger situations but, in large measure, you will know only that you talked about many issues that somehow became nonissues, and that somewhere in the middle of all this you began to feel and behave differently.

you develop a tolerance for the sort of dependency that each patient goes through in the course of his therapy and how it feels to be propelled from the therapist's office, at the end of the session but in the middle of an unresolved issue, back into the workaday world, of how it feels to wait out the doctor's vacation or absence. Unresolved conflicts over dependency and their relation to self-esteem are probably the most common reasons for disdain of psychiatric patients. Patienthood means admitting you need help too.

5. Your own therapy will help you understand that what is in the patient is also in you. It assists you in reaching the point where nothing human seems foreign. Anyone who has been through a successful exploratory psychotherapy knows that he is capable of the most selfish, envious, murderous, perverted, bizarre, and incestuous fantasies, as well as of previously unsuspected heights of love, altruism, concern, and remorse. The ideal therapist should hear nothing from his patient that he has not himself felt or fantasized or that he could not imagine himself, with a similar situation and history, capable of thinking, feeling, or doing. The less distance you see between the patient and yourself, the better therapist you will be. The fewer illusions you harbor about yourself, the harder it will be for you to be judgmental toward your patients. "We are all," as Harry Stack Sullivan (1953, xviii) said, "much more simply human than otherwise."

6. Your own treatment will help you lead a more tranquil and fulfilling personal, as well as professional, life. Psychotherapy is draining work and the clinician who does not get refueled in his private life or, quite to the contrary, is sapped there as well, is living dangerously. Taking care of yourself is important for your patient, as well as yourself.

In short, although it is possible for certain gifted, socially savvy, and habitually introspective individuals to be good dynamic psychotherapists without having been in therapy, I do not believe any therapist can develop his potential maximally without having been a patient himself. One who has not known and come to grips with human suffering *first hand* will never be the best psychotherapist.

In summary, although each patient's problems stem primarily from unfortunate interactions between parent and child, he needs more than an improved edition of parents, grandparents, siblings, and best friends. You cannot give someone in the present that which he needed in the past, precisely when he did not get it. You can only help him come to terms with his feelings about it, to understand its effect on his life, to enrich him by the loss of the illusion that he ever will get it and, by so doing, to help him see his options in the real world. If kindly grandmothers and perceptive next-door neighbors were enough, then there would be no need for the laborious, systematic exposition of theory, knowledge, and techniques that constitute our profession. The exudation of good will and warm feelings is not only insufficient, but too much of it can, as previously mentioned, actually get in the way.

At the same time that you possess a strong commitment to the personhood of your patient, you should have an equally powerful dedication to your craft, to your development in it, and to the furtherance of the process of exploration in which you are both engaged. Otherwise, you will not enjoin the necessary sacrifices upon yourself or the patient. You will be tempted to hold out too much of yourself, to promise more than you can deliver, to rush in with reassurance or become sentimental in the face of his pain, rather than maintaining the difficult and depriving (for both of you) role of one who is simply trying to understand and assist him in doing so as well.

# 8

# Insight-Oriented Psychotherapy: Beginning the Treatment

Who are the candidates for insight therapy? How do you spot such denizens? In Chapter 5 we examined this briefly; let us return to it now.

## THE PATIENT

Generally, these are the patients who are most like yourself and with whom you would be likely to converse if you met them on a train or at a party. They are, above all, expressive—capable of using language, gestures, and mannerisms to convey a wide range of information about themselves. They are, in other words, desirous and capable of translating their private worlds into an intelligibly communicable medium.

Presupposed by this is a certain level of intelligence. They should be capable of thinking logically and linearly, at the same time that their minds are nimble enough to make connections, draw parallels, and spot patterns. They must be sufficiently loose and unafraid to let their minds wander, to free-associate.

They must possess defenses sufficiently strong that they need not fear being overwhelmed by hitherto unconscious fantasies and feelings, that they can discuss them without (or rather than) acting on their impulses, and yet sufficiently weak that they are hurting, hence motivated to strenuous work the like of which no level-headed, comfort-loving individual would otherwise engage in.

They must have some respect for the internal life and an ability to recognize emotional states and talk the language of feelings and fantasies. Or, they must at least demonstrate that they are capable of learning

**251**

that language. This is in contrast to those patients, hardly a few, who simply have no grasp of what you mean when you ask "How do you feel?" and who respond by telling you about their belly aches, back pain, constipation, or diarrhea.

They must be capable of a certain amount of regression to more childlike and dependent (historical, or transferential) modes of behavior, but at the same time be able to resurrect their defenses and reintegrate enough to leave your office and contain themselves until the next hour. Likewise, while permitting themselves to enter into a regressive transference neurosis, they must possess sufficient observing ego to be called back to observe and process their behavior—to do, in other words, some of the work a therapist does.[1] This is part of what Kris (1952) called "regression in the service of the ego." A firm grounding, and some success in, at least one area of reality (work, school, family, friends, leisure, community) is a good sign that the patient has some sandbags to carry along on his flight.

They must not be too infatuated with their modes of being in the world, their idiosyncratic styles of indulging and defending against their wants—with their characters, in other words. They must see this character as ego dystonic enough to want to change it substantially or be rid of it altogether. They must be capable of recognizing that their pattern of interacting with the world is in some measure responsible for their pain and predicament and that to alleviate and ameliorate the latter, they must reconstruct the former. Those who habitually externalize the source of their distress (e.g., "the devil made me do it") do not make the best candidates.

They must possess patience and the abilities to endure considerable discomfort and to postpone gratification. They must be capable of abiding your deprivation of them in the form of refusing to enter into a "real" relationship (by analyzing, rather than indulging, their transference wishes) and of shearing them of their defenses against pain.

They must have experienced a sufficiently benign, or at least minimally malevolent, childhood to allow themselves to trust in your basic goodness and competence enough to gradually and progressively bare their souls.

If you have performed a good evaluation, then you can predict, with some assurance, whether your patient can enter into what Greenson (1967) calls the "working alliance" and Zetzel (1956) the "therapeutic alliance." This alliance is the union between the patient's healthy, self-observing and problem-solving ego and the therapist; it is in part a function of identification with the therapist. It entails the ability to

---

[1]Of course, too much of this, as with some obsessionals, and you have two therapists, and no patient!

participate in the treatment in both experiential and investigative modes. Although many patients cannot collaborate in an insight-oriented enterprise, it is a rare human being who cannot profitably develop at least some insight about himself.

## STAGES OF PSYCHOTHERAPY

For pedagogical purposes the continuous, organic process that is psychotherapy is divided into early, middle, and termination stages. Of course there are no red flags signaling where one stage ends and another begins—only a somewhat different "feel" to each. Similarly, although there are general guidelines to the therapist's behavior in each, there are no foolproof formulas or recipes. Indeed, the danger in writing about psychotherapy is that the student will take what he reads as the gospel and use it mechanically with every patient he meets. The principles enjoined here, for the most part, require subtle modifications from patient to patient and situation to situation. Ninety percent of intervening involves *timing* and *manner,* and no book or library will teach you this. It is learned only by falling flat on your face in supervised clinical practice.

Broadly speaking, the opening phase is characterized by *"getting to know the patient"*—his characterological style, defensive maneuvers, that which he defends against, and the danger situations that rule his life—and by *establishing rapport.* "Rapport" means that the patient is beginning to understand you and to feel understood, and to feel that you are genuinely interested in fostering his development. Rapport is established, from the patient's end, by the positive transference and the therapeutic alliance (the union between the healthy, self-observing part of the patient's ego and the therapist). It is assisted from your end by conveying understanding. "Understanding" means not merely intellectually knowing his history and dynamics, but empathically resonating with him (which latter will, if it occurs, almost invariably be perceived by the patient) whether or not you verbalize it. There have been treatments in which the patient's dynamics have been accurately understood, and to some degree communicated to him, but which have failed for want of empathy.

The middle stage is characterized by the blossoming of the transference that was only germinating and budding in the first phase and by the therapist's gradual peeling away of the patient's defenses against awareness of the origins and purposes of this transference. "Working through" begins after the important interpretations have been broached and overlaps the middle and termination stages. It involves the repetitive linking of past, present, and transference themes through the subtly different twists and turns in which they recur. Termination entails the resolution of the transference neurosis (into which the patient entered in the middle phase) such that the patient can take his independent, adult leave of a person who was formerly the most important in his life.

Each stage requires a different level and type of activity on the part of the therapist, as I shall demonstrate in this chapter and in Chapters 9 and 10. Remember that my comments in these chapters concern only the relatively verbal, psychologically minded, and adapted patients who are amenable to an insight-oriented approach and do not necessarily apply to work with severely disturbed and ego-compromised patients.

## OFFICE PROTOCOL

Let us begin with some mundane, but important, issues before discussing the early treatment itself. You have completed the evaluation interviews, arrived at a formulation, taken the patient's desires and abilities into account, and recommended insight-oriented psychotherapy.[2] Next you must establish the frequency of meetings. Here, as in the choice of modality, you rely heavily on the patient's inclinations. For some frequent sessions will be supportive and will facilitate the treatment. For others they would be too anxiety-provoking or dependency-fostering and hence inimical to it.

You must also have some idea of what it would mean to a patient to be seen once instead of twice a week, or thrice instead of twice. Suggesting more, rather than fewer, sessions may mean to some that you view them as "sicker" or "needier" than they thought they were. This could heighten their anxieties about themselves and cause them to lower their opinion of their coping abilities, both of which could contribute to the undermining of ego functions and/or to scaring them out of treatment. Others, by contrast, would feel supported and interpret this as a sign of your interest.

---

[2]Optimum therapist-patient fit—what personal characteristics in the therapist mesh best with those of the patient—has been discussed often. Some seem to contend that only a woman should treat a woman, a man a man, a black a black, a white a white, a native American a native American, an obsessive-compulsive an hysteric, and so forth. This might be the case with psychotic or severely borderline individuals or in brief treatment where, because you want to minimize the intensity of the transference, you might want to choose a therapist diametrically unlike certain problematic characters from the patient's past. In long-term insight-oriented therapy with reasonably well-adapted and reality-oriented individuals, such concerns are, however, usually unfounded. In skillfully handled treatments, the transference will radiate its various hues no matter what the sex, age, or race of the therapist. My foreign residents have been surprised to find that most of their patients who requested a therapist change, because of nationality, ended up changing their minds if the resident was able to resolve his own countertransference issues sufficiently to deal with the negative transference. In short, what most patients need is a *good* therapist, not one with any particular shape, size, color, or personality.

In setting the optimum number of sessions per week, you should take into account the intensity of the patient's resistances to affect and fantasy, his ego strength, and the general principle that for psychotherapy to be truly effective it must be placed temporarily at the center of the patient's life. For example, with an obsessive-compulsive patient with powerful resistances to experiencing affect and any dependent strivings, you might schedule two or three back-to-back sessions per week, making it more difficult for him to avoid his feelings, defend against the developing transference, and keep you and the therapy at the periphery. A patient whose anxiety level you want to decrease and whose ego strength you are less certain of should have his two or three sessions spaced throughout the week. This would be less anxiety-provoking and would require him to tolerate shorter separations from you than with the same number of sessions one atop the other.

When you are in doubt about the optimum number of meetings it is best, as Saul (1972) advocates, to start with fewer and add more if it appears indicated, being especially careful, again, if and when you increase the frequency, to gauge what it *means* to the patient at that point in time. One patient, with whom I increased the frequency of sessions, in hopes of sapping what appeared to be insurmountable defenses against experiencing any dependent and intimate strivings toward me, took this change to mean that she really was disturbed. The walls toppled down to reveal the raging dependent and erotic transference behind them. I had inadvertently contributed to a precipitous regression. More is not always better.

The sessions should be of equal duration. They are generally 45 or 50 minutes in length to give the patient time to make his reentry into the therapeutic ambience and for the issues to unfold, while leaving yourself a few minutes at the end to write process notes, clear your mind before the next patient, and attend to your own needs. You should neither shortchange your patient of his purchased "hour" nor habitually allow him to run past it. If he customarily brings up important matters in the last minutes, then you should treat this as a communication and a resistance to be understood like any other.

Once you have established appointment times you should cancel or change them *as seldom as possible*. If you want a patient to drop out, the surest way to arrange it is to break this rule. Long vacations should be announced at least a month ahead. The patient should be apprised of shorter absences one or two weeks in advance. The idea is to give the patient several sessions to work on his feelings about the forthcoming separation and what it may mean to him. The announcement should be matter of fact and unapologetic. The less you tell the patient about your plans or destination, the more you leave to his fantasies and the more you make him work in the treatment.

If you announce your impending absence or need to reschedule him at the beginning of the hour, you should know that it will inevitably influence what follows—that his first utterances can be viewed virtually as associations to your communication. If, on the other hand, you tell him at the end, you allow him no time to "process" it during the session and you run the risk of his feeling, unconsciously, that your decision to leave was related to his behavior during the hour. Either way he is entitled to his fantasies. Choose what feels best to you.

My comments about your office and bearing follow from this general principle: in order to allow the development of a maximally uncontaminated transference, you wish to minimize the determinants which *you* introduce into the situation. Your dress and office are extensions of your body ego and, as such, convey to the patient all manner of information about you. The less eccentric and the more consistent you are, the safer you will be in attributing the patient's behavior to the unfolding of historically based dynamics, as opposed to any reaction to real factors in you. You are the control, his behavior the variables. This means keeping the same times and places of meeting, not dressing outlandishly or in kaleidoscopically changing fashions, and keeping your own mental status as consistent as possible, because of its impact both on the patient and on how you perceive him.

For example, the male clinician who wears his shirt unbuttoned to the navel or the female therapist who favors short skirts and low-cut blouses should not be surprised if his or her patients of the opposite sex continually show early, intense erotic "transferences." Likewise, if you do not characteristically practice under the influence of three martinis at lunch, then do not do so occasionally, because of the impact both on the patient and on your perceptions of, and cognitions about, him. If noises from the hall, waiting room, or your secretary's typewriter continually barge into what should otherwise be a quiet sanctuary, then you may discover you are treating an inordinately large number of "paranoids." People are resistant enough without your providing them with good reasons to be so.[3]

---

[3]In considering style of dress and arrangement of office, you should remember that as a therapist you participate, whatever your discipline, in the socially prestigious role of physician or healer. This adds additional charge to the patient's transference valence to you and leads your interventions to carry more clout than they would otherwise. If, in the interest of "trendiness" or obeisance to the youth culture, or out of the mistaken idea that you must be a carbon copy of your client to help him, you convey an image incongruous with that of a health professional, you may forfeit some of your therapeutic charisma. Although the adolescent or lower socioeconomic class client, for example, must feel that you can speak his language, he does not necessarily expect you to be wearing love beads or work clothes. Patients who are seeing a physician or therapist generally feel more comfortable if he dresses and behaves like one rather than pretending, in a misguided effort to establish rapport, that he is something he is not.

Once you have established the fundamentals of this collaboration, you should ensure that it remains an endeavor into which the patient's friends, family members, attorney, or employer do not intrude. It should be understood that they are not even entitled to a communication from you that he is in treatment. Attempts by him to bring them bodily into the therapy or to coerce you to somehow intervene in his relationships with them should be avoided at all costs and treated analytically. The idea of getting his spouse's, mother's, best friend's, or boss's perspective on his behavior might be tantalizing. However, whatever is gained would be more than offset by damage to the rapport and by the message that you feel his friend or relative is capable of bringing something to the session that he himself cannot. In those rare instances where it does seem indicated to honor a patient's request that you communicate with a third party, any communications should be delivered with the patient *present* to obviate any fears and fantasies about what is said.

Last we must consider the crucial matter of the fee. Unfortunately, it is the exception rather than the rule that the trainee deals directly with the patient in its determination and collection. All interchange regarding the fee generally occurs between the patient and the billing office. Some therapists retain a lifelong inability to deal with such matters. One clinician, out of training for at least ten years, *boasted* to me, "I never discuss money matters with my patients. My bill and their payment never cross our hands. My secretary handles it all and we are free to deal with therapeutic issues"! Money is an important part of day-to-day adult living in our society and is a commodity fraught with meaning for each individual. That he is paying you for his contacts has a different meaning to each patient. If all his monetary transactions are with the business office, this allows him and you to politely and conveniently ignore that it is, after all, you whom he is really paying. His fee goes to the operating expenses of the institution among which is *your salary* or stipend.

I have had patients with whom the discussion about the fee was a large part of the therapy. Ms. Y., in particular, felt alternately dejected or angry about paying me to see her—the former because it tied in with issues of low self-esteem and with her expectation that no one would want to spend time with her unless he was being paid for it, the latter because money represented adult independence and she wanted to plop in my lap like an oedipal daughter and because she viewed me as exploiting her as did her mother and sisters. Another factor in her ambivalence about the fee was her sense of entitlement to special dispensations because she felt she had already suffered, and been deprived, enough. Often, rather than talk about these issues she would act them out by not paying her fee, by being inordinately late in sending the check, or by periodic protests that I was charging her too much. When she eventually disclosed to me something about her financial status that she had previously withheld, I revised her fee upward to the customary one. Although there was much complaining about this and threats of quitting, it brought home to her that ours was a contractual relationship between two adults, each of whom had certain obligations. It also had the beneficial side-effect of eliminating much of her attention-seeking, hostile acting out toward me between the sessions, in part because the fee was also applied to her phone calls. Therapists whose patients deal directly with the billing office often do not know when a patient is several months in arrears and hence overlook what amounts to acting out of transference and historical issues.

Trainees are generally content to let the billing office set and handle the fee for a number of conscious and unconscious reasons. Among the most common seem to be: conflicts over aggression; the view (for various reasons) that money is somehow "dirty" or bad ("filthy lucre"); unresolved issues around dependency versus independence; low professional self-esteem, i.e., the fear that one has nothing to offer the patient and that hence any paying is overpaying; guilt over profiting financially and professionally (you are, after all, learning from the patient) from your contact with him; and misguided intentions to give him something that will make everything all right—to be, in other words, the omnipotent, indulgent, and protective parent that everybody secretly wants. This is by no means an exhaustive list. The reasons vary somewhat from trainee to trainee depending on his history, his particular conflicts, and his parents' attitudes toward money. For one woman resident, for example, taking a fee had a sexual connotation: "I feel like a prostitute."

Once you have set the fee, and this should be done, of course, in the evaluation, you should treat it in a matter-of-fact way. Do not be embarrassed or apologetic about your charges. You are, after all, a highly educated apprentice professional who deserves to be paid for your time and effort. Therapy is your livelihood and although the patient is offering you the opportunity to practice it, you are giving him much in return. At the same time that you are not defensive about, and cannot be manipulated around, your fee, you make it plain that the patient is entitled to discuss any feelings he may have about it.

## WHAT DO I DO NOW?

Having completed the evaluation, established the frequency of meetings and the fee, and furnished yourself and your office, your next question is likely to be "What do I do now?"

Although, as I mentioned previously, there is no clear separation between the evaluation and the treatment, there are important differences between the two. Though in the former you allow the patient to freewheel as much as possible, while you take a back seat, you are inevitably more active, and the evaluation sessions more structured, than in the psychotherapy itself. You have an explicit aim in mind during the evaluation: garnering enough data to arrive at a preliminary formulation and treatment plan.

Once this is accomplished, an overly strong goal orientation, which characterizes much of Western man's behavior most of the time, is precisely the wrong attitude to adopt. There will be pressure from the patient and within yourself for you to ask many questions and to focus the hours, because unstructured time is anxiety-provoking for both of you. It takes considerable practice and self-knowledge before you can "just" sit back and see what happens, providing a safe atmosphere for the emergence of your patient's (and your own) fantasies and feelings.

Probably the most common mistake is to respond to one's self-doubt and frantic desire to be of assistance by becoming too active and leaping in to help the patient. The danger here is that you will assume too much responsibility for the treatment. Associated with this, you may become too much of the authority (to the detriment of the patient's self-esteem), implicitly hold out or promise more than you can deliver, imply that the treatment will be carried out quickly and that you will be impatient with dawdling, become so real to him that you sully the purity of the transference, and be so oversolicitous that you superheat his dependent and erotic strivings for you and for those whom you unconsciously represent.

This realization dawned on me one day, like the long-awaited answer to a vexing Zen *koan*, only after I had completed my residency. A long-term patient had missed two sessions in a row without phoning. After he called to say that he would be in for the next meeting, I found myself anxiously obsessing about why he was absent. It suddenly occurred to me that it was *he* who was going to tell me, and not I him!

Related to the frenzied desire to be of help is an equally intense fear of making mistakes. Both result in the same misguided attempt to "cure," rather than collaborate with, the patient. To begin with, you should know that you are allowed to make mistakes! If even the most experienced therapists err occasionally, how can you not expect to do so as well? It is some consolation to know that a few well-intentioned errors rarely harm the patient. The human psyche is resilient. If it has managed to survive a lifetime of making mistakes and of being subjected to them, then how damaging can your occasional *faux pas* be? For the most part, your technical clumsiness will be more than offset by the enthusiasm with which you encounter your task. This can even be powerful enough to make your results comparable to those of more experienced therapists—those who may have become overly pessimistic about certain types of patients or jaded in the pursuit of their craft.

Having the patient's history and your preliminary clinical hypothesis securely in mind helps you diminish your anxiety and make sense of what the patient says. It is wise, especially in the beginning, to review this history and update the formulation periodically. The course of each session should be summarized *immediately* after the hour. These notes can then be briefly consulted before the next hour so that you will have the work of the previous meeting fresh in mind. This helps you, and through you the patient, appreciate the continuity of the sessions, that they are a single treatment, and not a disconnected series of insulated treatments, in which you are involved. A failure to do this turns psychotherapy into a "presentistic" blur or "fly-by-the-seat-of-your-pants" enterprise.[4]

Writing process notes is a chore at first but, as explained earlier, you soon develop a remarkable facility for remembering the form and content of sessions. The sheer act of writing these notes helps fix the memories in mind. In time you become able to capture the red thread and particularly significant comments in five to ten minutes of concentrated reflection and writing. Pay especial attention to that which you forget while writing the notes, but which occurs to you later. This often indicates countertransference or mirroring of the patient's resistance to this material.

The therapist's activity level is the most important factor in the opening phase. Good therapists are less verbally active in the early stage of treatment, as in the beginning of each hour itself (which is, in some respects, a microcosm of the entire treatment), than in the middle and later ones for three reasons: 1) to emphasize, behaviorally, to the patient the awesome role that he plays in the process; 2) to allow the transference feelings and fantasies to unfold, maximally determined by the patient's historical dynamics, and minimally determined by you; and 3) to help you determine which behaviors are more defensive, and which more expressive—about the true significance of the patient's productions, in other words.

In short, you want the patient's preoccupations, defensive maneuvers, fears, fantasies, and feelings to sprout and grow before you jump in with confrontations, clarifications, and interpretations. Otherwise, you may mistake the weeds for the garden. For example, a patient who

---

[4]In an attempt to maintain continuity between the sessions, some therapists even advocate wrapping up for the patient at the end of each hour, pointing out the red thread. While this is useful with all patients occasionally, I do not see how it would be beneficial to anybody all the time (except, perhaps, in the most supportive of supportive therapies). If a patient in insight-oriented therapy is having trouble maintaining the continuity from session to session, broaches issues and then never returns to them, then this should be treated like any other resistance. To give your patients something at the end of the hour is to foster dependency and the expectation that you are in charge.

has had prior therapy or who is psychiatrically savvy may plunge right into his Oedipus complex and other "deep" issues presuming that this is what you want to hear. If you rush in with correspondingly "deep" interpretations, then you will either increase his resistance to meaningfully dealing with this material or provide him with another intellectualized defense against a genuine and affective appreciation of how his own special Oedipus configuration operates *in the present* and *vis-à-vis you* as well.

One young man entered therapy wishing to discuss his father's death ten years before and what he termed his "father complex." This was in fact a legitimate issue, part and parcel of the central one, as it turned out. However, at that particular point in time it functioned as a smoke screen for a more real concern: whether to become a patient and accept the particular negative connotations which this carried for him and to open himself up to the conscious and unconscious dangers that this entailed. By not taking the bait and diving into a deep discussion about fathers, the student therapist allowed this man's ambivalence about becoming a patient to develop fully. He was then able to work *backward* from this to the conflicts over, and fears around, dependency and intimacy which led to this ambivalence—fears and conflicts which *were* related to his father's death and his prior relationship with him.

## THERAPEUTIC NEUTRALITY

Discussing the therapist's activity level involves speaking to: the idea of therapeutic neutrality, listening, silence, and intervening. Beginning with the first, I have found that students have many misconceptions about what it means to be "analytic." Some feel that it means turning into an expressionless block of wood or a highly polished and rotating metallic reflecting device. I assure you that maintaining therapeutic neutrality, or an analytic stance, does not entail the sacrifice of your personality and humanity. It is unfortunate, but perhaps inevitable, that in learning dynamic technique students seem to undergo a phase in which, in their zeal to ape some caricature of the analyst, they lose access to the naturally intuitive and therapeutic aspects of their personalities. They go through a phase, in other words, in which they are probably worse therapists than they were before they had ever heard of Sigmund Freud! It takes time to integrate theory and technique with your personal style.

It is true that the insight-oriented attitude is unlike any to be found in normal social intercourse where one generally answers questions that are asked him, repays the self-disclosure of the other with his own, gives and receives advice, laughs at jokes, is occasionally judgmental, praises and blames, offers and accepts cups of coffee, lends and borrows books, and so forth. By refraining from these things you may feel that you are being depriving, even sadistic, to your patient. Indeed, you *are* depriving him of a normal social relationship, but you are offering him something more valuable in return—something which can, if it is successful, improve his entire way of being in those relationships. You know that you accomplish this by understanding his history as it is manifested in the transference and by minimally intruding your own dynamics into the picture. Keeping in mind this good theoretical and therapeutic rationale for your neutrality will help you come to terms with your guilt over what Malcolm's (1980, p. 77) Aaron Green calls your refusal to do "the things that decent people naturally and spontaneously do."

Because your mode of operation is so different from that to which the patient is accustomed in normal social encounters, he deserves a brief explanation of it *at first*. Otherwise, if he is offended, then you cannot merely assume that it is transference rather than a reaction to the novel situation in which he finds himself. You should inform him that the treatment is carried by what he, and not you, brings to the sessions, that the aim is to understand *his* issues and preoccupations, and that this is facilitated by your interfering as little as possible and by not intruding your personal life upon his fantasies and fears. You should also warn him that you will not necessarily answer his every question, but will often turn it back on him in an attempt to understand the whys and wherefores of his query at the same time that you remind him that he is entitled to have and express any feelings whatever about your procedure.

Answering personal questions is particularly inimical to the insight-oriented process. Apart from providing information about your professional training, you should seldom depart from this rule. If you answer any personal questions, however seemingly innocuous, you miss the opportunity to find out what motivates the question and the patient's fantasies about the answer. Furthermore, you have no way of knowing what your answer will mean to the patient, you foster the expectation that you will answer other, more personal questions, and when you do not the patient will be perplexed. In other words, once you start answering, rather than exploring the meaning of, questions about your age, whether you are married, where you live, where you vacation, whether you fantasize about him, then where do you draw the line? If you feel it is therapeutically indicated to answer a question about your life or your reaction to him, it is best to say, "I'll be happy to answer that question, but first I'd like to understand what goes into it, what you think about it."[5]

The most common reasons for unthinkingly and precipitously answering personal questions are probably the resident's conscious and unconscious guilt over "depriving" the patient and his reaction forma-

---

[5]See page 263.

tion against unconscious anger at the patient for posing them. Some trainees, worried about what personal questions a patient might ask, act as if they fear that the patient can actually make them answer a question they prefer not to. They then, in their anxiety, forget that their task is the same with such questions as with any other communication: to understand the affect-laden fantasies behind them.

Finally, you should know that it is possible to be silent and yet be perceived as very much present by the patient; to convey empathy, attentiveness, concern, and understanding without being a magpie; and to refuse to disclose intimate personal details about your life or private fantasies and feelings without being dishonest or being perceived as such or as withdrawn.[6] Thus, being a dynamic, insight-oriented psychotherapist is not incompatible with being human. Indeed, although certain aspects of your demeanor (lack of self-disclosure and analysis, rather than gratification) are highly *un*natural, insofar as being present, sensitively receptive, and understanding are peculiarly human traits, then yours is the most *natural* of attitudes. This is conveyed largely nonverbally through posture, gaze, facial expressions, nods, grunts, gestures and, when you do speak, with tone of voice. Indeed, it is probably true that the most important and most therapeutic transactions between patient and therapist are nonverbal.

## LISTENING

Listening is unequivocally the most important function of the therapist. Osler's dictum, "If you listen to the patient he will tell you what ails him," is truer in psychiatry than in any other medical discipline. It is a sort of "passive activity," or "active passivity," a mode of participant observation that allows you to remember important details and yet see the forest for the trees, to discern the theme(s) and red thread(s) of the hour. This manner of listening is unsurpassedly described by Freud (1912, pp. 111-112):

---

[5]The same holds true for requests such as increasing the number of sessions, lowering the bill, or filling out forms for disability determination. A patient may ask ambivalently for any of these without really wanting them or to test out your ideas about him. For example, a patient, whose deepest fear is that he is disabled, may give you such forms, in part, to see whether you agree. *Always* explore the meaning of such requests before deciding whether to comply with them.

[6]I have heard students argue that the therapist's lack of self-disclosure *is* dishonest. This has led some of them to discuss subjects as inappropriate as their own depressions and suicidal feelings in the past; their doubts, as novices, that they will be able to help the patient; or their revelation that, indeed, they would enjoy sexual relations with the patient. There is, however, nothing dishonest about not babbling about your personal life when you have been honest with the patient at the outset about the policy on answering personal questions. Being dishonest to patients means lying to them.

It consists simply in not directing one's notice to anything in particular and in maintaining the same "evenly-suspended attention" . . . in the face of all that one hears. In this way we spare ourselves a strain on our attention which could not in any case be kept up for several hours daily, and we avoid a danger which is inseparable from the exercise of deliberate attention. For as soon as anyone deliberately concentrates his attention to a certain degree, he begins to select from the material before him; one point will be fixed in his mind with particular clearness and some other will be correspondingly disregarded, and in making this selection he will be following his expectations or inclinations . . . [Otherwise,] he is in danger of never finding anything but what he already knows.

In short, Freud says, your task is simply to listen, without strenuously attempting to keep in mind anything in particular. This attitude, on your part, is the counterpart to the task set before the patient to disclose what occurs to him with a minimum of prior criticism or selection.[7] It is sufficient to mentally tag key statements immediately after they occur and your memory will do the rest, provided of course you do not have organic brain syndrome or conflicts around the particular item. Paradoxically, as Freud (1912) notes, too strenuously attempting to hold on to a point is more likely to result in its slipping away than in its retention. Nor do you need, if you really know them, to keep reminding yourself in the session of the patient's history and the record of the previous hour. It is sufficient that such information be available preconsciously. When a communication impinges on a relevant item in this memory store, it rises to consciousness and a connection is made. Nor need you be concerned about instantly divining the meaning of the patient's every communication and its impact on your clinical hypotheses. This often becomes apparent only after—sometimes considerably after (e.g., in one's study, while at lunch, or immediately upon awakening in the morning)—the session itself. Many of your understandings are prepared by perceptions and cognitions concealed from understanding itself. In other words, you must accept that part of your work (a very creative part) reflects activity that has been taking place preconsciously and unconsciously. If you are not beset by strong, unresolved, unconscious conflicts and resistances around the issue at hand, then your

---

[7]Nevertheless, true "free association" is an ideal which is never attained. There are always, even in analysis, several lines of conversation which could be pursued and the patient consciously and preconsciously chooses one of them for reasons sometimes more expressive, sometimes more defensive. Even more selectivity is exercised in psychotherapy because of the time limitations and less ambitious goals. In Chapter 9 I shall describe a patient who actually used his particular understanding of the idea of free association as a defense, as a means of disowning that his thinking was self-initiated, and as a way of avoiding his responsibility in the treatment.

consciousness will be heir to the fruits of your preconscious and unconscious elaboration upon the patient's material.

In writing process notes you should follow this same mode of letting your mind wander back over the hour's interchange and recording key statements and trains of association. If you take these notes right after the hour, you will find that "evenly suspended attention" is a net that catches a phenomenal quantity of data, as well as the all-important red thread.

Thus, therapeutic listening involves a sort of "negative capability"—of letting go, of relinquishing control, of suspending activity. It also entails dropping, insofar as is humanly feasible, conscious concerns and preoccupations from one's private life. You cannot be simultaneously with your patient and at the beach or in a heart-to-heart talk with your spouse.

The last two aspects of therapeutic listening to consider are 1) what I call "double bookkeeping" and Reik (1948) terms "listening with the third ear," and 2) "listening for form as well as content." Both are dependent upon the maintenance of Freud's "evenly suspended attention."

The first involves listening to the subtle voices in both the patient and yourself. This includes not just listening but observing in general, attending to that rich nonverbal medium through which so much (and often the most important) conscious, preconscious, and unconscious communication passes from the patient to you: changes in posture and muscle tone, glances, gestures, grimaces, frowns, smiles, blinks, sighs, blushes, coughs, subtle changes in the pitch and timbre of the voice, and so forth. This also entails being struck by that which is not said, as much as by that which is: i.e., the ability to recognize when a communication is not accompanied by the affective state that would seem appropriate to it; when a crucial topic from the previous session or a crucial event of which the patient has previously apprised you is conspicuously absent; when a significant individual in his life never comes up, or is not referred to by name; when *non sequiturs* point to a missing phrase or sentence; and when a complaint about a parent, spouse, or friend seems also to be directed toward you.

This is one side of the "double bookkeeping" function. The other is directing that same attention toward yourself, of monitoring your own behavior and reactions at the same time you monitor those of the patient. You should not retain an excessive and anxious self-consciousness that would hinder the therapy. Rather, the object is a quiet receptiveness to the soft voices from within. This requires some courage since many of these voices will be saying things that you would as soon not hear, messages from your own countertransference.

For example, you may find yourself thinking and feeling, "The whiny son-of-a-bitch. What does he want from me anyway?" Rather than, or in addition to, a communication about your own historically based conscious and unconscious unresolved issues about dependency, it might well be a sign that the patient is simultaneously bidding you to rescue him and chiding you for not having done so sooner. If this is the case, you can be sure that he is evoking similar reactions in friends, family, and colleagues—reactions that account for much of his distress.

My irritation, rather than continuing empathy with, Ms. Y.'s droning self-accusations and proclamations of her worthlessness and incapability first awakened me to the possibility that this was more than simply the expression of an historically determined low self-esteem. I began to recognize the accusations (leveled against her parents and me) beneath the self-accusations and the implicit demands that I do something for her. She was, in other words, "throwing her problems in my face." In addition, I became aware of her delight in foiling my too-strenuous efforts to assist her. Only by listening to these still voices from within was I able to help her understand her not-so-unconscious purposes and help turn the treatment around.

Likewise, sexual, affectionate, competitive, moralistic, paternal or maternal, and a host of other impulses toward the patient may tell us more (or as much) about him than (as) about us. Indeed, as noted in Chapter 1, intense reactions toward, and feelings about, patients are generally neither purely countertransference nor purely an appropriate response to them. Since none of us ever completely resolves the conflicts to which we are all more or less heir, neurotic responses are inextricably interwoven with more "realistic" ones. It is not necessary that we be rid of the former, only aware of them. Indeed, since some neuroticism is an unavoidable accompaniment of the human condition and since it is necessary for you to resonate with the patient as would his neurotic fellows (in order to appreciate the *intent* beneath his *effect* on you), then would any therapist want to be rid of it? As Goethe said, "If the eye were not sunlike, it could not see the sun."

Until the courageously self-disclosing work of Harold Searles (1965, 1979), generations of therapists sat nervously and guiltily, each thinking himself the only one unanalyzed enough to want to kill, seduce, tease, and moralize against his patients. Consequently, therapists ended up owning too much of the responsibility for these feelings or suppressing them as rapidly as possible. Either way they could not utilize them as important information about the patient.

Information about a patient may also occur to you in the form of associations, fantasies, images, and memories. Many experienced therapists maintain that *most* of their important insights into their patients first emerge as images and fantasies. For example, when I was listening to Mr. E., who usually arrived several minutes late, the silly tune "Call me Mr. [Dr.] Wonderful" kept running through my head. Reflecting on this, I realized that I wanted to withdraw from him. Shortly after, I became aware of the anger which the impulse to withdraw defended against. "Call me Mr. Wonderful" was thus a derivative of my hitherto unconscious desire that he acknowledge my importance to him. The anger was in response to my frustration at his failing to do so. It was this fantasy that first alerted me to one of his most important defensive maneuvers: keeping his distance and minimizing others' importance to him as a way of coming to terms with a number of unconscious dangers associated with intimacy and dependency.

"Listening for form as well as content" entails being aware of the patient's *style* of speaking. Does he, for example, favor the active or the passive voice: e.g., "I think," "I felt," "I did," versus "the thought came to me," "a feeling came over me," "I found myself involved in." A penchant for the latter can reflect a desire to disown the responsibility for his behavior, thoughts, and feelings and/or an expression of the view of oneself as powerlessly buffeted about by forces around him. Does he speak in a stilted, jargonistic, affected manner designed both to impress you (and perhaps scare you) and to keep feelings at bay? Does he refer to people by role, rather than name ("my spouse," "my brother," "my best friend") thus attempting to keep some distance from his feelings about them. Does he qualify his statements excessively, hedging them round with "but," "maybe," "probably," "perhaps," and so forth? Or does he do quite the opposite and deliver them as pronouncements? Either extreme could be a way of dealing with various self-esteem issues and fears of you. Does he habitually use profanity and if so, what sort? This might represent a "macho" maneuver. The list is endless.

Be attentive to favorite figures of speech. These are not to be taken simply figuratively but, at least on the unconscious level, literally as well. With these the patient discloses some of his most remotely historical and deeply unconscious body-based desires and modes of organizing and interpreting his perceptions of self and world. One patient, for instance, constantly referred to the fantasies, feelings, and memories he was bringing me as "shit." This was, as it turned out, not merely an unconscious derogation of himself, me, and our work together, but an expression of a concern with alternately pleasing and frustrating parent imagoes that went all the way back to his toilet training, where he would give, and withhold, gifts of feces to his meticulous and highly obsessional mother. Thus, this infantile meaning of the very act of talking lived on in his unconscious. Another man, Mr. P., whose most powerful issues centered around his deficient sense of masculinity and wish-fear of sexual-emotional submission to father figures, favored expressions like "being one down," "getting screwed," "being f___ed over," "being ridden," and "getting it from behind."

Closely related to the aforementioned is the patient's manner of communication. Often important aspects of this are not appreciated until
well into the therapy, and are not communicated to the patient until
later still. For example, it was some time before I realized that Mr. E.
frequently spoke in an elliptical manner and that, when I spoke to the
content or asked for clarification, he would gleefully reproach me for not
understanding him. It eventually became apparent to both of us that a
part of him did not want to be understood for a variety of reasons,
including: the fear that I would gain the power to manipulate him to my
own ends; the feeling that I would then be superior to him; the fear that I
would feel I had totally explained him and view him as a static and
prosaic entity; and, most important of all, the fear that, if I understood
him, he would then feel closer to me.

The nonverbal manifestations of a patient's style are just as, or more,
important. They can function defensively, expressively or, more often,
as compromises. What we mean when we refer to verbal and nonverbal
patterns of coming to terms with drives and defenses is "character" of
course. Refer back to my discussion of how Mr. E's character manifested
itself (in Chapter 3) and to the mental status examination section in
Chapter 5.

Symptoms may "talk" to you as well. If one of the patient's symptoms
is a nervous cough that embarrasses his public speaking, then pay
particular attention to it when it arises in the therapy. Note what you
were discussing before the cough and what arises after it. This, coupled
with the history of the symptom (which you have presumably already
obtained), will tell you a good deal about its function. Mr. P. would
describe transient depersonalization, like clockwork, when he found
himself in a submissive position vis-à-vis authority figures—a symptom
going back to the times when his father would "belt" him for "misbe-
havior." This, it eventually turned out, was a way of warding off
unconscious murderousness, as well as the actual desire to passively
acquiesce to the father and his imagoes (including me). Psychosomatic
symptoms may also speak to you in the course of the session. One
woman often wheezed toward the end of the hour or when dealing with
issues of loss and separation.

Finally, you must oscillate, when appropriate, between the more
experiential mode of evenly hovering attention and double bookkeeping
and a more problem-solving and theoretical mode. It is in this latter that
you review and analyze what you have gleaned from experience and
observation and prepare it for communication to the patient in a theoretically correct and intelligible form. Similarly, when you intervene in
this mode you are recalling the patient from his experiential position to a
momentarily self-observing and investigative one. You will save yourself heartache if you accept that learning to function smoothly in these
various modes takes considerable time.

## SILENCE

It is impossible to discuss the patient's communications and the therapist's interventions without first considering the ground against which they appear—silence. One of the novice therapist's supreme fears, like his patient's, is that of silence. The student's reactions to this fear are often responsible for inappropriate interventions. A few seconds' silence can seem, literally, to both patient and therapist, like many minutes or, in the case of the supervisee who said "none of our silences lasted for more than 10 or 15 *sessions* [he meant to say *seconds*]," even longer. "How do I keep things going?" you ask.

Apart from its psychodynamic roots, which vary from therapist to therapist, this concern about silence stems from normal social intercourse where the aim is to keep the conversation going (albeit often to avoid direct and honest communication) and where silence is viewed as a failure on the part of one or both parties. The resultant anxiety would then, like all anxiety, have what Sullivan has termed a "disjunctive effect" on the relationship. The need to "keep things going" is also a function of the traditional doctor-patient relationship, where the former assumes an inordinate amount of responsibility for the interaction and treatment.

It is in fact the *patient's* responsibility to bring the material to the session, and do so he will in one form or another. He does not always have to be talking in order to communicate. He also "talks" with his silences, his facial expressions, and gestures. As Freud (1901, pp. 77-78) said:

> He that has eyes to see and ears to hear may convince himself that no mortal can keep a secret. If his lips are silent, he chatters with his fingertips; betrayal oozes out of him at every pore.

Thus, a patient's silence is a communication to be understood just like any other. It is also, as discussed subsequently, a defense or resistance and, like all resistance, is as much the "content" of therapy as that which lies beneath it. The treatment of silences involves a division of labor. The patient brings the material. "All" you do is listen and get him to teach you what it means.

By not rushing in to fill up a silence, you convey to the patient his awesome responsibility for the treatment. If he is uneasy with the silence, as he will invariably be, whether or not he is conscious of it, then ask him to help you understand, first, the nature of his discomfort and, next, the fears and fantasies behind it.

The patient is entitled to an empathic appreciation of the difficulties of a silence. This should be acknowledged explicitly in the beginning: "Yes, I understand you feel uncomfortable. People commonly feel uncomfortable during silences, but the discomfort is never exactly the same from person to person. What I need to know is what *your* discomfort is like." If he looks to you to fill the silence you might add that the aim is not to prevent silences from developing but to understand his current preoccupations, and that this is best done by your interfering as little as possible with *his* work. You can reassure him that, when you have something to say, you will communicate it to him.

After the first few times no explanations are indicated and you should proceed directly to an attempt to understand the nature and origin of the patient's fears, fantasies, and feelings. Usually it is best to wait out a silence unless it appears the patient's anxiety might drive him out the door. If you do so you can then treat what emerges as an untainted manifestation of his internal dynamics rather than a response to any particular stimulus from your side. Pay especial attention to the form and content of the silence-breaking communication. When you couple this with your remembrance of what was said immediately before the silence began, then you have two powerful clues to the nature of the affect-laden complex that was impinged upon and that led to the silence.[8]

When confronted with a silence you ask yourself the same question you pose to every one of the patient's behaviors: "What does it mean that he, with his particular history, is doing this with me right now? What are his purposes?" Keeping in mind what you have learned about conflict theory will help you get your patient to answer this question.

A silence is, in essence, an unconscious resistance to appreciating the full affective and cognitive significance of an unconscious intrapsychic conflict. It is, at the same time, often a more conscious "resistance" or, more accurately, "refusal," to communicate what one already knows about the derivatives of this conflict. This is invariably because full conscious awareness of the material and its communication to you are associated with one or a number of danger situations. Freud believed that a patient's conscious and unconscious feelings, fears, and fantasies about his clinician were lurking somewhere in the background of every silence. The patient splits off and projects a part of his own intrapsychic life onto you and then reacts as if the danger comes from without rather than from within. He may, for example, project a bit of previously

---

[8]Of course there are times, apart from any concerns about a too rapidly escalating anxiety level, when you might want to break the silence yourself. If it appears, particularly in the early stage of therapy, that the silence is going to last the whole session, it might seem to the patient that you are uninterested if you do not query him. In such a case you would say, "What sort of silence is this?" "What has been going through your mind?" Another case would be when, in the midst of an otherwise uneventful silence, a patient appears struck by a particular thought or feeling. If he does not spontaneously share this with you it is good to ask, "What is on your mind just now?" lest it be lost.

internalized parental judgment (of superego, in other words) onto you and act as if he could expect, if he disclosed what he was thinking or feeling, the same treatment from you.

How you deal with this resistance depends on whether the patient is consciously withholding, out of conscious *and* unconscious fears of your reaction to any disclosure, or whether he is genuinely unconscious of the motives of his silence. No matter which, you begin by inducing the patient to elucidate the nature of his silence: what it "feels like." Then, if it appears he is consciously withholding, you ask him how he fantasizes you would act, and he would feel, if he told you. You speak, in other words, to the danger situation that motivates the defensive maneuver of silence. If you do so, the patient will usually begin to talk. If not, then be patient.

If the patient makes it plain that he is consciously aware of the derivatives and associated dangers that he is warding off and he says, "I *can't* talk about it," then you should convey an empathic appreciation of his plight. "This must be a very difficult issue for you if you feel you can't talk about it."

The other case, that in which the patient is unconscious of the danger, the fantasy and feeling, and the defensive purposes of his silence, is more difficult. You approach this by asking him what was in mind during the silence—not "Was *anything* in mind?" or "Does *anything* occur to you?" but "*What* was in mind?" or "*What* occurs to you?" In other words, you assume *something* was in mind. To do otherwise would be to abet his resistance. If the patient says "nothing, absolutely nothing," you can inform him that the waking (and the sleeping) mind is always at work, thinking, feeling, and receiving and processing information from the environment. You can apprise him that his perceptions, thoughts, and feelings are often delicate and fleeting and can be experienced and recalled only with difficulty, but that at other times he is quite aware of them and yet they are adjudged too trivial, silly, or embarrassing to mention. Invite him to reflect back over his silence and tell you whether he found himself daydreaming, thinking of someone or somewhere else, or merely looking around your office at the books, a particular picture, out the window, and so forth. Failing this, ask him to sit back and talk about whatever comes to mind.

If your patient responds to a direct question with silence, it is particularly advisable to wait it out. If you immediately re-pose it, he may interpret this as a sign that you are impatient or irritated.

If your discomfort with silences—whether in general or with some patient in particular—does not abate with time and practice, then you must launder your soul to wash out the conflict-laden fantasies and feelings, coming from your own history and stimulated by the patient, that are making you anxious.

## INTERVENTIONS

I shall begin this section with a discussion of the therapist's counterpart to the patient's silences: knowing when to keep quiet. This is more important than knowing when to speak. To appropriately refrain from speaking is, as Schafer (1976) points out, a strenuous activity and not merely the absence of action. The young therapist must constantly fight the tendency to blurt out the first thing he thinks of. Again, the most important theoretical reason for this is to permit the development of a maximally internally determined transference neurosis. The most important "practical" reason is to emphasize to the patient his responsibility in the treatment.

I have often observed a well-intentioned novice tramp down in the midst of a beautifully budding garden of affect, heavily laden with ill-timed observations and interpretations. Unless it appears the patient is utterly unaware of the feelings that are unfolding, you need not jump in immediately to label them. Rather, allow them to blossom, permit him to savor them, nonverbally empathize with him, and then you can, if it appears appropriate, comment on them and invite him to help you understand their roots. You must first get the *feelings* out in the open before you can pursue motives, defenses, danger situations, and such. To do otherwise makes therapy a sterile, intellectualized procedure.

Although there are times when your patient will feel relieved when you inadvertently crash into a fledgling feeling, at other times he will feel irritated and intruded upon. The commonest reason for barging into your patient's affects will be your own discomfort with the corresponding feelings in yourself. If you cannot tolerate warm, sad, angry, sensual, and other affects in yourself, then you will consciously and unconsciously try to forestall their emergence in the patient.

Another important reason to keep silent is to avoid abetting the patient's defenses by giving him a premature interpretation or comment, which can then function as a new defense (an intellectualization) against a genuine and deeper understanding. This not only brings the discussion to a false and premature closure, but panders to his conscious-unconscious illusion that he has at last found the omnipotent parent-healer-guru. If you are or have been a patient, you will recall times when you have longed for your clinician to murmur the magic word and banish your conflict and discomfort, thereby obviating the need to go into embarrassing detail and to stay in the patient role and spend your money. When he does not, and you, despite your righteous indignation at his "malicious deprivingness," find yourself surprised and overwhelmed by what emerges, then you will be thankful many times over that he had the presence of mind to be quiet, to stay out of the way of your work. It is only through the therapist's judicious silences that patients become aware of some of their most powerful conflicts.

In general, as stated previously, good therapists are less verbally active earlier in the hour, more active toward the end. It is best to allow the patient to begin the session in order to form a clear idea of his immediate concerns and to influence the direction of conversation as little as possible. What arises often presages the red thread of the hour and continues one from the prior one. Even when important issues remain unresolved from the previous meeting, it is best to wait and see whether he will bring them up. If he does not, then you will have a gauge to the charge of the conflict, danger situation, and resistance and can then bring them up yourself (or not, as the situation warrants) along with a comment to, or query about, his failure to do so.[9]

When therapy is going well the patient's associations are flowing, he is making connections, and there is no need for you to say anything. It is like midwifery in which, in normal presentations, the clinician stands back and lets the patient do the labor, coming in only when there is some obstruction to an otherwise natural and spontaneous process. In the ideal delivery, as in the ideal psychotherapy, the clinician intervenes little. You come in only when there is a block in the train of associations—in the experiencing of ideas and affects. Even then you do not always intervene right away, as I illustrated in the discussion of silences.

You are, preeminently, a *facilitator*, more so in the earlier phase of therapy than in the middle and later. To reiterate, this is so because you wish to interfere minimally with the germinal transference, with the emerging drive derivatives and defensive patterns. This is also true for at least three more reasons: First, until you come to know the patient you will have no idea what any given intervention will *mean* to him, how he will react to it, whether it will decrease or increase his resistance. Furthermore, you cannot make the same comment to two different people in the same way. What is acceptable to one might be deplorable to the other. You must learn how to talk to each patient in turn, and if you listen he will teach you. Second, you must establish rapport *before* doing much clarifying and certainly before confronting and interpreting. It is easier to hear things about ourselves from those for whom we care and who we feel care for us than from enemies or total strangers.

Third, the patient is psychologically unprepared for confrontations and, especially, interpretations in the beginning. We address the patient's resistances and conflictual feelings only as he indicates his will-

---

[9]Pay particular attention to comments that a patient drops as he walks out the door, if he meets you in the hall or happens upon you between sessions, and as he enters the office. This applies also to his verbal and nonverbal manner of greeting and taking leave of you. Such comments are often especially revealing of his expressive-defensive style since he mistakenly considers them off limits to the therapy and hence may drop his guard a bit. However, this is information you store away for use at an appropriate future date. To comment on it too early is definitely countertherapeutic.

ingness to deal with them. To do so prematurely is to heighten the resistance, delay the unfolding of the work, and hamper the development of the therapeutic alliance.

Speaking prematurely to these defenses, the danger situations that motivate them, and the fantasies and feelings beneath them is futile anyway since they are *unconscious*. Material does not move directly from unconsciousness to consciousness, but rather from preconsciousness to conscious awareness. To speak directly to a totally unconscious issue will elicit no response at all at best, and anger, ridicule, or panic at worst. Whatever the patient's reaction, you can be certain that you have increased his resistance to dealing with the item in question. You have put him on his guard and made him suspicious of you. For the same reason you should not comment upon the patient's characterological style, expressive-defensive mannerisms, and nonverbal communications. This augments his self-consciousness and decreases his spontaneity. Such comments, if made at all, should be reserved for the later stages of therapy. Nor should you speak to the dawning transference too soon lest you have the same effect or scare him out of treatment. (When you do begin speaking to it, do not immediately connect it to its historical determinants because you will defuse the intensity of his feelings in the present and make him think you are trying to explain them away.)

For example, Mr. E., to whom I have referred several times, had powerful defenses against acknowledging warm and intimate feelings for people. His self-esteem was so low, and sense of vulnerability to rejection so great, that he refused to acknowledge the importance of anyone to him. He treated me arrogantly, became indignant whenever a question or comment implied someone was significant to him, and generally attempted to avoid experiencing any feelings whatsoever. It was some months before I felt he was dropping his shield sufficiently to begin viewing me as important to him. Had I labeled his behavior at this point I would have destroyed the incipient rapport. It would have been too great a threat to his self-esteem. By waiting patiently I was eventually able to gingerly offer observations and comments speaking to his need to avoid feelings and to minimize the role of people in his life.

Apart from the theoretical rationale for soft-pedaling interpretations early in therapy, there is a quasi-moral one. To wit, it has taken the patient years of hard work to erect his defenses. They are not merely psychopathological, but represent the patient's best effort, on his own, to come to some sort of equilibrium within himself and with his environment. You do not crash into such cherished and time-honored possessions. It is a cruel imposition to ask the patient to relinquish them prematurely, before he no longer needs them. Above all you must not view his resistances as a recalcitrant affront, as a challenge to your competence as a therapist.

It is common, for example, that apprentices to our craft present to a therapist announcing they wish to enter "treatment" (although they almost never use this word) for "professional" reasons, to learn about transference, conflict, the unconscious, and so forth. This is virtually always a rationalization for the more important, conscious and unconscious, underlying reasons. However, you gain nothing by rushing in to make the patient cry "uncle," to own up to his "real" motives. Such a patient is implicitly telling you, "The very idea that I might need *treatment*, like my patients, is so threatening to my self-esteem right now that I must cling to a partial truth *without which I would feel too uncomfortable to enter therapy with you."* It is sufficient that you take a history, listen to him, and provide such a safe and empathic environment that he will eventually give you the custard beneath the meringue.

For all these reasons your early comments are generally limited to facilitative ones. These can be divided, roughly, into *reflections, questions, confrontations,* and *clarifications.* When a therapist begins to engage in the latter two, it is a sign that he and the patient are moving from the opening to the middle phase. Before discussing each of these in turn, I shall mention talking to patients in general.

If you are in doubt about the propriety or timeliness of a particular intervention, then the rule of thumb is to *refrain from it.* Errors of omission are far better than those of commission. It is easier to comment upon something the second time around (and the important subjects *will* turn up again) than to attempt to undo the effects of something once said. Another good rule of thumb, as Kernberg suggests, is to avoid intervening when you are angry at the patient. Wait until the anger subsides. The novice's most common response to the first mistake is trying to undo it with others, to save face by means of a flurry of erroneous verbiage, thus appearing more foolish and abrasive, not less.

Since unexpressed or misplaced affect is the single greatest problem with which the insight-oriented therapist is faced, any style of talking that facilitates expression of feelings is good, any that interferes with it bad. You should not use stilted words or psychiatric jargon. Such words rip the guts out of feelings. Speak plainly. Say "mad," not "irritated"; "sad," not "melancholic"; "frustrated," not "discommoded"; "hard," not "difficult." The more you do this, the more difficult it will be for the patient to avoid his feelings.

Your interventions should be clear and succinct. A good therapist, like a good writer, makes his point as graphically and with as few words as feasible. Count your syllables. By so doing you not only minimize your determination of the patient's behavior but make the words you do deliver as thought- and feeling-provoking as possible. In line with this, *cultivate a vocabulary of nonverbal communications:* nods, gestures, grunts, knowing and questioning gazes, and so forth. They will take you a long way.

Your comments, clarifications, confrontations, and interpretations should not be dogmatic and yet, when you are fairly certain of them, they must carry some ring of conviction. Otherwise, you allow the patient to escape too easily from your observation. When the evidence suggests he is angry at you and you feel it is probably not unconscious, then do not be put off by his first lukewarm denial. Follow it up. If, on the other hand, your idea is tentative, put it forward in that spirit and yet in one that invites the patient to seriously consider it.

Although you wish to minimize your intrusiveness upon, and structuring of, the patient's conversation (particularly in the early stage), you cannot, nor should you wish to, avoid this altogether. The most verbally passive psychoanalyst exercises selectivity in what he comments upon and what he requests clarification about, when he focuses the patient's attention to a topic the analyst feels he is avoiding, when he reminds him of something he said earlier, and so forth. And you are involved in a more verbally active interchange than psychoanalysis.

## Reflections

I shall begin with the least intrusive interventions and proceed to the more intrusive ones. *Reflections* and *questions* are undoubtedly the most useful maneuvers in the opening phase and throughout the entire therapy as well. They encroach the least on the patient's dynamics and implicitly convey that the answers will come from him and not you.

*Reflection* of the patient's key words and phrases or of whole sentences back to him is the least intrusive of all the modes. It is a way of demonstrating your interest in his elaborating on a certain score. When doing so you must be careful to be an accurate reporter. There is nothing more irritating than to be misquoted by one's therapist. Quoting your patient accurately, on the other hand, conveys that you take him seriously enough to remember and value his own words. For example, "You say she told you she couldn't go," "You say you felt strongly about that," or "You didn't know how to take what he said." Reflections uttered with a rising inflection border on questions or even confrontations. For example, "You didn't feel *anything* about *that*?" "You don't care one way or the other?" Of course, if reflections are overused they can lose their effectiveness and lead you to sound like a parrot.

## Questions

There is something to be gained from likening your patient to a literary text and yourself to the interpreter. He is a "living human document," as Boisen (1939) has termed him, with whom you are in dialogue in an attempt to discern the maximum possible meaning from the passages in his life. In this never-ending quest for meaning, questions are your primary armament.

Questions accomplish more than inviting your patient to teach you more about himself and about human nature in general. They also convey your empathy and understanding of the ramifications of any given issue. They communicate your interest in, and valuing of, his inner life. They also inform the patient about the nature of the treatment and the sort of information that is necessary for its furtherance.

Like all other interventions, questions should be used only when necessary to facilitate a patient's discussion of a particular issue. Indeed, when the resistances are diminished and the therapeutic alliance is strong, then you do not need to ask questions or do anything except listen empathically. Every question is to some extent addressed to a resistance, however minor. In other words, the frequency of questions is directly proportional to the strength of the resistance and inversely proportional to the strength of the therapeutic alliance. When the resistance is down and the therapeutic alliance is up, the patient is doing most of your work for you.

When the patient is in the midst of an important topic, about which you want to know more in general or to be apprised about some piece of information in particular, first wait awhile and let him talk. He may spontaneously reveal that which you are seeking. (It is always better when he does so because you want to avoid a question-and-answer format in which he continually looks to you for cues about what to discuss.) If he does not, then by all means ask for it. Many trainees forget that the most common reason a piece of information is not available is that it was not requested in the first place. There are important matters which a patient will never disclose to you unless you ask.

Initial questions are keyed toward understanding the *phenomenology* of the patient's world. You want him to paint as graphic a picture of it as possible. You want him to tell his story with as much nuance and richness of detail and feeling as possible. At this point you are interested in *how it feels* to be him and not in what *causes*, or *motivates*, his behaviors (in what his purposes and intentions are). Because of this you should, as I mentioned, minimize "why" questions in the early treatment. There is plenty of time for cognitive understanding *after* his experience has been revealed. We shall discuss questions about motivation or purpose in Chapter 9.

Such interventions can be phrased as direct questions: "What was that like?" "How do you feel?" "What else [not *"was anything* else . . ."] was going on then?" They can be presented as statements, or implicit requests: "I wonder if that's all there is to it." "I'd like to hear more about that." Or they can be benign imperatives: "Tell me more about that." They may even be communicated nonverbally with a grunt, gesture, glance, nod, or change in posture.

In order to stay as close as possible to the patient's productions, without intruding your own, it is helpful to incorporate *his own words* into your questions (as in your *interventions in general*) as much as possible. Often this can be done, in a manner bordering on reflection, by merely repeating his last words with a rising inflection. For example, the patient says, "He wasn't trying to humiliate me with that remark. At least I don't think so," and you respond "At least you don't think so?" This is particularly useful in those numerous cases where patients leave off before the end of the sentence. Get them to complete the sentence by posing the conjunction, substantive, or whatever words at the end of the phrase back to them. For example, the patient says, "I was hoping he would have dropped by or something," and you reply, "Or something?" He says, "I would have told you that before but . . . ," and you respond, "But?" He says, "The woman in the dream was probably my wife or somebody." You say, "Or somebody?" The patient says, "It probably had something to do with my ambition or whatever," to which you query, "Or whatever?"

To return to the metaphor of patient as text, you can use questions as a tool with which to unpack the wealth of meaning and feeling in communications which the patient otherwise takes for granted, as self-evident, and as if they were the final word on the matter. In the evaluation section I discussed the need to unpack deceptively communicative words like "depression," to induce the patient to elaborate on them as much as possible. This is even truer in the treatment itself. Indeed, *clarifying communications is 90% of the business of psychotherapy.*

You will continually encounter words like "upset," "bonkers," "embarrassed," "bored," "intimate," "dependent," "relationship," and "confrontation," which contain whole paragraphs, even chapters, of meaning. Since such partial communications work in the service of the resistance, often the patient will not enrich their meaning for you unless you request it. Whole treatments can come to a close without the therapist really understanding what the patient means by some of his most cherished words and phrases. The *key* is to assume that you understand as little as possible about such communications.

For example, the patient says, "I would be embarrassed if I told you about that," and you respond, "What would that be like?" He says, "I was 'mortified' by his comment," and you reply, "Help put me in your shoes. How did that feel?" Possibly you continue with queries like, "What else does that situation remind you of? When have you felt that way before? Tell me about the first time you felt that way." He says, "My wife is domineering." You say, "How? What is that like? How do you feel about it?" He says, "I was afraid I would go crazy." You ask, "And what would being crazy consist of?" If you pursue such statements, both you and the patient will invariably be surprised by what emerges.

The other primary reasons to ask questions are to test out, to confirm or disconfirm, tentative clinical hypotheses and to catalyze the patient's awareness of something that is already in preconsciousness. An example of the latter is my query, "What else was going on then?" to the man in Chapter 1 who had failed to make the connection between his parents' divorce and his childhood distress.

The usefulness of questions does not end with the close of the early phase. They continue to be your most useful tool throughout the therapy, though the manner in which you utilize them changes somewhat in the middle and later stages. We shall return to their role in Chapter 9.

## Confrontations

It is important to know when to move from questions to confrontations. *Confrontations* are verbal communications of your observations and empathic resonances to the patient. In some ways the term "confrontation" is unfortunate because of its legalistic and pugilistic connotations. If they are based on accurate understanding and delivered in a sensitive and timely manner, they do not have the jarring and abrasive quality usually associated with the word "confrontation." Confrontations and *clarifications*, which restate what the patient already knows about himself but in a deeper and richer context, and in clearer focus, often go hand in hand. Together, confrontations and clarifications function to identify and sort out the threads that are eventually woven together into interpretations. We shall begin by discussing confrontations and then consider their handmaidens, clarifications.

Confrontations increase in frequency as you learn more about the patient and as rapport is established. You utilize them more often as you move through the middle and later phases of the opening stage on into the middle stage itself, where the actual interpretations begin. Correct and timely confrontations augment rapport—the patient's sense of being appreciated and understood. Incorrect or premature ones interfere with rapport or increase resistance. Correct confrontations delivered in a critical or patronizing tone are worse than incorrect ones presented benignly. The use of confrontations, clarifications and, especially, as we shall see, interpretations exemplifies that in psychotherapy *knowing when (and how) to say it is more difficult than knowing what to say.* An accurate sense of timing, once more, cannot be taught in this volume.

For example, with Mr. E. I erred once or twice by speaking prematurely to his withdrawal and arrogance and inviting him to help me understand what they warded off. He responded with derisiveness and ridicule. As a result of my ill-timed confrontations of his characterological defensive maneuvers, it was some time before we could again discuss the matter. Ms. Y.'s sense of emptiness and blandness was a defense against powerful feelings and fantasies but, had I pointed this out to her too early, it would have driven her out the door.

Like questions, confrontations function as facilitators and should be used no more than necessary. They are primarily utilized to make the patient consciously aware of an affect or defensive maneuver that was hitherto *preconscious* (not unconscious). If, on the other hand, it is plain that he is consciously aware of something, then it is usually redundant to label it.

Confrontations are used to avoid questions that would lead the patient to feel he is being quizzed for the right answer by a professor. In general, you should not ask questions the answers to which you already possess or are virtually sure that you possess (based on information he has already given you). There is a certain dishonesty in this, and if the patient realizes your ploy, it will disturb the rapport.[10] You should either wait until he comes to the understanding of it himself or communicate it to him in the form of a confrontation, your tone of voice indicating the degree of tentativeness or assurance you feel and want to convey. He can then agree or disagree with you. If your understanding is accurate and you have timed your intervention correctly—when the material in question is in the patient's preconsciousness—he will nearly always agree and/or respond with confirmatory associations and memories.

For example, in one session Mr. E. went from his concerns about how therapy was progressing and his fantasies about my views on the matter, to a disclosure that he edits and reedits his personal correspondence, to his preoccupations with his grade in a sculpture course, to his indecision about asking a certain woman out. We had been talking about his low self-esteem and insecurity in people's affections for some time so I did not ask, "Is there a connection here?" or "What is the connection here?" That would have contributed to his concerns about being evaluated or tested. (Nor did I spell out the connection for him because that would have adversely affected his low self-esteem.) Rather, judging that these apprehensions were preconscious in him, I said, with a tone of conviction and the expectation that he would understand me, "It's no accident that you go from talking about how therapy's going, to editing your letters, to your grades, to whether to ask Molly out." He responded, "Yes, it's the rejection thing again, whether I'm interesting enough, and just what the hell it is you expect from me." A train of affirmative associations and hitherto repressed memories followed. I had dissected out the red thread that was buried in 40 minutes of conversation and had invited him to look at it. It was still many sessions before I was able to make complete interpretations that linked his apprehension with

---

[10]The exception is when you ask a question you are virtually sure the patient can answer and about which you are prepared to acknowledge you have a hunch, e.g., my aforementioned query to the man in Chapter 1, "What else was going on then?"

Molly, his professor, his friends, and me to much earlier ones related to his parents, but these confrontations were paving the way.

In their zeal to please their supervisors and to pursue feelings, young trainees often repeatedly ask, "How do you feel?" This is another question that should not be asked when it is plain to you how the patient feels. If you believe that he is totally *unconscious* of his feeling, then it is probably premature to speak to it at all. If, on the other hand, you feel that he is most likely preconsciously aware of it, then you might ask a closed-ended question (e.g., "Do you feel sad?"), but a confrontation, not a question, is generally appropriate (e.g., "You look sad"). If he is telling you about a situation in which you know, from Sullivan's "one genus hypothesis" (i.e., "We are all much more simply human than otherwise"), that he must have been angry or hurt, even though he seems not to be (or have been) consciously aware of it, you would be less likely to ask, "What was that like?" than to say, "That must have been hard." The latter empathically and implicitly conveys that he is entitled to such feelings and that you expect him to be able to talk about them.

If the patient already knows how he feels and is expressive about it and you ask "How do you feel?" then he will think you are incompetent or insensitive. The cartoon that springs to mind is that of the therapist who responds to his patient's upraised knife by querying, "How do you feel?" Furthermore, if it is obvious that the patient is consciously aware of his feelings, then it is superfluous to try to induce him to verbally label them or to label them yourself. (That would be equivalent to saying "You're angry" to the patient in the cartoon.) The correct response is a nonverbal communication of empathy or else a question that presumes the mutual awareness of his feelings such as, "What are you mad about?"

Thus, to recapitulate, in dealing with feelings you begin your interventions with an open-ended "How do you feel?" As the patient makes his feelings progressively obvious, move successively on through "Do you feel such and such?" and "You look [sound] such and such" to "What do you feel such and such about?"

I have been primarily considering the confrontation of feelings of which the patient is at least preconsciously aware and the identification of themes and parallels (e.g., Mr. E.). The other primary mode of confrontation, that of resistance, is crucial but has little place in the early treatment. It can occur profitably only when a strong rapport has been established, when there is some development of a positive transference and therapeutic alliance, and when the patient's "resistances" to acknowledging his resistances have eroded somewhat largely out of his decreased fear of you. The time will come when you can tell a patient "You don't seem to want to talk about yesterday's experience with your boss" or "I notice that every time we start talking about your mother you change the subject" or "It strikes me that in our year of work together you haven't said a word about your brother." For example, the time came with Mr. E. when I could point out to him that his arrogance and withdrawal were means of avoiding feelings about me and other people. With Ms. Y. I could explain that her blandness was a defense against experiencing strong affect. Because such comments are more character- istic of the middle stage of therapy, I shall reserve further discussion of them for Chapter 9.

Confrontations often shade into clarifications or else the two accompa- ny one another. In the gray zone between them are those confrontations which restate something a patient has said, or a feeling that was obvious to him, but in a more focused way. For example, the patient says, "I was uncomfortable with your remark" and you respond, "Yes, you looked angry to me." He says, "I've been in a blah mood since my meeting with the supervisor yesterday," and you respond, "You sound hurt to me." Such interventions are particularly useful in moving patients from the diffuse, vague, affective wastebasket often called "depression" to the awareness of the specific anger, sadness, hurt, frustration, guilt, low self-esteem, warmth, and fear that lie beneath.

### Clarifications

*Clarification* is the most active and intrusive of the interventions de- scribed thus far. Its occurrence marks the setting of the early stage and the rising of the middle. It is a bridge between the rapport-building and information-gathering tasks of the opening stage and the interpretive and working through of the middle. It is the first phase in the process of amplification and enrichment of meaning that culminates in the so- called "complete interpretation" (which links past, present, and trans- ference motivations for a given symptom or behavior). One of the prime functions of clarification is to move the patient closer to *a pragmatic understanding of the operation of unconscious conflict and the danger situations in his life.*

This is illustrated in the following interchange, where the patient is moved first to a conscious awareness of her ambivalence and then to an understanding of the conflict beneath it.

*Patient:* I don't care for him and didn't really want to go to the dance with him at all.
*Therapist:* And yet earlier you had mentioned you were attracted to him.
*Patient:* Yes, yes. I guess so. But I can't stand the son of a bitch.
*Therapist:* Sounds like you have *mixed* feelings about him.
*Patient:* [Angry] All right. I guess I kinda wanted to go with the bastard [tears]. I guess I kinda wanted to go and kinda didn't. I guess that's why I wasn't at home when he said he was going to call. I was anxious about it all.

*Therapist:* It seems that you wanted to go and yet for some reason were afraid to.

Thus, she was introduced to the notion of intrapsychic conflict and her curiosity about her fears and fantasies was aroused. We shall return to the topic of clarifications in Chapter 9.

Finally, there comes a point in the early phase which is particularly hazardous to the therapeutic process. Freud (1937, p. 231) spoke of it as the enmity of the "better" to the "good." By this he meant that the positive transference, catharsis, and acquisition of new defenses that occur in early treatment often produce a sense of well-being that, coupled with fear of the unknown and fear of learning something that may dash this newfound sense of contentment, may lead the patient to drop out of treatment. When this occurs you must decide whether you are satisfied to have effected what is largely a transference cure or whether you feel that it is overwhelmingly to the patient's advantage to continue therapy. If the latter, then you can speak to the defensive function of dropping out and the danger which it is designed to avoid and/or inform the patient that you feel he can profit from continued therapy and your reasons for thinking so. If he remains adamant, then you must part from him with good will and good wishes and apprise him that you are willing to resume work should he so desire in the future.

# 9

# Insight-Oriented Psychotherapy: The Middle Stage

In psychotherapy, as in chess, the contest is won or lost in midgame. The crux of the middle moves is your handling of the resistance and the transference phenomena which are, if you have played a skillful opening, coming to plain view. Learning to treat the transference and resistance is undoubtedly the hardest part of becoming a psychotherapist. If your patient is to win more than a new, intellectualized set of defenses, then his understanding of the links between past and present, which have forged his *viewpoint of self* and *mode of operation* in the world, must go *through*, and not *around*, this transference. He must experience himself not merely remembering but repeating, or desiring to repeat, his history with you. His neurosis must remove itself from the outside world and set itself up with a vengeance in your office. As Freud (1912, p. 108) said, you cannot slay a demon in effigy or *in absentia;* you must first resurrect him.

By now you have established rapport; obtained a good longitudinal history and conception of his current environment and preoccupations; become increasingly aware of his defensive maneuvers, character style, and dawning transference; and learned a great deal about some of his most enduring fantasies, feelings, and fears. The patient, in turn, is moving you progressively closer to the center of his life and is beginning to set up lasting internal representations of you—to think about you occasionally between the sessions, to wonder what you would have to say on particular matters, and perhaps even to carry on a sort of internal dialogue between self and his inner picture of you.

**284**

The middle stage is characterized by an intensification of the search for meaning that began in the first hour. To return to the metaphor of the patient as text and the therapist as exegete, you are progressively unpacking, in ever finer detail, the meaning embedded in his verbal and nonverbal communications and noncommunications. Meaning encompasses that person-related nexus of fantasies, feelings, and fears that lies behind, and leads to, each of the patient's communications and defensive maneuvers. Your goal is to understand the patient's characteristic preoccupations and behaviors in their fullest possible historical, current, and transference context.[1]

This chapter outlines the steps in this enrichment of meaning in the patient's life. I shall begin by picking up a thread from the last chapter: your dogged attempt to understand, maximally, the patient's productions. This involves, above all, a continuation of the expert listening and questioning of the first stage. Second, I shall discuss gauging how much of a communication is expressive and how much defensive, and how one extracts the meaning from each pole. Third, I shall examine that paragon of the therapeutic craft, the "complete interpretation," which ties current and transference behavior to their historical meanings and motives. Finally, I shall examine that mysterious process of working through, of following the red threads in their multifarious twists and turns in the patient's life and treatment, of unmasking the central dynamics as they crop up, in manifest disguises and disclosures, in one area of a patient's life after another. A consideration of transference runs throughout the chapter.

Although it is artificial to separate them one from the other, I shall, for didactic purposes, divide the chapter into sections on listening, resistance, transference, interpretation, reconstruction, and working through.

## LISTENING REVISITED

First, you are always listening for the affect-laden fantasy or fear behind each communication. You are not to assume you comprehend optimally any of the patient's verbalizations or behaviors. In the previous chapter I emphasized your getting him to explain his terms, such as "dependency," or "control." Out of servitude to his resistance, the

---

[1]This meaning is not static. Not only does each symptom or behavior pattern mean multiple things (i.e., overdetermination or multiple function), but the chief meaning can vary over time. Old meanings can move from center stage, and new ones take their place. For example, tardiness may mean one primary thing at the outset of therapy, another in the middle, and still another toward the end. A woman's agoraphobia may serve one function in childhood and take on new ones (while still retaining the original) in adolescence and adulthood.

patient is always eager to take his first, facile statement as the final description or explanation of the matter, to consider, for example, that by muttering "bored" he has fully explained his discomfort at a recent social gathering or by muttering "depressed" he has fully described his affective-cognitive state.

Consider the following interchange with Mr. P. which illustrates how, with every utterance, the patient confronts you with the task of deciding whether to stop there or go forward.

*Therapist:* What were you thinking or feeling when you paused?
*Patient:* Oh, nothing.
*Therapist:* [Having decided to pursue the matter] Nothing at all?
*Patient:* Well, nothing worth mentioning.
*Therapist:* Oh?
*Patient:* Well, it was pretty silly, I mean. Not the sort of thing to waste time with here.
*Therapist:* Silly?
*Patient:* Yes.
*Therapist:* Is that all?
*Patient:* Yes.
*Therapist:* How do you think it would feel to tell me about it?
*Patient:* Hmm. I don't know. I would probably be embarrassed.
*Therapist:* And what would that be like?
*Patient:* Hell, you know, I would turn red, get jittery, sweat, and choke up—what happens when I do the sales meetings at X. I'd be nervous.
*Therapist:* It sounds like there's some sort of danger connected with telling me what's on your mind.
*Patient:* All right, dammit, that you would laugh at me, I guess, lord it over me or something. [He revealed at this point how his father would laugh at him as a child and tell him how inept he was at baseball and other sports at which his father excelled. He then connected this with a similar set of expectations vis-à-vis his colleagues and, especially, supervisors, at work. *Finally*, he disclosed the "silly" fleeting fantasy—that his penis would grow so tall that it would pierce through the roof of my office and destroy it.]


Consider, also, the following interaction with Mr. E.:
[This was the first session of the summer and the tenth month of treatment. He was then attending his graduate school's summer studio in the mountains and had to drive an hour and a half to make our sessions. He spent the first half hour berating several figures before he became aware that he was displacing transference anger from me.]

*Therapist:* What are you mad at me about?

*Patient:* I'm mad at you because, because, because—well, simply because I come here. When your office was a five-minute walk away it was easier to believe these sessions aren't all that important. I could even pretend coming here was mechanical, out of habit, rather than from free choice. But now, now that I have to drive an hour and a half, three days a week, for these sessions at this ungodly early hour, I can't believe that any more. You see, every time I drive down here it reaffirms your importance to me.

*Therapist:* And what's troublesome about that?

*Patient:* [Silence] Well, partly because now you know about it too [silence—shifts nervously].

*Therapist:* Yes, and what is it about that?

*Patient:* Because I'm *vulnerable,* because I'm putting all my eggs in one basket, getting close to you to the exclusion of others, that makes me feel vulnerable. It's not safe. It's not good for me [silence].

*Therapist:* Will you talk more about the dangers?

*Patient:* Well, it's not safe to get too close to one person. Then you're kind of at their mercy. I mean, you can be affected by what they do. Like if they leave or don't like you [silence].

*Therapist:* So, you're telling me that if you draw too close to me I might leave or not like you.

As important as asking questions to discern meaning is simply listening, following the flow of associations. The following is an example from a session in the ninth month of the thrice-weekly psychotherapy with Mr. E.

[He arrived 15 minutes late for the fourth session in a row.]

*Patient:* I was reading an article on a home for the retarded. It was funny but it wasn't supposed to be. I mean I was reading about a girl who couldn't put two sentences together [silence]. It reminded me of how I ramble. I don't want to talk that way. But conversations are the *most important things* in the world [his emphases]. And I can't help but talk disjointedly.

*Therapist:* I don't see it as a matter of ability. I suspect you talk that way for various reasons.

*Patient:* [Silence for several minutes] Well, it may be a way of being close and not close at the same time, of being close and not touching.

*Therapist:* Yes.

*Patient:* My mumbling too [silence]. You know, I was thinking about Joe [his best friend]. I was angry at him for asking me to talk with his girlfriend while he made some phone calls, to keep her entertained. Later he came in and said, "It sounds like you're not doing a bad job of it." Like with Al, who asked me, when we went on the skiing trip, if I would go out on the slopes with his girl, Marie, since his leg was in a cast. I guess in a way it's a compliment, but in a way it disregards me.

*Therapist:* In what way do you mean?

*Patient:* As a man. I don't know. I feel excluded in all these relationships [e.g., the threesomes in which he is involved with male friends and their girlfriends]. Like it seems they want me around, but then sometimes I'm not sure. Like I get double messages. But I don't know. I don't guess anybody wants other people around all the time [silence]. I don't know. It's hard to explain, but it seems like it might have something to do with the fact that I was the third person in our family.

*Therapist:* What was that like?

*Patient:* We-e-ell, a little like how I feel with my friends and their girls— the double message thing. Kinda in and kinda out [silence]. What comes to mind is the way I feel sometimes when I walk into the student union. I look at the tables to see where the oddball is, the misplaced domino, the piece of the puzzle that doesn't fit in. At times when I sit down I feel like that piece. But I guess everybody does from time to time [silence]. I guess I only felt that way every time I sat down at the table at home or went on vacations [including skiing trips] with my parents [laughs].

*Therapist:* Yes [said in a slightly rising inflection with the tone of "Please go on"].

*Patient:* No, I was only joking. I'm not sure I felt that way at all. Just joking. The same way I joke when people ask me what therapy is like [silence].

*Therapist:* Would you tell me about that?

*Patient:* [Shifts nervously in his chair] Oh, nothing to tell, just jokes [silence—he looks lost in thought]. You know, I was thinking about those conversations my father and I used to have and how I was never too sure if he really liked them or was just humoring me. Sometimes he did look bored [silence]. You know, when I called your office yesterday to cancel the appointment I was surprised when *you* [his emphasis] answered the phone. I was expecting your secretary. I was also a little surprised when you offered me this make-up appointment.

*Therapist:* You felt I wouldn't?

*Patient:* [Silence] It's the end of the session. When did you say your vacation starts?

*Therapist:* In two weeks. [Silence for several minutes. Then he rose from his chair as if to go].

*Therapist:* We've got ten minutes left by my watch.

*Patient:* Not by mine. Mine says we're through.

*Therapist:* We need to talk about what you're feeling that makes you want to come late, cancel appointments, and leave early. [He rose to walk out and then changed his mind. By checking his acting out, he permitted a hitherto repressed, preconscious complex of sorrowful memories related to his globe-trotting parents' frequent jaunts to come to consciousness.]

All I had to do was listen, and make a few facilitating remarks, to know that he was preoccupied with acceptance (by male and female friends, by parents, and me), with his sense of vulnerability in relationships, and with his feelings about my (and his parents' before me) leaving him. If you simply pay attention, the patient will show you the red thread virtually every time.

## RESISTANCE

The patient is talking. You are listening. Suddenly he stops, shifts nervously in his chair, or changes the topic abruptly. A resistance has announced itself. The flow of communication has been disrupted by anxiety or by the threat of anxiety. You are then, if you have been paying attention, in a position to recall what was occurring immediately prior to the point of change—what *he* was discussing and *you* were saying or doing. You then have a clue to the current danger situation which, depending upon the strength of the therapeutic alliance and the intensity of the resistance, you will either file away for future reference or inquire into or comment upon at the present moment.

This is perhaps the most important section of the chapter. Knowing how to deal with resistance is crucial to one who presumes to master this craft.

First, to reiterate, the defense mechanisms (the "resistances," from your point of view) are the patient's time-honored and cherished possessions. You would rob him of them no more than you would divest him of his wallet or watch. They are his way of making the best of an unpleasant situation, of coming to terms with self and environment in the most creative way he knows. As Fromm-Reichmann (1950) wrote of the obsessive-compulsive hand-washer, his rituals, while we might consider them debilitating, may be the one thing that stays his impulses and anxieties sufficiently for him to engage in human social intercourse at all. You ask him to relinquish his defenses only *after* you have given him something in turn: an *empathic relationship. Confronting defenses without an empathic appreciation of the anxieties motivating them is disastrous.*

Second, rarely, if ever, is any verbal and nonverbal communication simply an expression *or* a resistance. Most communications, within or without the therapeutic situation, simultaneously disclose *and* withhold.

Transference is the supreme example of this. It is *both* a resistance (an acting out rather than a remembering of conflict-laden historical issues) and a veiled expression. It is a resistance and yet it is the vehicle of treatment.

Patients tell you something about one subject to avoid telling you something about another. At one time they talk about the past to avoid looking at the present, at another about the present in order to dismiss the past, at others about the past or present to sidestep the transference, and at still others they talk about the transference to escape from the present or past.

The following interchange, between a resident just returned from vacation, and his hysterical female patient, illustrates the bimodal nature of human communication.

*Patient:* How was your vacation?
*Resident:* It was nice, thank you.
*Patient:* Are you on call much?
*Resident:* I'm curious about why you ask.
*Patient:* [Shifts nervously and smiles] Oh, I used to date a physician and he was on call a lot. I just wondered if you have it as bad as he did [silence]. We stopped dating a couple of years ago. He had just left his third marriage and wasn't ready to settle down [silence]. By the way, I saw my boyfriend over the weekend. He says he's not dating Sally any more, but I'm not so sure. June told me she saw his car at her house on Thursday. What am I going to do with him? [silence] I stayed at my parents' over the weekend. As usual, they didn't have anything of substance to say. My Dad hardly talked with me, except to give me hell about turning up the heat in the house. He keeps it so cold in there [which should of course be taken symbolically, as well as literally]. I explained to him how cold-natured I am. But he should know that. After all, I grew up in that house! He didn't seem to understand a word I said [silence]. And Mom, into her depression as usual. You know, I had a dream about her. She was sick and I rushed to the hospital to tell her I love her, to hug her, but she died before I got there. You know, since she's been depressed it's like she has died to me [silence]. Maybe I do wish the bitch would die. If Dad goes first, I'll have hell to pay with that woman. It'll be awful. I don't need a load like that [silence]. I think Dad's depressed too, trying to deal with Mom the way she is and all. I don't know, he could die before Mom. I just don't know. [She talked on about this for several minutes and closed by saying, with a faint laugh, "If he died it would be bad enough, but I guess I would buy a Jaguar!"]

She began with a polite reaction formation ("How was your vacation?") to her unconscious sense of abandonment by, and concomitant hurt and anger at, the resident. The subsequent question about his call schedule and the comments about her former physician-boyfriend and her current untrustworthy beau were all derivatives of her frustrated neediness for her therapist, at the same time that they defended against consciously acknowledging it. She then went on to discuss *legitimate* current issues (themselves a continuation of historical ones) with her parents, but in large measure as a way of *not* discussing these same feelings toward her resident. The red thread of frustration, disappointment, hurt, and anger wound its way through the hour, but she remained unconscious of the person to whom it was most immediately tied. Because the resident intuited that her frustration in the transference was unconscious, not preconscious, he did not comment upon it. He accepted what she had to offer without asking her for more than she was then prepared to give.

Knowing when, and when *not,* to speak to resistance is one of the most important and, unfortunately, one of the least teachable skills in psychotherapy. Although it is learned largely by making mistakes, there is at least one rule of thumb that will prove useful in your stumbling. From conflict theory you know that where there is resistance there is danger, and where there is danger there is anxiety. The closer to consciousness the danger situation, the safer it will be for you to intervene. The closer to consciousness the danger situation, the more likely the patient will be to manifest the overt signs of anxiety and/or be subjectively aware of it. When either of these is the case, your confrontation of the resistance is more likely to gain results than if the patient is relatively placid or dealing with his anxiety symptomatically.[2]

For example, Mr. E. had been railing out against a couple of obnoxious Southerners in his dormitory without consciously realizing he was also talking about me. [I am from the South, as my accent reveals.] At some point in his harangue he began to shift in his seat and glance up quickly and nervously. Since at this point I suspected that he was *preconsciously* aware of the danger (i.e., that I would be offended and leave), I said, "You sound like a man who is treading cautiously." Following this he sighed in relief and began to directly discuss his feelings and apprehensions about the various differences between us. This is also another good example of how, if you speak to the resistance and the danger situation motivating it, the preconscious will surface automatically. If, by contrast, I had spoken directly to the content ("Mr. E., are you aware that when you talk about these students you are also talking about me?") I would have heightened the resistance and he

---

[2]Here again, I am referring only to the relatively intact patients of insight-oriented psychotherapy and to anxiety that is moderate in intensity. With a psychotic or ego-compromised individual, the greater the anxiety the more likely you would be to reinforce, not sap, his defenses.

would more likely have responded with ridicule and irritation than with confirmatory associations.

A patient's *manner* of communicating is often an example of the simultaneously revealing and concealing nature of communication. Mr. P. would communicate in a slow and deliberate manner, giving the impression that he chose his words carefully. Furthermore, he would hardly allow me to get a word in edgewise. As related subsequently in this chapter, this was a defensive maneuver—an attempt to cover up an underlying sense of inadequate masculinity and to protect himself from an unconsciously longed for, and yet feared, homosexual penetration. Mr. E., ostensibly to please me, would come in and begin "free-associating" immediately. He would sit back and report the cascades of ideas, recollections, and (hardly ever) feelings that poured over him from, as he saw it, "out of the blue." He did this with the distant objectivity of one who was simply reciting the numbers on passing boxcars. Granted, he was bringing me interesting, often "deep" material, but he was doing so in such a disjointed fashion, and it was so sequestered from the vital issues of his everyday life, that it was impossible to use it in any meaningful way. In effect, he was talking about everything in order to avoid talking about anything (and at any depth) in particular, using expression in the service of repression. Mr. E. utilized the idea of free-associating to pretend that he was not a self-thinking, self-feeling individual with his *own* burning issues that he sought desperately to avoid. He was also surreptitiously expressing his dependency, his conflictual unconscious desire that I pull it all together for him.

This *bimodal* nature of resistance has implications for the manner in which you confront it. It is important that you do not give the impression that you view his resistance as bogus behavior trying to pawn itself off as the real thing. For example, take the case of rationalization. When a patient with a pattern of tardiness and absences apologizes that he missed the previous session because he had to catch up on paperwork at the office and meet with his accountant and that he was late to the present session because he had to stop for gas, you do not say, "No, you are wrong. You did not miss because you had to do your paperwork and see your accountant. Nor were you late today because you had to stop for gas. You did all three as a way of avoiding dangers associated with certain feelings about me." To do so would be not only tactless and disrespectful, but actually erroneous. The patient *is* right: doing his paperwork, seeing his accountant, and getting gasoline *were* reasons for his behavior—reasons which were motivated by the desire to avoid more important, more troublesome, and less conscious ones. In other words, when people rationalize, they are usually clever enough to rationalize with a statement that does have some basis in reality.[3]

---

[3]See page 293.

This can be illustrated as well with other defensive maneuvers. For example, with a patient who displaces his anger at his father and you onto an older colleague, you do not say, "No, you are not angry at your co-worker. You have no reason to be. You are *really* angry at your father and me." In all likelihood, he may well have some real basis for irritation at his colleague—only one insufficient to account for the magnitude of his response. What you want to convey to him is that some anger at his father and you seems to be getting a free ride out at his associate.

Third, and in line with point two, *resistances are not simply obstacles which impede the course of treatment* and which must be cleared away as soon as possible. They are not simply that which prevents the "real" material, the "content," from emerging. Not only do they disclose as well as withhold but, in and of themselves and in their purely defensive mode, they are as much the *content* of the personality as that which they defend against. It is, in other words, *just as* (sometimes even more) important to know the defensive purposes of a symptom or character trait as it is to know what it obliquely expresses. It is as important to know the danger associated with a fantasy or feeling, that which summons up the defensive maneuver in the first place, as it is to know the underlying fantasy or feeling. In the case of the hysteric, Mr. T., it was as necessary to know that any expression of anger was associated with so strong a danger of losing the loved object, castration, and superego condemnation that he had to obviate it by crippling himself, as it was to know that he was defending against anger. Unfortunately, you will remember, I did not realize this at the time.

The mistaken idea that your challenge is to slip around, or batter through, the resistance in order to rescue the affect-laden fantasies is a heritage from the early, cathartic days of psychoanalysis. Then Freud viewed the psyche as a drum in which were stored X gallons of hurt and frustrated infantile dependency needs, Y gallons of anger, Z gallons of incestuous sensuality, and so on, and that the therapist's task was, somehow, to drain them. To aid and abet this cathartic process, Freud at times resorted to hypnosis in order to bypass the resistances. He soon discovered, however, that only temporary relief was obtained, and that it was just as important for a patient to know why he is so afraid of dependency, anger, or sensuality that he has to repress them, as it is for

---

[3]Resistance may even crystallize, after the fact, around something over which the patient has absolutely no control! Let us say that he misses a session because of an unforeseeable mechanical failure of his car or because you have to cancel owing to illness. Although he can logically be held accountable for neither, they can take on the subjective meaning of resistance, come to function in the service of the resistance, the patient perhaps feeling not only disappointment but also relief at missing the session. (In the case of your illness he may also feel, unconsciously, that he has somehow caused it.)

him to know that he *is* dependent, angry, or sensual. The most important part of your work is neither swamp drainage nor treasure seeking, but alerting the patient to his *mode of operation* and the *historically based view of self and world from which it derives.*

An occasional patient finds it easier to jump over the resistance and danger situation to the "content" itself. Ms. Y., for example, had a habit of obsessing silently for 15 or 20 minutes about whether or not to disclose some feeling or fantasy to me and then blurting it out at the end of the session, never to return to it again. She acted as if mentioning it magically banished it. After this had occurred several times, I was able to inform her, the next time she repeated it, that it was as helpful to know why she was anxious, what was dangerous about the idea of telling me, as it was for her to disclose the fantasy itself. By leaping over the former she was denying us both important information about herself. Mr. P. would hesitate nervously for a few moments, remind himself, "Well, after all you're only a therapist," and then disclose the matter at hand. It was necessary for me to find out the concerns that reminding himself I was a therapist helped him to overcome.

Also, this is an example of the aforementioned dictum "interpret resistance before content." If you can help a patient understand the motive of his avoidance, what he is avoiding will emerge as a matter of course. When Ms. Y. understood the nature of her fears with me, and how they were related to earlier experiences with her parents, she then disclosed her fantasies and feelings.

The precise way in which you speak to the resistance varies of course from patient to patient and situation to situation. At times, as I just illustrated, you speak to the resistance and the danger situation associated with it. At times you speak merely to the resistance itself: "You seem to be avoiding something." "Perhaps your talking philosophy with me is a way of avoiding your feelings about real people." Often, you speak to the resistance and to that which is resisted in the same breath, e.g., "Talking about your anger at your boss is a way of avoiding your anger at me for being away last week"; "You loaned him the money as a way of keeping at bay your resentment for him"; "You find it easier to focus on your career decisions than on how much you dislike feeling dependent on me."

I shall close this section with a brief discussion of the wording of your interventions when the resistance is a conscious, rather than unconscious, decision not to talk about something. When you are both aware that this is the case and when the therapeutic alliance is *well established* and the patient says, "I *can't* talk about that," it is good to emend this to, "You mean that, for various reasons, you don't *want* to." When rapport is well established and he has become acquainted, operationally, with the notion of resistance and intrapsychic danger, there comes a time when you want to "personalize" his avoidances. For example, he says, "I don't want to talk about that right now." You respond, "With me," thereby bringing home to him that there is a danger associated with his discussing it, not just with anybody, but with you (and with those whom you unconsciously represent) in particular. He says, in response to your invitation to talk about a certain matter, "Doctor, don't you get tired of this work some time? Doesn't it drain you?" You ask, "Are you afraid that I get tired of you?"

In other words, as the patient's defensiveness subsides, you arrive at the point where you can be a bit bolder, where you do not have to take his first, feeble denial of your confrontations and clarifications as the final word. With Mr. E., for example, it was finally necessary for me to say, "It's hard for me to believe that you didn't have *any* feelings about what she said"; "You have a positive phobia against the slightest hint that someone might be important to you." When I felt that, as in these cases, his resistance was a more purely conscious one and that the danger situation and fantasy defended against were close to consciousness, I could at times "outwit" his defensiveness with statements like, "I suspect you're going to reject this out of hand, but it does sound as if you wanted to move closer to her"; "You probably won't want to hear this, but I think you're actually afraid to feel like we're accomplishing anything in here because then I would become important to you." Timed correctly and used judiciously, such tactics enabled Mr. E. to talk about that which he would sooner avoid. When such maneuvers are used, your voice must not express the slightest hint of irritation or impatience.

Finally, you need to know that your interventions do not diminish the resistance in a smooth and linear fashion. Rather, the process is more like two steps forward, and one and a half backward. The patient drops his guard a bit one day, and then becomes frightened and redoubles it the next. Diminution in resistance, if graphed over time, would produce a jagged, gradually downsloping curve rather than a smoothly declining one.

## TRANSFERENCE

We shall turn now from resistance in general to that special instance of it without which there would be no dynamic treatment—*transference*. Throughout this book I have provided copious examples of the remarkable phenomenon of the reenactment, rather than recollection, of the past in the present. The capacity to form a complete transference neurosis (and, in some cases, psychosis) is present in all of us. Our patient comes to us with a transference just waiting to happen. It is all there, at some level, though it takes many months or years for it to unfold. It is a more or less accurate replication of his history, depending upon how much, and in what way, the real aspects of your personality impinge upon him.

It is essential to realize that this transference is not something that is taking place merely in the patient. You are unrolling your own set of feelings, fantasies, and fears vis-à-vis him as well, and not merely in reaction to his, but as a manifestation of an historical agenda that you bring to the session. You now feel inclined to use the patient sexually, now aggressively, now affectionately, now dependently, now paternally or maternally, and so forth. At times you are tempted to use him less expressively than defensively—to project unacceptable impulses upon him and then feel judgmental, to be overly solicitous as a way of avoiding your anger at him, or to withdraw from him out of the intrapsychic danger posed by your fantasies about him.

All this is known as "countertransference." It is your fastest friend and fiercest foe. It is the latter because, as Tarachow (1963) tells us, a pressure is within both of you to *act out* your transference issues with one another, to turn the therapeutic relationship into a "real" relationship. To the extent that you are unaware of your countertransference, it is to that degree in danger of being acted out (gratified or inappropriately defended against) or of interfering with your perceptions and understandings of the patient. It is not, however, incumbent upon you to be conflict-free! The completely "therapized" clinician is as much a myth as the completely "therapized" patient. You only, it is hoped, diminish the intrapsychic dangers associated with your historically based conflicts sufficiently to be aware of them, stay in the room, listen, and avoid acting out expressively or defensively when the patient's communications impinge upon them.

Evidence pointing to hitherto unacknowledged countertransference acting out might include: 1) forgetting a patient's appointment; 2) finding frequent "good reasons" to change or cancel a particular patient's sessions; 3) feeling excessive solicitude toward, or constant worry over and preoccupation with, a patient; 4) feeling overanxiety about helping and being liked by the patient; 5) not taking process notes with a particular patient (may also be a case of transference acting out vis-à-vis one's supervisor); 6) consistently receiving a particular reaction from all your patients, such as the complaint that you are critical and judgmental or cold and unfeeling; 7) being unable to empathize with a patient; 8) persistently forgetting to bill a patient; 9) perennially sharing the case with your colleagues, out of either a search for help or exhibitionism; 10) persistently feeling perplexed about or failing to understand a patient; 11) feeling marked anxiety before, during, or after meetings with a patient (relatively direct evidence that conflict and danger are associated with your feelings and fantasies about the patient and those he represents); and 12) experiencing difficulty staying awake in sessions.[4]

Unrecognized, countertransference is your enemy. Acknowledged, it is your ally because it is only through your own responses (feelings and fantasies) to the patient that you come to know him. As I have asserted, these responses are more often an *inextricable combination* of what the patient realistically evokes in us (and would in anybody—what some call "counter reactions") and of that which comes from our own particular history. The countertransference often first alerts us to the nature of the transference.

For example, I refer the reader to the case of Mr. E. I have already apprised you of my fantasy, "Call me Mr. Wonderful." That was but the first in a chain of three associations, the second being a concern with whether I was making a contribution with my clinical work, and the third a puzzling over how my physician father would feel on the matter. In other words, I was alerted to Mr. E.'s defensive minimizing of my importance to him by a fantasy that was a momentary derivative of an unconscious complex about acknowledgment by my father. I had come to know the patient's behavior as it impinged upon this complex. Because of my own therapy, this particular issue, though still active to some degree, was sufficiently nonthreatening that I could have conscious access to it and use it to help me understand the patient.

In short, a transference totally uncontaminated by our *mishegoss* is an ideal toward which we strive, but know we shall never attain, nor would we perhaps want to. Sullivan (1953) acknowledged this by calling the psychiatric mode one of "participant observation." We know our patient, never directly, but only as he impinges upon our historically conditioned perceptual-affective-cognitive apparatus. We see his neurosis through the lens of our own. We, in turn, with our particular interventions and physical and psychological characteristics, impinge upon his. Thus, every behavior of the patient must be viewed as a *vector*, or compromise, between historical-current intrapsychic determinants and those issuing from the environment (the therapist and his milieu). In a correctly handled case, the role of the latter is minimized, but never removed altogether.

---

[4]One manifestation of parental countertransference, the "Pygmalion complex," is especially unlikely to be noticed and can be correspondingly troublesome. There is some of the conscious-unconscious desire to clone ourselves in all of us. This intermeshes with the tendency to identify with the therapist which operates in each patient. Nevertheless, we must be cautious about transmitting the expectations that our particular solutions to the problems of life should also be his.

The particular fashion in which a transference unfolds depends of course on the patient. The early environment of most who survive childhood has been sufficiently nonmalevolent that they approach us, as I have said, with some initial positive evaluations and expectations. This is the *positive transference* that plays so great a role in bringing the patient to the office in the first place and keeping him coming. Others, whose upbringing and past experiences have been less favorable, enter cautiously and suspiciously, keeping their distance from one who may turn out to be "just like the rest."

Some mixture of 1) love and approach, and 2) hatred, fear, and avoidance, with the former predominating in consciousness is the most common presentation. Often there is an initial "honeymoon" in which the patient basks in the warm glow of your "omnipotence," "benevolence," and "wisdom." This inevitably begins to wane when he discovers you are not the godlike figure he imagined you to be. It is then that you and he become uncomfortably aware that his transference, like all transferences, is an *ambivalent* one.

Here again, the transference is not something you make happen. It has already happened. It has been happening all the patient's life. The complete transference already exists, as a sort of homunculus, within the patient. It merely has not yet unfolded itself to you. You can perforce, initially, have little or no knowledge of it, other than what you can predict from the history. In the reasonably healthy patients of the insight-oriented therapist, the early transference is characterized more by its resistances, or defensive aspects, than by its expressive ones. Consider, for example, the arrogant aloofness of Mr. E., behind which cowered an overwhelming emotional neediness.

The transference of Ms. Y., as well, was characterized by its initial defensiveness. I shall expand at length on its evolution to illustrate some principles about transference in general.

She entered treatment with a bland and colorless look, unsuccessfully disguising the considerable physical attractiveness beneath. She complained of "no feelings" and "emptiness," with a total sense of alienation from, and lack of desire for closeness with, other human beings. She decided to enter treatment after learning of the death of a woman who had been her only close friend in childhood but whom she had not seen for years and who, as I later discovered, had disappointed the patient in many ways. Ms. Y. was perplexed over her inability to grieve this loss (which resurrected a host of issues related to prior deprivation and rejection).

Past history revealed that she was the product of an unplanned, undesired conception by a couple who already possessed one child. The mother was chronically depressed, had previously given what little she had to the older child, and was doing poorly in her fashion career. She had the utmost resentment for the patient, whom she regarded as yet another obstacle to realizing her dreams of success in her vocation; the mother alternately railed out against and withdrew from Ms. Y. The father was a professor, a cold and distant scholar who gave what little he could to the patient's older sister, with whose academic abilities and ambitions he identified. Neither parent esteemed Ms. Y. or encouraged her academic or social interests and abilities. They reacted to her tears and tantrums, frantic bids for attention, by abusing her or by withdrawing still further, ultimately using her turbulence as the excuse for their behavior. From her tenth to eighteenth years her parents separated and reunited several times. She was shuttled back and forth between her father and mother. At age 20, during one of her parents' reconciliations, she was told she would have to go her own way.

The next ten years were a chaotic odyssey in which she tried to keep one step ahead of her pain. During this time she went through a brief, traumatic marriage, managed to earn a cosmetologist's license and practice her trade sporadically, and saw several therapists in short encounters. Because of her low self-esteem, she had kept herself out of many situations where she would have learned crucial skills about navigating in an adult world. Although 30 years old she was, in many respects, psychologically a preadolescent. Shortly before reentering treatment with me she had moved back in with her parents in, as it later emerged, an unconscious attempt to go back and wrest from them (particularly her father) what she had been denied in the past. Especially striking was the continual competition between mother and patient for the distant father's attention.

The first three months were characterized by aloofness and her persistent protest that she "feels nothing and has no thoughts." She contemplated dropping out frequently ("because I can't do this work") and tested my willingness to see her by requesting changes in appointment times and a postponement in payment of two of the monthly fees.

By the fourth month of twice-weekly psychotherapy, this facade of emptiness began to break down and she gradually became aware of erotic and dependent longings for me that had been germinating for some time. Her initial response was to withdraw still further, to miss and come late to sessions, and to again contemplate dropping out altogether. Only after three more months was she able, as a result of my exploration of her defensiveness and the dangers associated with disclosure, to begin expressing her fantasies to me. This was facilitated by my countering her protestations that "my feelings are too silly, too unjustified by this situation, to talk about" with some information about the logic of the emotions—that, in other words, feelings have their own good, internal *raison d'être* and she is entitled to them. At a few points I made the mistake of prematurely linking some of her transferential feelings to their historical determinants rather than, as I should have done, allowing them to develop. She responded as if I were discounting and taking lightly her feelings for me.

Since I remained her therapist and empathized and sought to *understand*, rather than *gratify*, her transference strivings, she began to feel that I was spitefully and maliciously depriving her, as she accused her parents of doing, and for the same reasons: that she was a "worthless, stupid, unattractive, no-good person." She responded with hurt and rage, which latter she either internalized as depression or displaced (back to its original object!) onto her father by drawing him into fights with her. For a time she acted out the positive pole of her ambivalence toward me in an abortive affair with a physician about my age.[5]

She began to experience dreams in which she was having sexual intercourse with male figures who would kaleidoscopically change back and forth between looking like her father and me. She began to speak of her father's sexually provocative behavior and subsequent frustration of her during childhood and accused me of acting similarly. Toward the end of the first year she dealt with her anger. She phoned me at times between the sessions, throwing what were essentially tantrums and evoking in me an internal response that must have resembled that of her parents. It was some time before we both realized (because *I inferred an intention to push me away on her part from my desire to withdraw from her*) that this turbulent behavior was not merely expressing her frustration, but also designed to *distance* me. In other words, she not only longed for intimacy with me, but was afraid of it, in part because of the rejection she had experienced, in part because of her sexual abuse at the hands of an older male neighbor and unscrupulous pediatrician, and in part because each time she experienced warmth toward me and felt my empathy it sadly reminded her how much she had missed and caused her to fear losing it. Her turbulent acting out was also a way of refusing to sit quietly and feel her more painful warmth and sadness, a way of circumventing it. The time came when she was preoccupied with my physical and emotional health which, as it turned out, was not merely an expression of her caring for me (and a reaction formation to her hatred), but a derivative of her childhood concerns about her patently depressed and withdrawn mother. She also discovered that her repetitive accusation that I was a liar and my caring a farce was a displacement of her earlier complaints about her parents' behavior. As she was transferring her neurosis to me and as the therapy became stormier, her outside relationships with her parents and sister actually improved and she resumed her trade, which she had been afraid to do for some time.

By the eighteenth month this woman, who feared she had no feelings, was finding that she was full of affection, dependency, hatred, sensuality, and guilt. She who was afraid that there were no real persons in her life had found that people were all too present. In some respects she was feeling worse than before entering treatment, but she was *feeling*. Indeed, it was necessary for me to *empathically acknowledge this* and to point out that this was the way psychotherapy worked—that she was in midstream where the water is most turbulent and that, to get to the other shore, she had to swim through, and not around, this pain. *Repeatedly* conveying my empathic appreciation of her plight (patients do not always hear you the first time)—that the man who was stirring up her long-repressed neediness was refusing to gratify it—was as important in resolving this transference neurosis as my interpretations themselves.

---

[5]Some writers distinguish between the acting out (rather than recollecting, recognizing, and verbalizing) of historically based transference issues which occurs *within* the hours from that which occurs *between* them. The former they term "acting in," while reserving "acting out" for the latter. For example, Ms. Y.'s eventual altercations with her employer were a form of *acting out* her transference hostilities, her repetitively asking me personal questions a form of *acting* them *in*.

She was *in treatment,* although it was some time before she would fully realize the link between her feelings toward, and behaviors with, me and her disappointing past. It was also some time before she could appreciate that what she experienced as my deprivation of her (my refusal to do other than consistently empathize with, and understand, her) was actually my ultimate way of expressing concern. She came to see, in other words, that she had been imposing her historically determined categories of perception and interpretation on to my behavior (i.e., she felt that I refused to gratify her needs not because it was incompatible with the therapeutic enterprise, as I had explained to her, but because I simply did not want to, as seemed to be the case with her parents). Eventually she also recognized that her turbulent and self-destructive *defenses* against affect were actually causing her more pain than the underlying feelings themselves.

There were many times when I felt, in my dogged maintenance of a therapeutic stance, deprived myself—when I wanted, out of my own countertransference and her provocativeness, to give her what she desired. On other occasions she elicited in me the wish to reject or, even, thrash her.

With Ms. Y., as with all patients, I was watching for manifestations of transference from the outset. The therapist must be a bit self-referential if he is to spot the transference in its many guises. There is a facetious story about one famous supervisor who required his students to wear an identification bracelet with a "T" on it, constantly reminding them to think "transference."

Nevertheless, although transference is always a consideration, you are hardly always speaking to it, and certainly not in the beginning. Recall the case of the resident just returned from vacation and his hysterical patient. Because he had learned to look for subtle manifestations of transference, he was aware of it though he knew that to speak to it would be premature. It would cause her, if anything, to pull back from him. Addressing transference issues early in the middle stage is generally indicated only when a negative transference, or the need to defend against a precipitously upswelling and conflictual positive transference, threatens to drive the patient from treatment. Indeed, much of the nonconflictual positive transference is never addressed at all since it is one of the factors that not only keeps him coming but, in the form of the desire to please the therapist, actually contributes to his recovery.

When you do begin commenting on it, you should not leap right away to the interpretation of its historical roots. To do so would be insulting to many patients, as it was with Ms. Y. There is plenty of time, after the transference has begun to take shape, to link it to historical and current environmental issues.

Most residents find the negative transference most difficult to manage. Most of them like to be liked, though I have encountered an occasional one who seemed more comfortable when his patients were angry at him! Trainees have ways of cutting a patient's anger off at the pass: acquiescing to unreasonable demands and requests in order to avoid frustrating him or speaking to the anger prematurely such that his defenses heighten. Saying "It's O.K. if you get angry at me" or inviting him to be angry at you usually have the paradoxical effect of choking off anger. In addition, some patients interpret such comments to mean that you will not take their anger seriously when it does occur. You can also quash the anger by interrupting to ask the patient to explain it too soon. The most common reason to try to defuse the patient's anger is to avoid feeling angry (with any conflicts connected thereto) oneself.

The positive transference can be trying as well. The overwhelming sexual, affectionate, and dependent neediness of the schizophrenic or severely disturbed borderline is tailor-made to incite any of our own unresolved conflicts around such issues. The net result, if we are not careful, may be our withdrawal from the patient.

In reenacting the past in the present, it is important to know, the patient does not merely treat you as the significant other but, at times, as a representative of himself. Through a combination of what Anna Freud (1936) termed "identification with the aggressor" and the attempt to go back and actively master the passively experienced traumata, the patient may attempt to do unto you what was done unto him. For example, Mr. E., who ordinarily had great problems with eye contact, undertook on several occasions to observe me minutely and critically, remarking, in the process, on a real characteristic of my personality (his perception of which I consensually validated). After several sessions I realized that, at least in part, he was critically examining me as he had felt observed by his parents and, in the transference, by me. In other words, he was unconsciously communicating his affective state by eliciting in me an experience similar to his own. When I interpreted this to him, a wealth of previously repressed memories and feelings poured forth.

In dynamically based insight-oriented psychotherapy, the transference is resolved by *interpretation*, to which we shall turn in the following section.

## INTERPRETATION

To reiterate, the patient will push you to gratify the transference derivatives of his unconscious, historically determined wishes, to behave in a way that conforms to his fantasies, fears, and expectations. He has been more or less adept at getting everyone else to do so and wants to include you as well. He strives to make you treat the transference as "real," rather than analyzing its meanings and motives, rather than extracting the troublesome recollections embedded in it.

Since interpretations can occur only in an ambience of "therapeutic deprivation," I must first address this before turning to the mechanics of interpretation. At each step you must decide whether to gratify his transference strivings or to pose, as Tarachow calls it, the "therapeutic task" and deprive him. The former may make him feel better temporarily; the latter forces him to labor, often painfully, and paves the way for that maximum of all deprivations—the interpretive work, in which you divest him of his illusions about his relationship with you and his cherished ways of avoiding himself. The following vignette illustrates this concept:

> Mr. S. became a childhood comic as a way of overcoming a low self-esteem and depressive affect secondary to the death of his mother and the cold inattentiveness of the surviving father. He discovered that telling jokes was usually the only way he could get the attention of this chronically depressed man and, he feared, of his friends as well. By early adulthood he had developed into an accomplished raconteur and had even, at one point, considered becoming a professional comedian. It came as no surprise when he dealt with his depressive affect, low self-esteem, and fear of rejection in the transference by lacing the hours with jokes and anecdotes. After laughing at the first few, for they were genuinely funny (and not to have laughed would have disturbed the incipient rapport), I had to decide whether to continue to laugh, and gratify his transference acting out, or to sit quietly and deprive him of the much-needed attention of the father imago that I was. I opted for the latter and, after a few times, he became quite nervous. When queried about it, he discovered that beneath this discomfort was a sense that I had neglected, hurt, and deprived him. "I got the impression that you didn't like my stories, that you weren't interested in me."

> As we pursued this over the next several sessions, it emerged that his anxiety was a manifestation of conflict between his rage at me for depriving and disappointing him on the one hand and his defenses against it on the other, the dangers being loss of the loved object and superego condemnation. Eventually he was able to relate this, as well as his current behavior with friends and associates, to a constellation of fantasies, fears, and feelings related to his mother's death and his father's distance. Had I continued to laugh he would have continued to *act out*, rather than *recollect*, the historical issues that led to his behavior. By depriving him (but continuing to empathize), I helped us both to understand.

The same principle could be illustrated by several other situations, such as when Ms. Y. asked me to call her by her first name or when Ms. H. asked where I lived and whether I had children. In all of these situations I elected to explore the meanings and motivations behind these comments and questions rather than to indulge them. To do so is to painfully remind the patient that, however close the two of you become, you will never be involved in a "real relationship," in the usual sense.

Furthermore, by refusing to gratify the transference derivatives of deeply unconscious desires, by frustrating the latter, you cause them to gather in strength, to clamor more loudly and move closer to consciousness, where they will one day be interpretable.

From the outset you engage in a series of activities that break the ground for sowing "complete interpretations." First of all, you listen. You learn enough about the history and current *modus operandi* to be able to identify patterns of behavior, central affects, desires, and defenses against them, and to begin to infer some meaning about the most prominent danger situations.

You continue to promote this process with reflections and questions. Since many of the affects and issues are out on the table, these questions have a different cast from those in the early stage. They are designed to elicit *motives, meanings, purposes,* and *intentions.* For example, the patient says, "I'm angry at you." You say, "What's that about?" She says, "I found myself wanting to withdraw from him?" You say, "For what reason?" She says, "I wonder if you really want to keep seeing me." You say, "What leads you to say that?" She says, "I wouldn't want to talk with you about that." You say, "Why not?" He says, "I think I'd like us to get in an argument." You say, "What purpose would that serve?" He says, "I don't know why, but it almost seems like I wanted to make a fool of myself." You say, "To what end?" In exploring meanings and motives it is important, once more, not to take the first, often facile, answer as the final one, but to continue unpacking.

Second, the confrontations and clarifications of preconscious material continue. Giving the patient an *operational* understanding of conflict and danger is, as I have said, particularly important. (For example, "You want to assert yourself with Mary but, for some reason, are afraid to, such that you end up avoiding her.")

Third, you strive to give your patient an operational understanding of the idea of psychic causality or psychic meaningfulness. Initially, this is done in short steps, linking actions, situations, and events to subsequent behaviors and affective states. For example, the patient tells you, casually and in passing, that his girl friend had to cancel their weekend in the mountains, and adds, "But that gave me a chance to catch up on my paperwork." A few minutes later he complains of "feeling in a funk" but he doesn't know why, and you point out that he had just finished talking about his girl friend (thereby also confronting his defense mechanism of isolation). Mr. E. rails out at me, closes his eyes, and looks up a few minutes later out of the fleeting fantasy that my silence indicated I had left the room. I point out the temporal connection between his anger at me and this fantasy, and he concludes that he was afraid his anger had driven me away. A patient remarks about his anxiety over the weekend and you remind him that Friday he had told you his mother would be visiting.[6]

When a patient is talking about a particular symptom, in addition to knowing its history and the context of its most recent occurrence, you

[6]See page 305.

should pay particular attention to the context in the session in which he tells you about it, to the associations that both precede and follow it. These too are clues to the unconscious complex underpinning the symptom. Occasionally, it is useful to ask the patient to associate specifically to the symptom, to talk all around it and see what emerges.

Instructing a patient about psychic causality involves making him aware of the red thread winding its way through what otherwise seems a chaotic skein of an hour, of saying, "I think it is no accident that you went from talking about feeling intimidated by your father, to your public speaking anxieties in grammar school, to your fears of sexual impotence, to your concerns about how well you are doing at work, to your anxieties about keeping conversations going, to your fantasies about how well I think you are doing in here." To another patient you say, "Your fears of being found out by the IRS, your boss, and your wife seem similar to your concerns about disclosing yourself with me." To still another you say, "That you go from talking about your affair, to your girl friend's abortion, to the issue of confidentiality in here suggests that you have more concerns about the two former than you would care to admit." With some you might occasionally share your own associations to their material, e.g., "What you said about how you feel with Bob and Mary reminds me of the time when you and your parents were at X." "When you told me about Y I found myself thinking of what you had said about Z." Much of the work with Mr. E. involved helping him attain a sense of the meaning and purpose of his behavior such that he could no longer disown responsibility for his thoughts, feelings, and actions.

From identifying themes and temporal contiguities it is a short step to making *partial interpretations:* connecting current outside behaviors to historical *or* transference motives, transference preoccupations and behaviors to historical *or* current issues, and historical behaviors to more remote historical motives. You direct such partial interpretations to the most immediate affect and to conscious or preconscious preoccupations. For example, with the same patient you might say, at various points, "You are afraid that if you get close to John he'll treat you as your father

---

[6]In exploring the relationship between situations and distress or maladaptive behavior, you must not give the impression that the patient's feelings and behaviors are somehow mechanically *caused* by the other person. Ms. Y., for instance, went through a phase when she understood my linking of her self-destructive and turbulent behaviors ("fits") to arguments with, and abandonments by, her father to mean that she was passively buffeted about like a billiard ball by him. It was necessary for us to also discuss the role she was playing in creating the situations to which she then reacted, to look at her conscious and unconscious intentions in, and interpretations of, those situations.

did." "You're afraid that if you move too close to me I'll walk out on you like your Dad did." "You never told your next-door neighbor how much you liked him because you were afraid he would have turned away like your father did." "You're afraid that if you open up to John and me that we won't like what we see." You might have to say all this and more, during many different times and contexts, *before* you can begin to communicate complete interpretations like, "You want to draw close to John and me, just as you wanted to with your neighbor and father, but you withdraw from us because you are afraid we will push you away, like your Dad did."

The *complete interpretation* should speak to the *historically determined affect-laden fantasy, the intrapsychic danger, the defensive maneuver,* and *the current and transference behaviors in which they are manifested.* For example, to Ms. Y. I was eventually able to say, "You want to be close to me, as to a father and lover, to get from me what you have been denied in the past. But you hold back because you fear that I will feel as bad about you as you do, that I will either turn away like your father or abuse you as did your neighbor and doctor." At other times she actively tried to push me away by making obnoxious phone calls between the sessions, dropping bombshells in the hours and then refusing to elaborate on them (a form of sadistic teasing), threatening to drop out of treatment every other day, badgering me with repetitive personal questions she knew I would not answer, and constantly protesting that I did not care for her. Then I was able to say, "You want to be close to me but you push me away because you are afraid that I will reject or abuse you, as you have experienced with others." At other times I pointed out that her self-destructive threats were ways of retaliating against her parents for their past deprivation of her and against me for currently refusing to meet her needs, and that her fear of losing me was so great that she dared not express her anger more directly. In addition to these and other interpretations, it was necessary for me to *empathically acknowledge* her frustration in the transference. "I understand how hard it is for you, having suddenly become aware of needs which you have previously denied, to want things from me that I refuse to give. You interpret my consistent commitment to help you, as no more nor less than a therapist (which is what you need most), as meaning that I am as indifferent to you as your father appeared to be." This last is also a good example of clarifying reality (see Chap. 11).

In your interpretive resolution of the transference it is important that you do not pretend and convey that you are trying to "explain away" all the patient's feelings for you as nothing more than recapitulations of an infantile past. Rather, you must accept that you are not merely a father, mother, sister, or brother imago, but also a flesh-and-blood person, with a particular personality and physiognomy. The reality of your presence and your empathy cannot be analyzed away. Although therapists do not often mention it, a special relationship develops between two individuals involved in as emotionally intimate an enterprise as psychotherapy. Recall that Ms. Y. was insulted when I prematurely related her feelings toward me to her history. She felt that I was thereby devaluing and discounting them. To reduce all aspects of the therapist-patient relationship (including the therapeutic alliance) to transference is as egregious an error as the opposite extreme, viewing it all as current and "real."

Complete interpretations should be delivered only when you feel there is ample evidence for the clinical hypotheses, only after you have encountered and addressed the issues many different times and ways and have received confirmatory responses from the patient. Only after hearing the central themes and preoccupations of Ms. Y. for hour after hour, only after witnessing her alternating approach, withdrawal, and turbulence in the transference, only after seeing the clockwork connection between her parents' weekends away from her and my absences on the one hand and her self-destructiveness on the other was I able to link her behaviors to feeling deprived and abandoned by her parents and me.

How does one know when a confrontation, clarification or, especially, interpretation is correct? What are your criteria? First of all, it is necessary to understand that accurate (and correctly timed) interpretations result in a *diminution* of the resistance to conscious awareness of the matter under consideration. Consequently, the most common validation of an interpretation is the patient's production of hitherto repressed, preconscious memories, affects, fantasies, and fears—associations, in other words, which are consistent with, and amplify upon, the issue in question. An interpretation may be confirmed by a simple assent, nod of agreement, or a comment such as "it rings true" or "it feels right." Of course, an assent or too ready agreement followed by no more attention to the matter may mean the patient is agreeing just to quiet you and to shelve the matter. Or, it may mean that you are actually incorrect or premature and that he is simply complying with you out of fear or the desire to please you.

This sapping of the resistance, and concomitant saving of the energy previously tied up in countercathexis, may issue in a laugh, a sense of relieved pressure, the lighting of a cigarette or a change in posture or, more rarely, an "Ah-ha" experience or mild sense of euphoria. (Upon the recognition of particularly pivotal connections and their communication to the patient, the therapist sometimes undergoes his own "Ah-ha" or "Eureka" experience, a mild intellectual intoxication or, at times, an aesthetic appreciation of the beauty of the psyche and of his craft.) The reduction in resistance may eventuate, though it need not, in symptomatic improvement. Or, quite to the contrary, it may lead to a worsening in symptomatology, the result of the ego's frantic effort to resurrect its defenses against the onslaught of dangerous preconscious and unconscious fantasies. Or, it may resurrect old symptoms or construct new ones as a final defense against the forbidden impulses. Recall Mr. T.'s substituting, following our pillaging of his defenses, an illusion for a paralysis. Mr. P.'s impotence, long dormant, flared up temporarily as he became aware of a hitherto repressed castration complex related to positive and negative oedipal issues, in particular related to discomfort with the discovery that his concern with castration was not simply a fear, but a wish (to submit sexually and emotionally to his father). This is the case of a symptom bucking itself up, fighting harder in the face of your advance, just like the army of a beleaguered nation when the enemy approaches its capital. It is, unfortunately, necessary that most people, like Ms. Y., "get worse" before they "get better."

If your interpretation is correct, but ill-timed (i.e., when the material is *un*conscious rather than *pre*conscious), you heighten, rather than lower, the resistance, and you encounter phenomena such as a violent denial, a complete block in the train of associations, an indignant silence, ridicule, nervous and uneasy coughing and shifting, changing the subject (although even here, the next topic tends to be obliquely related to the previous one), or acting out (getting up and walking out of the office).

If your interpretation is not merely ill-timed, but actually incorrect, then you may of course elicit any of the aforementioned responses, but you are more likely to provoke a blank stare, a puzzled look, or complete indifference and resumption of the previous line of conversation. In other words, it is rare, as we know from common experience, that people respond obstreperously to comments that are totally erroneous. Comments that are on target, even if they do not hit the bull's eye, are more likely to evoke our indignation than those that miss it altogether.

In addition, each patient has his own unique style of confirming or refuting interpretations or of alerting you to their prematurity. Mr. P., with central issues around dominance-submission and power-weakness, all of which he equated with masculinity versus femininity, experienced each interpretation as a violation of his masculine self-esteem, as a castration and homosexual penetration to which he reacted with hurt and anger. In order for me to intervene at all, it was necessary to eventually interpret this behavior (an example of how the *form* or *style* of a patient's communication is as much the substance of therapy as the content of the communication). He confirmed my interpretation by answering with a string of associations about "belittlement" at the hands of his father and employer and by expressing that one of his deepest fears was that he might actually bring this upon himself and enjoy it. Thus, he discovered that much of his anger at the interpretations, which represented little rapes, was a way of reacting against his underlying enjoyment of them and of preserving his masculinity. Other patients respond to interpretations as magical milk from an omnipotent mother and care less about what you say than that *you* are saying it. This, too, can be counterproductive and must eventually be commented upon.[7]

In the final analysis, if a line of interpretation is correct, it eventually issues in behavioral change because it accurately addresses the unconscious conflicts and dangers that have impeded it.

Interpretations should be couched in plain language, free of jargon, and should incorporate the patient's own words as much as possible. They should be highly polished and crafted, well thought out and precisely formulated, *before* you express them to the patient. The *manner* in which they are delivered is as important as the wording and content. They must be clinically correct and yet accompanied by empathy. There must be a ring of conviction in your voice and yet your interpretation must not sound like an *ex cathedra* pronouncement. You must recognize that no complete interpretation, or whole barrel of them, ever totally captures the rich complexity that is a single human being, that you can never completely extract the meaning from even the most prosaic of lives.

Be careful not to sound like a detective or prosecuting attorney on the trail of a criminal. Avoid an attitude that suggests, "I've got you now." Refrain from interpreting, like intervening in general, when you are angry. Do not appear too triumphant or pleased with yourself. Remember and implicitly convey that you can give the patient only what he has given you. Indeed, he will occasionally arrive at his own complete interpretations and should be allowed to do so as often as he can. For example, it was Mr. P. who alerted me to his masculine-feminine issues and the fact that, for him, my interventions were sexual penetrations and power plays.

You should never interpret along more than one or two lines at any given time. The patient will be in the midst of a tangled forest, seeing only a few trees and the underbrush. You must give him his bearings, show him the path, and help him sense the lay of the land. To point out every little side path, in addition to the main one, will detract from the

---

[7]Similarly, your interpretive and therapeutic work will have unconscious meanings for you too: voyeurism, aggression, dominance, sexual exploitation, masochism, vicariously giving to yourself that of which you have been deprived, raising a child, procreating a new self with the patient, magically seeking solutions to your own problems, and so forth. To the extent that you have been successfully "therapized" you will be consciously aware of, and uncontrolled by, these and other elements of your personality.

power of your message and hopelessly confuse him. Eventually you will see that many of the peripheral issues intertwine and intersect with the central ones. Indeed, it is often possible to trenchantly summarize the red threads, the central dynamics, of an entire life in a few sentences from which radiate all your interpretations of the infinite variations upon this theme. For Ms. Y. one of those sentences would be: "I have already suffered enough at the hands of my parents and shall now return home to get that of which I have been deprived, and to punish them for their mistakes; however, since I am deathly afraid of the consequences, I must woo and batter them in a self-destructive way."[8]

## RECONSTRUCTION

*Reconstruction* is another important species of intervention, and it bears a close and complicated relationship to interpretation. Reconstructions can lead to interpretations, can form part of interpretations, or can follow from the patient's response to an interpretation. Greenson's (1967) discussion of this type of intervention is excellent.

Broadly speaking, to reiterate, psychodynamic therapy is a largely reconstructive procedure. You and the patient are involved not so much in uncovering his pristine pure history and prehistory as in reconstructing it from a combination of accurate recollections of actual events, defensively and wishfully distorted reminiscences, and sheer fantasy.

However, "reconstruction" proper means the therapist's substituting his own hypotheses for missing details in the patient's story. For example, when Ms. Y. was at the height of her oedipal transference, she had recollected several dreams in which her father and I exhibited ourselves to her. I suggested that there were perhaps times in the past when her father actually was exhibitionistic to her. She then recalled that he often wandered around in his underwear. Then, after several minutes of uncomfortable silence, she remembered that there were occasions when, while he was hugging the patient in bed, her mother would tell him to put on his underwear.

---

[8]Although I advocate limiting your interpretive work, at any given time, to no more than a dynamic or two in the patient's life, I do not intend for you to fall into the trap of viewing him reductionistically. Because you acquire, for transferential and social status reasons, much authority in your patient's life, it is easy for him to adopt your interpretations as the gospel. Indeed, what can result in some so-called insight-oriented treatments is that the patient acquires a few reductionistic interpretations (partial truths at best) from the therapist and uses them to build himself a new defensive structure. From a pragmatic point of view (in many supportive treatments) this may be acceptable, for the new level of compromise formation may allay anxiety and permit the patient to establish a more adaptive equilibrium. However, it may do so at the expense of his autonomy and the richness of his experience of self and world.

Not all reconstructions are so easily confirmable. With one patient there was considerable evidence, from his adult relations with women, to support the hypothesis that his preoccupation with being esteemed by women and his sense of incapability when separated from them were functions of his mother's withdrawal of her acknowledgment of him upon his dawning assertion of his own autonomy in childhood. This rang true to the patient and produced a chain of affect-laden memories of her failure to acknowledge him in adolescence and early adulthood and her constant message that he could not manage on his own and that he should return to the parental home and work in the family business.

## WORKING THROUGH

Isolated complete interpretations are transformative only in Hollywood. In real life it is necessary to speak to the central dynamics again and again, each time in a slightly different context and with a different nuance. In "working through" the real changes occur; this is where the patient progressively feels his way into his insights. He learns, through your interpretations of his transference and current behaviors, that he has been living in an intrapsychic, historically determined world, rather than the real one, and that the dragons he fears are but shadows from the past.

Working through is a process in which the patient becomes aware not only of previously unconscious matters, but of conscious issues whose significance he never appreciated: "I seem to have always known that but never quite like I do now." "I always thought that was true, but I never dreamed *just how true.*" Working through is following the red thread through its twists and turns in the skein of the patient's history and his relationship with you.

For example, with Ms. Y. I had to continually address, in sometimes exasperating repetitiveness, her alternate approach to and withdrawal from me and her father, her self-destructiveness, her negative self-image, her conflictual love and hate, her sense of entitlement, her need to distance people and the various intrapsychic dangers that led to this, in all the different guises in which they manifested themselves. Sometimes it seemed that we were getting nowhere, but my line of interpretation was correct and eventually bore fruit.

Mr. P. was less resistant than Ms. Y. in that the working through was less strenuous, though still difficult. It was necessary for him to understand not simply about his strong, antithetical desires to overcome the father on the one hand and submit to him on the other, and the castration complex associated with both. He had also to learn that this polarity manifested itself, in one form or another, in virtually all his fantasies, endeavors, and relationships—that he equated strength and sexual potency with masculinity and weakness and sexual impotence with femininity; that every interaction, whether with males or females, was a battle in which there would be one superior and one inferior, one castrater and one castrate. Working through showed him how he applied these infantile categories of interpretation, derived from his early relationship with a seductive, smothering mother and a domineering but emotionally distant father, to all his perceptions of self and world.

It involved tracing these categories through his relationships with his wife, employer, friends, colleagues, and me. They were expressed in his need to control and dominate his conversations (including those with me) such that any interruption or comment by the other was viewed as a penetration; in his inability to be sufficiently passive to be receptive to his feelings, and to relinquish control enough to optimally free-associate (i.e., he viewed any upsurge of preconscious and unconscious material as itself another penile intrusion); in a tendency to first "analyze" his own material before then "reporting" it to me (i.e., a way of "covering his bases," as he put it); in a preoccupation with deadlines and "pushing his work through" to completion lest he find himself unable to do so, just as in intercourse he would insert his penis the moment he had an erection out of fear of losing it; in a preoccupation with athletic prowess, with oscillating viewpoints of himself as powerful and weak; public speaking inhibitions and stuttering related to conflicts over masculine assertiveness and to castration anxiety; in what he called "pee shyness," a difficulty urinating in the presence of others; in his habit of leaving sales reports undone such that his employer would "have something" on him and could "come down on" him; in his taking control of what he feared most—mortification (a castration equivalent)—by behaving in a manner unconsciously calculated to make him appear the fool and, as I expressed in the last chapter, in his figures of speech ("being one down," "getting screwed").

For him, working through also entailed seeing how his positive and negative oedipal (expressive and defensive sexuality and aggression) issues were intertwined with his preoedipal, especially oral, ones—related to early loss, deprivation, repressed dependency needs, and fear of rejection. This latter functioned as a sort of minor melody or harmony throughout the treatment. The danger situations alternated back and forth between castration and loss of the loved object, often with both present simultaneously.

The all-important matrix in which the interpretations and working through occur is that of *empathy and consistent concern, acceptance,* and *attentiveness.* This should be the ambience in which your interpretations, like all your interventions, transpire. It is impossible to separate the therapeutic effect of the interpretation from that of the attitude that you convey. *Both* must be present. One cannot work without the other. Both are curative. It is impossible to overestimate the transformative potency of simply being there, attentively, day after day at the appointed hour, of simply sticking with the patient through fair weather and foul.

For example, Ms. Y. felt stupid, unable to think, worthless, devoid of interests and feelings, and viewed the world as a cold and malevolent place because of her parents' lack of esteem of her. By repeatedly seeking to avoid her feelings, by rapidly "forgetting" about crucial issues we discussed, by using her sense of inability as an excuse to avoid this difficult work, by being withholding, by saying, eventually, "I know I can do this work but, you know, I'm not going to try," and by being querulous and plaintive about my refusal to meet her needs, she tried to induce me to reject her and scream at her as did her parents in order both to protect herself from conflicts around intimacy and to "go ahead and get over with" what she feared most (my rejection of her). I assisted her *as much* by empathically staying with her and by refusing to respond like her parents as I did with any of my interpretations. She began to esteem herself as I esteemed her, to see herself as I saw her, to expect of herself what I expected of her, and to adopt toward herself the same tolerant understanding that I displayed. I was becoming, to speak technically, a benign and constructive part of her ego, ego ideal, and superego.

In addition to the patient's internalization of your benevolent and constructive attitude toward him, your esteem of him is important because it in large measure allows and induces him to undergo the deprivation and pain of therapeutic work. His sense of your unconditional positive regard also enables him to eventually talk about that which he otherwise fears would result in his eviction.

Being nothing more nor less than an empathic therapist, rather than adopting any particular prescribed, contrived, and "cooked-up" set of attitudes, is the real "corrective emotional experience" in psychotherapy, the real afterparenting, insofar as any occurs. Neither my interpretations nor my attitude alone was sufficient for change; both were required. (Recall my remarks on empathy in Chapter 7.)

# 10

# Insight-Oriented Psychotherapy: Termination and Other Issues

The first point to understand about termination is pessimistic: that you will never be involved in a totally satisfactory one. This is not merely because the overwhelming tendency of both patient and therapist is to avoid their feelings about the upcoming loss, but because no neurosis is ever completely analyzed and dissolved, no human being ever exhaustively understood, and no transference ever totally resolved. Finally, there is the fact, which is real and cannot be analyzed away, that two human beings have participated in an intimacy the like of which few people ever experience.

From the patient's side, he has been understood in a way that he has never encountered before. You know more about him than does any other human being, including his father, mother, spouse, or best friend. In some respects you even know him better than he knows himself. You have patiently listened to, and empathized with, him about material so painful or embarrassing that he had never dreamed he could disclose it to another. You have helped him become aware of secrets that he kept, not merely from others, but also from himself. And, throughout his disclosure of what he deemed the worst parts of himself and of humanity in general, you have stayed with him, thereby reassuring him of his basic worth. As anyone knows who has successfully completed his own therapy, one's therapist is fondly and permanently ensconced in one's heart. He will always be a special person.

From your side, it may seem less obvious why the patient's leaving should pose any special difficulties. After all, you have rarely mentioned your personal life and private feelings and fantasies, have assiduously limited your contact with him to the prescribed hours, have received payment for what is basically a contractual relationship, and have consistently refused to gratify his needs for the ideal parent, spouse, or friend. Nevertheless, even though you have have not spoken of yourself or taken the patient onto your lap or into your home or bed, you have felt, tried to understand, and stayed with him every step of the way. To be sure, this much of yourself you have revealed to him. A bond of closeness develops between us and our patients which, though physically severed at the close of treatment, does not end with it. I continue to have nostalgic memories of those whose treatments I helped carry to a reasonable completeness, and bittersweet recollections of those whose failed or did less well. Finally, as Jung was fond of saying, every therapeutic encounter is a *mutual* transformation. Your patient impinges upon you, just as you on him and, if you resonate with him you often hear voices in yourself you never dreamed existed or thought long silent. If you listen to him he instructs you not merely about human nature in general, but about yourself—your mannerisms and ways of being with patients (and people in general). Wise is the therapist who can say, in paraphrase of the Talmudist, "From all of my patients have I learned."

How do you know when a patient has entered the final, or termination, stage? Does the patient himself announce it or do you? Or is it some sort of an osmotic, telepathic, or mystical interaction between the two of you?

The answer is that *the patient himself will tell you,* not by proclamation, but gradually and quietly, verbally and nonverbally, wittingly and unwittingly.

The working through that began in the previous phase will continue, but the threads are by now being woven into a tapestry with a discernible pattern. In termination you tighten up the weave, filling in the gaps in figure and ground, and smooth the edges. To express it more prosaically, the patient is by now aware of the major dynamics and their role in his psychopathology. He is gaining a full appreciation of how he is reacting to you and the world, not as you really are, but as he wants and fears you to be. He recognizes his strenuous attempts to induce those outside his head to conform to his expectations of those within it. He catches himself reenacting the old dramas of the past—the troublesome triumphs and bitter defeats—at home, at work, at play and, above all, with you. He understands that he has been living in a world whose treasures and traps are historical illusions which cast, however, real shadows on the present.

When the patient himself begins to take the initiative in making and amplifying upon the connections in "working through," it is a sign that you are entering the final stage. When he begins to adopt the same tolerant and understanding attitude toward himself that you do, when he exhibits the same curiosity about, and reflectiveness upon, his feelings, fantasies, and behaviors that you do, and when he stops assuming responsibility for that over which he had and has no control and starts assuming it over that for which he does, then you have, again, a reliable milestone to the termination stage. These newly acquired intellectual and affective-attitudinal abilities are not the same as the personified intrapsychic dialogue and recollection of your physical presence that commonly occur in the middle phase. They are, rather, the function of a genuine identification in which your positive and therapeutic characteristics have become, to some extent, depersonified, and now serve as the bricks and mortar for a reconstructed ego, self-image, ego ideal, and superego. In short, the patient has obtained not merely previously inaccessible information about his personality, but a new way of looking at himself through identification with you.

He does not wallow in self-reflection and self-analysis to the detriment of living his life, but he does remain capable, when appropriate and in the times of crisis to which no one is immune, of knowing how he feels, of identifying and understanding his behavior and something about its purposes, and of charting his course accordingly.

When the patient's resistance has withered to the point that he begins to approach that ideal of free association—honest and minimally self-reflective and selective talking—then you have another clear indicator of the approaching end. In other words, when patients become able to obey the fundamental rule, it is time for them to leave treatment!

As you approach the destination of your voyage the pace slows and the waters become less turbulent. There is more stillness and tranquility, less sense of urgency, more quiet sitting together. The hitherto prepotent complexes rear their heads less frequently and awesomely. You may find yourself running out of things to say and being tempted to talk about the weather or sports. Superficially, this may resemble the resistance of the earlier treatment, but it has a different "feel" to it. It is still a resistance, that is, an avoidance of dealing with separation issues related to termination, but at the same time it is an oblique communication to you that it is time to address them.

At this point the patient often reports that the therapy "feels" different. To express this in the metaphor of a long hike, the early stage feels like a gentle slope, the first half of the middle stage a steep and strenuous climb, working through a plateau strewn with boulders, sinks, and periodic peaks and chasms, and the final phase as relatively smooth and level ground, though not without thorns and brambles. To use the analogue of a tunnel, entering termination is seeing the light at the end.

The patient nearing termination will report feeling better, experiencing fewer problems with spouse, friends, family, and colleagues, getting more engaged with life, feeling more productive, more solid, more balanced, and more securely anchored in both self and world. The old issues are losing their sting. He fears less and can risk more. He may begin to make and implement decisions over which he has vacillated for years. Often he apprises us that friends and family tell him he is somehow different, more relaxed, easier to be around. He begins to take a different perspective on self and world, which one patient expressed as "suddenly discovering that I had been walking about with one eye shut."

He is not diffident about the role he has played in his transmutation at the same time that he is able to feel, and express, some gratitude for your part in the process. Neither should you be shy about accepting any thanks. Although he has done the lion's share of the work, what was achieved could not have been without your tenacity and expertise.

In the termination of a reasonably complete insight-oriented psychotherapy, the patient's heated blame and hot pursuit of the malefactors in his life usually begin to cool. He recognizes that the foibles and failures of his caretakers, siblings, friends, and others were in large measure the tragic fruit of their own early histories rather than of maleficent attempts to warp him. He may even find himself in the position to forgive, a bit, those who have failed him and to realize that "there but for the grace of therapy would go he." Indeed, I have found that this ability and willingness to turn that same tolerant eye toward one's parents that he turns toward himself is a prime gauge of the completeness of the therapy.

Ms. Y., for example, went from an initial total (conscious) assumption of the responsibility for her problems with a concomitant refusal to look at her parents' role, through a stage in which she viewed the latter as malignant devils from whom she was determined to exact her pounds of flesh, to a point at which she could acknowledge that they, like she, had been in the grip of history (her parents had been deprived and abused in their childhoods). In the end, she accepted that though they shared the responsibility for her neurosis, she was no longer a helpless child at their mercy but an adult with the sole responsibility for extricating herself from it.[1]

---

[1]Daily we are made tragically aware of the ways in which people misuse one another. We are oftentimes tempted to chime in with the patient in blaming a malignant parent, friend, or spouse. By and large, particularly in the case of the first, such interventions are not indicated. We empathize, convey to the patient that he is fully entitled to his feelings, and encourage him to elaborate on them, but we stop short of blaming. Although, on the one hand, the patient might welcome our imprecations of the "malefactor," on the other he might unconsciously resent our attacking someone who, in all probability, he also loves and needs to see as to some extent loving him. What might it say to him, by implication, about himself if he viewed his parents' dispositions toward him as totally malignant? Also, to engage in blame with the patient strengthens any tendencies to externalization and sense of entitlement.

On a more pessimistic or, as I prefer to view it, *realistic* note, you and your patient will not have delivered a paragon of psychological virtue. Many of the same conflicts will still beset him, but with an important difference. They will be of diminished charge and he will be aware of them and can, in his navigation through life, sail round them as a pilot does a shoal.

Nor will you have removed (nor would you want to) all his defenses. Life in human civilization is impossible without them since the demands of the passions and of society are never totally compatible; the most we can hope for is an intelligent equilibrium that does not sacrifice too much of the one for the other. You will have helped him exchange his maladaptive defenses for more adaptive ones: intellectualization may replace projection; reaction formation may replace denial; suppression and sublimation may replace repression or displacement. For example, he may become a fanatical member of Alcoholics Anonymous rather than an alcoholic. He may consciously decide not to have an extramarital affair and risk hurting his loved ones (e.g., suppression) rather than repress these desires with the attendant loss of energy and danger of symptom formation. He may channel, appropriately, his oedipal aggression into his career rather than displace it onto his spouse and children. He may stop looking for the ideal parents and family and join a group dedicated to the advancement of constructive social, political, or religious ideals. He may give to his children what was not given to him as an adaptive way of actively mastering the passively experienced traumata.

One thing your patient will *not* have acquired is a pain-free existence. Mental, like physical, pain is an important signal that something is awry and needs our attention. Life is not without stress. The results of therapy will help your patient cope with stress more successfully, but will not eliminate it altogether. Reality, while it sometimes works for us, sometimes against us, can never be totally controlled nor analyzed away. You can protect your patient from the "slings and arrows of outrageous fortune" no more than Freud's successful analysis of the Rat Man could save him from the Juggernaut of World War I. Indeed, a part of human wisdom, to which therapy may or may not move one closer, is accepting that reality will eventually snuff out every last ember of our narcissism, while resolving meanwhile to burn as brightly and warmly as we can.

In sum, your patient's personality has been years in the making and is transformed only minimally in the handful of hours at your disposal. Nevertheless, most patients (and therapists) find what results to be worth the time and effort.

When the aforementioned is occurring, the patient usually will bring up termination himself. It is always preferable for him to do so. In those rare instances where termination seems indicated and yet he has not broached it, then either you are wrong (generally out of countertransference discomfort and distortion) or else there is a bit of unresolved neurosis (usually around issues of separation and dependency). If it seems that the latter is the case, then you might introduce the topic by saying, "In the light of the progress we've made, I find it curious you haven't brought up the issue of when we should stop."

The termination date should be mutually agreed upon and should be set far enough in advance for your patient to begin his grief work. Within a treatment of two to four years, this means allowing him from three to six months. You should not, as I once mistakenly did, allow a patient to walk in and announce it is his last session without strenuously attempting to convince him to go through a proper termination. (Largely because of this, it was necessary for this patient to reenter treatment several years later.) The patient needs ample time, not only to peel away his defenses against grieving, but to deal with the unresolved bits of neurosis that inevitably resurrect themselves (partly in the service of the unconscious desire to stay in treatment). If symptoms he thought himself freed of return, you should explain this to him and then analyze them in the context in which they occur. The patient should experience himself moving toward a previously agreed upon date, at which time he will walk in to take his leave of you.

Every termination, whether it be the natural and mutually agreed upon result of a therapeutic collaboration that has accomplished its goals, or the function of your relocating and transferring the patient to another clinician, is to some degree experienced by him as a *rejection*. If you are the one leaving, then this is easier for him to acknowledge, along with the accompanying hurt and anger (and correspondingly harder for you), than if it is he who is departing, but it will be present either way. In the latter case it is you, after all, who are encouraging and permitting him to leave.

You also need to be aware that the anticipation of this loss resurrects unresolved feelings about previous losses, separations, and rejections from the least, to the most, significant. Every leavetaking is a bit like a death and unconsciously reminds us (and prepares us for) that more or less distant occasion when we shall bid our final farewell to friends and loved ones. Terminating therapy is hence a microcosm of the most fundamental issue of human existence: that we are fully human only when we are connected to others and yet that we are destined to lose every last one of them, to depart this globe as we entered it—alone.

Once the date is set there is usually an initial period of denial in which the patient may not speak of it again for sessions or weeks. In some this denial takes the form of a mild hypomania. If the therapist is sufficiently uncomfortable with loss, then he will collaborate with this process and a grossly inadequate termination may vitiate the results of an otherwise satisfactory treatment. If, however, both patient and therapist are willing to come to terms with their feelings about this reality, then the next stage is usually one of vague and low-grade depression. The patient's isolation may be such that he does not consciously attribute it to the termination and hence needs reminding.

This depression is composed of hurt, warmth, internalized anger, guilt over this anger, and the fear that one will not be able to go it alone, that the consequences of separation will be disastrous. Your task is to help him sort out these and other painful and highly specific feelings from the smokescreen affect that is depression. Some people find it easier to deal with their anger than with the hurt and warmth that go hand in hand. Others deal with the latter to the exclusion of the former. Some attempt to circumvent these feelings altogether by bargaining for progressive postponements in the termination date. Virtually all will do some anticipatory grief work if you do not allow them to avoid the termination.

The patient grieves, not merely for you and for those whom you represent, but for the dying, psychopathological identity with which he has lived for many years. One does not discard an identity—even a neurotic one—easily. It is a bit like losing an unpredictable, often troublesome, but sometimes helpful, companion to whom one has grown accustomed. One is mostly relieved, but a little bit sorrowful and fearful that one may not find another.

You should apprise the patient that he will not do all his grieving before he leaves. Indeed, mourning is, by definition, something that occurs after the fact. He should know that this is likely to manifest itself after termination as a transient melancholy and irritation which he should not psychopathologize, but deal with like any other grief. Because of this, and because of the positive, alloplastic changes that will begin to issue from, and play back upon, the patient's transformed internal state, he should also know that it will take some time before he realizes how much therapy has helped him and before he reaps its full harvest.

It is important for you to recognize that it is not merely the patient's unresolved feelings about previous losses that will be resurrected, but also *your own*. This eventuates in a bit of sadness and anger. In avoidance of this you may invent all sorts of "good reasons" to prolong treatment. This is especially true of those patients whom you find particularly interesting and easy to cathect or identify with.[2] Departing from more troublesome and less rewarding patients may be equally hard, in part because of guilt over any relief you may feel. Of course any

---

[2]For an amusing example see Lindner's (1954) article, "The Jet Propelled Couch."

time it is we who are leaving, guilt will loom large, no matter how we feel about the patient, especially if he has major issues around deprivation and rejection.

Upon his departure, the implicit communication that you are experiencing a loss as well, a fond handclasp, genuine wishes of good will, and perhaps a statement that you have enjoyed and valued the work that the two of you have done are all in order. You should not, however, burden him with a maudlin show of sentiment or the feeling that he remains somehow accountable to you.

Finally, be reassured that every therapy, even the most successful, is carried out in the face of an infinite number of blunders and missteps, and an often appalling obtuseness, on the part of the therapist. At times it seems that patients recover despite, not because of, us. Patients will, however, if we pay attention, correct our errors. And by far the majority will forgive us our mistakes, our humanness.

## CONTACT WITH PATIENTS OUTSIDE OF TREATMENT

Every patient harbors the conscious-unconscious fantasy that your mutual involvement will not end with termination, but that it will resurrect itself in its old form or that you will at last reward him for all his effort with a real relationship. At times you will feel a corresponding inclination; Searles (1965) has confessed to marital fantasies with his terminating patients.

If you are handling the termination properly you will be cognizant of this issue and looking for any indication to address it. Most patients with intense "continuation fantasies" will broach them long before the actual day of termination. If a patient has not talked about it at all and raises it importunately in the last session, this indicates that something has gone awry in the timing and/or the analysis of the termination.

You should have your own feelings and philosophy worked out in advance—both in general and for each patient in particular—of the occasions on which such issues might arise. With some adolescents and certain schizophrenic or ego-compromised individuals it is helpful and indicated to leave the door open for letters and phone calls in particularly stressful times. For many of them, the mere knowledge that they can phone or write is sufficiently supportive that they never feel the need to. However, for patients who have completed a course of insight-oriented treatment, more caution is advised.

A male therapist may, for example, in the case of a woman who retains certain of her dependent and histrionic features, fear that refusing to comply with such a request might lead her to feel rejected or insignificant. Nevertheless, the fantasies that he might stimulate otherwise and the unintended wheels he might set in motion may end up calling for limits that would prove far more devastating to her self-esteem than had he simply analyzed her fantasies and, if need be, kindly but steadfastly reasserted the boundaries between treatment and the real world.

First of all, no relationship between an ex-patient and his therapist can ever be anything like a normal friendship. There is too much water over the dam. You have occupied roles, vis-à-vis one another, so out of the ordinary that it is hypocrisy and self-deception to think you could just slip into a normal relationship as if all that has transpired had not. The interaction has been too one-sided, with too much exposure of one person, and not enough of the other, to turn it into a truly egalitarian friendship.

Second, *no* transference is ever completely resolved. Consciously-unconsciously the patient continues to view you as a bit godlike (and perhaps a bit devilish). Time with you is supercharged time. Your every utterance, every disclosure, and every gratification or deprivation are laden with significance. This poses as heavy, or heavier, a burden on the therapist as on the patient. The ex-therapist turned friend bears a responsibility for the impact of his behavior on the ex-patient turned friend borne by no other friend.

Third, it is always possible that, due to the unforseeable turns in the wheel of fortune, the patient might need to consult you again at some point. It is always easier and less time-consuming if he can return to his old therapist for a refresher than if he has to tell his story anew. If you have, meanwhile, become his "friend," then you will be useless to him in your former capacity.

In short, I advocate first analyzing the patient's desires for a continuance and then, if necessary, sensitively conveying to him the aforementioned and explaining that any inclination to return in the first months following termination will most likely be an attempt to circumvent the mourning and to avoid coming to terms with the full implications of his independence.

As for outside contacts with patients during the treatment, they should be minimized. In certain locales an occasional serendipitous contact with the patient is unavoidable, in which case you should understand that the same transference is operating there as in the treatment and that your every word will be suffused with meaning. A bit of discomfort about this is normal for any therapist, but if you are excessively anxious then you should ferret out your own conflicts and fears.

You should of course greet him and be polite and if, as at a bus stop, the contact is going to be for more than an instant, let him do most of the talking. Other than a general comment about the weather or a bit of superficial chitchat about the transit system or the world series, you should continue to hold fast to the rule about self-disclosure. You do not have to own the responsibility for any discomfort he may feel. If the patient does not bring up the contact in the next session, it is usually wise to ask him how he felt about it, thereby bringing home to him that yours is a therapeutic, not a real, relationship.

Unfortunately, therapists sometimes attempt an insight-oriented approach with friends, relatives, or associates. This can even occur in psychiatric facilities where one staff member is treating another or a faculty member a student. In any case in which therapist and patient are to be thrown into more than occasional contact, and particularly when they are called upon to work together as colleagues or supervisor and supervisee, this is *unworkable*. Anyone who believes in transference and the analytic way of resolving it cannot think otherwise. All this should be self-evident but, from the extent to which it occurs, it would seem not so.

## THE NEGATIVE THERAPEUTIC REACTION

Initially I thought that the "negative therapeutic reaction," the idea that a patient might actively, if unconsciously, sabotage his own treatment in the face of accurate interpretations and empathy, was a ploy cooked up by cranky therapists to explain their own ineptitude! One of my biggest surprises in this field has been that it is not, or at least that it need not be. It is impossible to believe, unless you have seen it, that people can actually be invested in remaining disturbed.

Patients may cling to their suffering and maladaptive behavior for a variety of, mostly unconscious, reasons (quite apart from what is known as primary gain): because the security and predictability of present pain and dissatisfaction are viewed as preferable to the risks of change (i.e., "out of the frying pan and into the fire"); because of the dependent benefits and decreased demands for adult responsibility accruing to their dysfunction; because their psychopathology is a familiar part of their identity; in order to punish themselves for a variety of conscious and unconscious, real or imagined, transgressions against superego ideals; as a way of chiding you, in your capacity as parental imago, for not giving them more and implicitly holding you responsible for their distress ("throwing it in your face"); out of the fantasy that, if they eventually suffer enough, you will give them what they want; as a relatively "safe" way (internalization) of dealing with anger toward you and those whom you unconsciously represent; as an oblique way of expressing this anger by attempting to defeat your efforts to help them; out of the sheer *enjoyment,* as Searles (1979) has noted, of foiling your efforts to "cure" them; out of a purely sexual masochistic enjoyment; and out of fears of gratitude and the insult to their self-esteem that your successful assistance of them would pose.

Two of my patients, despite considerable dynamic insight, did not begin to change until I addressed their sheer delight in defeating me and until I took sufficient distance to drive home that, although I greatly desired to be useful to them, I would neither be made nor broken by the outcome which they, in any event, and not I, controlled.

## TALKING WITH PATIENTS

Learning dynamic psychiatry involves three tasks: 1) learning the theory, 2) applying the theory in the organization and formulation of clinical data, and 3) intervening clinically on the basis of one's dynamic understanding. This last is by far the most difficult and is the facility this book will help you the least to attain. Some do relatively well in the academic task of learning the theory and formulating history and yet, for various reasons (often characterological or psychopathological), fail in applying it.

Dynamic theory is, preeminently, a way of *thinking* about patients but not of *talking* with them. There is no place for talking id, ego, and superego with patients. All of dynamic theory is nothing more than a complex model or scientific metaphor, a tool for understanding; it is a way of making sense of reality but it is not that reality itself. The theory must remain subservient to that never totally analyzable or explicable *gestalt* of human flesh-and-blood interaction. If the fealty is reversed, dynamic theory becomes worse than useless.

If dynamic psychiatry is to eventuate in truly therapeutic interventions, then one must cultivate the technique of translating dynamically based understandings into a language that is meaningful to the patient. By and large, this means converting our metapsychological comprehension into the language of purpose and intentionality that is the common currency of everyday communication.

For example, we do not lecture the patient on psychic causality and historical determinism. We use our reflections, questions, confrontations, clarifications, and interpretations to facilitate his appreciation that his behavior is always *meaningful* within the context of his view of self and world and his history, that he is always purposeful and intentional even if at times he is ambivalently so and in ways in which he is consciously unaware.

Nor do we instruct him upon the analytic theory of conflict, danger, and symptom formation. Rather, we talk to him in terms, as I have demonstrated, of that which he wants and fears. You do not lecture a neurotically guilt-ridden patient on the "omnipotence of thoughts." Instead, you say, "You act as if, merely by talking angrily about your father, who is, after all, 1,000 miles away, that you are somehow capable of injuring or even killing him."

Above all, although you use the tripartite structural theory to conceptualize the otherwise bewildering complexity of his total personality, and although you speak of object representations as if there were crowds within his head, *at no time do you perceive or address him as other than a unitary and more or less integrated individual.* In line with this, you do not tell him he has a hostile superego which obeys the talion law; you convey to him that, although he has been away from his mother for years, he continues to berate himself for every thought and deed, as if he were an arch criminal, just as she did. You do not tell him his id wants one thing, his superego another, and his ego still a third. You tell him he seems to want, simultaneously, three incompatible things. In the case of the man who wants both to fail and to succeed, you say not that, "Your id and ego want success, your superego failure," but rather, "You feel so guilty about wanting to succeed in business, which for you amounts to triumphing over your father, that you need to sabotage your success at every turn."

Furthermore, you always speak to the level of conscious and preconscious control that the patient possesses. This is the place in which the therapeutic alliance is forged. To reiterate, you are not dealing directly with the unconscious. You do not foster the fiction that the patient is a passive automaton buffeted about by the forces of biology and his environment, but rather that he is an autonomous and self-determinative—even if not always consciously so—agent, and that he molds his world as much as it molds him.

Finally, as if matters were not already complicated enough, each therapist must develop modes of intervention and patterns of expression compatible, not only with the particular needs and sensitivities of each patient, but with his own inimitable personality style. What is right for me may not be so for you, and vice versa.

## INTERPRETING DREAMS

Dream interpretation does not carry the same weight in dynamic treatment that it once did. Since the resistance is at its weakest in dreams they, like hypnosis, provide relatively direct access to what is ordinarily unconscious. Therefore, dreams, like hypnosis, played a powerful role in the early history of dynamic psychiatry in convincing people of the unconscious, symbolism, and primary process. Indeed, the dream became the model, as I stated earlier, for the understanding of neurosis itself.

When dynamic psychiatrists shifted their focus from the id to the ego, the drives to the resistance, dreams lost some of their importance. Today's therapist is above all concerned with the preconscious resistance in the wakefully conscious human being, and dreams receive relatively little consideration or are viewed as diversionary exotica in many treatments.

Doubtless this is in some way unfortunate, for the dream is a light shaft into the patient's unconscious. There is no better way of forming an emotional conviction in overdetermination and psychical causality or meaningfulness, nor of obtaining a more rapid overview of a patient's dynamics, than by examining his dreams. A single particularly rich and complex dream has roots extending into every area and era of the patient's psyche and life such that it would virtually be true to say that the latent dream is the patient's personality itself.

Dreams can be utilized in several fashions. They can be interpreted in Talmudic detail, like the ones that Freud (1900) so brilliantly elucidated. This is not likely to occur outside psychoanalysis and in it but rarely. In the training analyses of apprentice psychoanalysts, it is invaluable to have undergone an exquisitely complete understanding of a dream. There is no surer way to appreciate the power of our science than to have experienced a significant dream from one's early treatment, about which one understood little at the time, grow progressively rich and antique in meaning until by the end it is a tapestry of phenomenal beauty and extent. Commenting upon and interpreting such dreams can play a pivotal role in the analysis.

By contrast, in a more supportive therapy, where one would be more concerned with shoring up, rather than analyzing, resistances, the dream could be used in what Saul (1972) calls an "ego-interpretive" way. In other words, you might interpret superficially, speaking especially to the more obvious and currently relevant meanings rather than to the deeper, historical aspects. For example, one borderline woman, terminating a reasonably successful outpatient treatment with me, reported a rich dream, full of symbolism and barely veiled allusions to dependent and oedipal issues, which ended with my jumping out of the car in which we were both riding. I chose to ignore the tantalizing labyrinths of meaning, in which we could have wandered for years, to focus only on her obvious feelings of abandonment and fears that she could not make it without me at her side.

The third and most common way in which dreams are used is simply to increase the therapist's understanding of the patient, even though he might not comment directly to, much less interpret, the dream. A dream can be used diagnostically, as I mentioned earlier. Previously unsuspected degrees of ego weakness can be revealed in dreams with relatively undisguised expression of primitive erotic and aggressive fantasies.

Pay particular attention to any dreams that occur the night before the patient's first meeting with you. These will at times give you an uncanny glimpse into his most salient, if unconscious, preoccupations about, and attitudes toward, treatment. It has been noted, for example, that dreams of going on a trip often express an unconscious wish to flee what the patient has only just begun.

It is well known that people dream every night whether or not they remember their dreams. That we recollect no more dreams than we do is a function of our resistance and of our inattentiveness and disinterest. It may be many weeks before a patient reports his first dream. Mr. E., with his rigidly obsessional defensive structure, did not mention dreams until almost the end of the first year of treatment.[3] When insight-oriented candidates begin to bring you dreams, it is a good sign for the therapy. It means that their resistance is declining and that they are becoming more interested in their inner lives. Since patients know that therapists like dreams, it also means that you are becoming more important to them and that they wish to please you. (The more interest you show in dreams, the more they will bring.) This last can lead to a phenomenal proliferation of dreaming, though it need not substantially influence the dream *content* itself. Patients may even use dreaming and their reporting of them in the service of the resistance, to avoid looking at any other facets of their lives.

You would be well advised to keep a record of the patient's dreams, in the contexts within which they occur, for it will be fascinating to turn back to earlier dreams in light of what you later know. They can presage major shifts in the patient's dynamic equilibrium and transference weeks or months before they occur. Also, as Saul (1972) advocates, you can sometimes pull a treatment out of the doldrums by looking back over the previous eight or ten dreams; you may spot themes and threads you had hitherto missed.

When a patient brings you a dream, keep in mind particularly the line of conversation that immediately preceded it, since there will be unconscious, associative links between them. Note also the patient's affective state and manner of relating it: agitated, sad, angry, urgent, hesitant, and so forth. If he brings in a written account, urge him to first report it to you off the top of his head before reading it. Any omissions or additions from the oral account to the written are clues to particularly affect-laden or conflictual issues. Indeed, some therapists always have the patient repeat the dream report, whether oral or written, for just this reason.

At the same time that you want as accurate a rendition as possible of the dream as actually dreamt, you should accept that you are not some sort of archaeologist who is going to unearth the perfectly preserved manifest dream, much less the latent one. The pristinely pure manifest dream is gone forever. The dream as reported *already* contains the patient's waking associations to it. It does not matter that you hear a

---

[3]His initial dream was a fascinating example of compromise formation between the desire for intimacy and the defenses against it. He dreamed that he slept through the session, but his anxiety about this was such that it actually awakened him from the dream and he arrived at my office on schedule!

mixture of dream and associations; you are not the curator of a dream museum but rather a therapist out to discern, for pragmatic reasons, as much as you can about the patient's dynamics.

Resist the patient's (and your friends' at cocktail parties!) attempts to draw you into interpreting dreams immediately. To do so, without any appreciation of his associations, would be engaging in what Freud called "wild psychoanalysis."[4] If you know much about dreams in general, you will appreciate that it would be presumptuous to think that you could *ever* completely interpret a dream, much less adequately explain it at first hearing. Second, to render an initial interpretation, even if it is basically correct, is both to foster the patient's passivity and belief that you are an omniscient wizard-parent and to make it easier for him to feel that the dream is over and done with, perfectly packaged and ready to be put on the shelf.

When the patient has finished recounting the dream, just sit back and wait. It is a common misconception that when he finishes his report you must say "free-associate." This is as unnecessary as telling the patient to breathe, since it is something that he will do anyway! In other words, you can treat whatever he says next as the first *association* to the dream. Indeed, the rest of the session might be profitably viewed so. Even apparently unrelated topics bear some relationship, expressive or defensive, to it. Only if you fear the patient is going too far afield should you bring him back to the dream itself and request him to free-associate, with the dream specifically in mind. If he responds by attempting to interpret his dream, you should point out that you said "associate" not "interpret." The former is the result of a genuine relaxation of the mind and comes from deeper levels of the psyche; the latter is an intellectual exercise coming from somewhere in the crust of the ego.

If you want to analyze the dream as completely as possible, and this should not be done indiscriminately with every dream with which the

---

[4]A word about so-called "wild psychoanalysis" is in order here. This entails totally bypassing (ravaging or ravishing, perhaps more aptly) the resistances and making highly speculative, "deep" id interpretations in the face of little evidence. This is a common parlor game for some trainees who ferret out the "symbolism" and "hidden motives" in the behavior of their friends and colleagues. Not only is this irritating to the object, but the hypotheses that result are meaningless as well. You can arrive at empirically based dynamic propositions in only one situation, the consulting room. Otherwise, you have insufficient history about the person in general and the behavior in particular and you do not have an unsullied transference to draw inferences from. Unfortunately, some practicing therapists are not immune from such behavior and use psychodynamics to analyze away the opinions of those with whom they disagree. Stanton and Schwartz (1954) found that senior clinical administrators were particularly likely to analyze or diagnose, rather than confront, opposing ideas in trainees and junior staff.

patient regales you, then there are several ways to approach it. You can ask him to begin associating to that segment which seems clearest or most important (to him) or you can simply pick a section or element of the dream and ask him to associate to that, moving gradually through the rest of the dream.

Finally, before leaving off any dream that you are attempting to understand optimally, ask the patient how he felt upon awakening and recalling the dream, whether it was a nightmare that snatched him from sleep, and about his initial associations to it. If he has not, in the course of his associating, given you a good idea of the day residue, ask him about the events and concerns of the previous day. In addition, if he has not gone far toward elucidating the identity of certain figures in the dream, you can ask him specifically, "Who [all] do you think X was?"

Symbols are not considered until after you have finished your more historical spadework. As set forth in Chapter 3, certain symbols appear to be virtually universal: snake for penis; left for feminine, right for masculine; houses, apertures, and enclosures for the vagina, and so forth. Others appear more relative to time and place. Nevertheless, even the so-called universal symbols may have highly idiosyncratic meanings for any given dreamer. In one patient, for example, a snake may symbolize objects that, for his particular historical and current context, are more important than the penis to which it may also allude.

Thus, you must be cautious about assuming you understand the nature of the symbols in any dream. Some of them will be obvious, some will not; and none of them, since they are overdetermined, will be completely understood. You generally use symbols only to elucidate that which is not otherwise explicated by the dreamer's history and associations.

If, after you follow these guidelines, the patient presses you for an interpretation, it is best to turn this back on him and find out what he thinks it means. It is extremely rare, in the early and middle stages, that you would feel secure enough in your knowledge to undertake a "complete" interpretation of a dream. If you feel sufficiently confident in your comprehension of certain pieces of it, and of their relationship to the patient's history, transference, and current life, and *if* you feel that it would somehow facilitate the patient's work if he were apprised of your ideas, then it is permissible to make certain limited statements which point as much to what you do not yet know as to what is known. You want to convey to the patient that his dream, as a part of his psychological life, is relevant and potentially, though not completely, intelligible. However, at the same time you want to impress upon him that both of you must be patient and tolerate a certain amount of ambiguity until you learn more about him. Rich though obscure dreams may not be interpretable, if at all, until the end of a treatment.

## ON BEING SUPERVISED

Dynamic psychotherapy is learned, above all, in supervised clinical work. It is transmitted and immortalized, like all crafts, primarily through the oral tradition. If you are to use this or any other book in a manner useful, and not inimical, to your work with patients, then you must participate concurrently in good supervision. It is the laboratory for which the literature is but theory. It is also the forum in which you learn the supervisory art that most of you will be called upon to practice at one time or another.

Good supervision must speak to both the forest (the red thread and overall drift of the hours) and the trees (the patient's specific communications and your interventions). In order to address both adequately, you must bring the sessions to your supervisor in a variety of ways: process notes, extemporaneous presentations, periodic written revisions of the case history and formulation, and audio and video tapes.

I advocate that you cultivate the practice of beginning the supervisory hour by presenting "off the top of your head" and only later consulting your notes. Doing so will both train your memory and give your teacher a better sense of the "feel" and flow of the hour. In your spontaneity you will often surprise yourself with new insights and with the discovery that you "knew" aspects about the patient of which you were not consciously aware. The process notes add a further dimension to the appreciation of this flow. Remember that your supervisor is more interested in a concrete account of your interactions with the patient than in your theories about him. Finally, periodic revisions of the longitudinal history and formulation often make the difference between a treatment that stagnates and one that advances.

Audio and, especially, audio*visual* recordings allow for an incomparably high-powered examination of the reality upon which your process notes are but commentary. This is the medium in which the supervisor can best comment upon those otherwise intangible manifestations of character and nonverbal communication. Observing and listening to a tape for a few minutes often alert the supervisor to aspects of the patient's and therapist's styles that might not otherwise be apparent until much later, if at all. This, the most anxiety-provoking of all forums, is also where the most detailed criticism of your interventions and attitudes occurs. Many of these latter are transmitted by subtle changes in posture, facial expression and, especially, tone of voice. While no one has the time or the desire (since you would lose the forest for the trees) to use it exclusively, periodic recording is an essential part of being supervised.

Being "supervisable" entails taking good process notes; honestly reporting the interactions of the hour (including your most unspeakable blunders and private reactions); being able to fall flat on your face and to be criticized for it; and listening to your supervisor and suspending disbelief long enough to profit from and test out his ideas without slavishly aping him and while retaining your own critical capacities.[5]

This, of course, is the ideal, and any number of processes, in either party, can interfere with its realization. This brings me to my central point: Although there are considerable differences between being in supervision and being in therapy, and although any confusion between the two on the part of supervisor or supervisee will be worse than unproductive, there are important similarities between the role of supervisee and that of patient.

Like the patient, you are enjoined to absolute honesty in your reporting of the sessions and your internal responses to, and interventions with, the patient. Also like the patient, you will find yourself tempted to withhold and distort information about your interaction. This is so, most superficially, because of your desire to avoid criticism and make a good impression. These overt concerns will rest on psychodynamic, unconscious underpinnings concerning your particular conflicts and danger situations.

In other words, you will see your supervisor, as your patient views you, as an authority figure with all the unconscious baggage attendant thereto. You may have either unrealistically great expectations, or correspondingly intense fears, of what might result from your collaboration with him. To the extent that the former is the case, you will be disappointed; to the extent that the latter is true, you will view disclosure as carrying certain potential dangers, depending upon your history and personality configuration.

As for the expectations you might, for example, out of a sense of inadequacy and idealization of the supervisor, long for him to do all the formulating and suggest all the interactions rather than producing any yourself. This might be less stressful than having to formulate your own ideas, but it would be less profitable as well. If your supervisor is a good one he will give you enough to model something about thinking and intervening dynamically, while depriving you sufficiently for you to experience doing it yourself.

As for the fears, you might, for example, see making mistakes as carrying 1) the danger of so disgusting your senior that he will abandon you altogether or evict you from the program; 2) the possibility that you will retain his presence but forfeit his liking and respect; 3) the potential

---

[5]Do not, as some trainees have done, mention your supervisor within the therapeutic hours. To do so interjects a sort of shadowy meta-therapist into the situation. Only if the patient directly asks you whether you are supervised should you bring it up, and then merely acknowledge, matter of factly, that this is so and ask him about his concerns and fantasies regarding it.

for your being shamed, mortified, and exposed as therapeutically impotent; and, finally, 4) the danger that you will be reviled for your self-indulgence, insensitivity, obtuseness, and cruelty with the patient.

On the other hand, any desire to impress, and perhaps even outdo and triumph over, this respected authority figure and parent imago can lead to varieties of acting out if you are not careful. For example, you might find yourself persistently forgetting to write process notes, forgetting the contents of the supervisory hours, or misapplying your supervisor's suggestions to ensure they will not work.[6]

Among the occupational hazards of being supervised are two that deserve special mention. The first involves the resident's oscillation, in response to the supervisor's criticisms and suggestions, back and forth between extremes. For example, the supervisor says you are talking too much and heating up a dependent-erotic transference in an hysteric and you respond by becoming silent, letting important material pass by, and inadvertently giving the patient the impression you have withdrawn and are insensitive. The teacher then criticizes you for this and you secretly accuse him of engaging in double-talk or one-upmanship. The second (and related to the first) is adopting a general attitude or approach with a particular patient, upon the supervisor's advice, and then failing to notice when the situation demands that you modify it or assume a different strategy altogether. The interaction between therapist and patient is dynamic, not static, and a stance appropriate at one stage is not necessarily so at another. It is the supervisor's appreciation of this that so often makes his suggestions appear whimsical or sadistic.

To the degree that you can accept that you do not yet know how to do this work, and that nobody expects you to, then to that extent will your supervision be feasible and profitable, if never quite enjoyable. And remember, you will learn most from those supervisors who spare you least.[7]

## THE TELEPHONE

Although each therapist must develop his own policy for the use of this blessing and bane, I shall offer a few suggestions from my own experience. To begin with, every patient is entitled to a number through

---

[6]There is one fascinating way in which you will sometimes bring the material of the sessions to your supervisors. This involves an identification with the patient, an acting out with (rather than reporting to) the supervisor that which the patient is acting out with you. If the patient, for example, is "catastrophizing" and demanding, then you may find yourself frantically pressing the supervisor for magical and foolproof advice. If he is boring and confusing you, as a way of avoiding affect-laden issues, then you may find yourself doing the same to your supervisor.
[7]See page 333.

which you can be reached between sessions or after hours. During my residency and for several years thereafter I had a publicly listed home telephone number and gave it to my patients. However, experience with several borderline clients caused me to reconsider the wisdom of this policy. Some patients react to the possession of your home phone number as a stimulation of their erotic and dependent strivings. Some respond to their sense of deprivation in the transference by attempting to wreak havoc over the wires and destroy your life on evenings and weekends. Eventually such calls elicit your anger and thereby impair your therapeutic effectiveness.

To give certain patients what amounts to an avenue into your home is to give them more power over your life than they can handle and than is good for the treatment. Consequently, I advocate that your home phone number be unlisted but that you be reachable through a 24-hour desk at the clinic or an answering service. You can then return the patient's call.

As for handling the calls themselves, there is no hard-and-fast rule. For some ego-compromised individuals, with grossly impaired reality-testing, self-restraint, and object-constancy, an occasional phone call to you is their lifeblood. These people are reassured and their egos strengthened by these contacts. For some patients, simply knowing they can call if necessary allays their anxiety sufficiently that they seldom need to. During times of crisis, otherwise well-functioning individuals may also be supported by a call to you.

For others, however, use of the phone becomes countertherapeutic. They may use it as a vehicle for the acting out of hostile, erotic, voyeuristic, dependent, and many other fantasies. For example, some patients of the opposite sex derive sensual pleasure from talking with you over the

---

⁷The supervisor can behave in such a way as to facilitate or impede the supervisory process: being too dogmatic or too active, being possessed by a Pygmalion complex, treating the supervisee like a patient, and so forth. The focus of the hour must consistently be the *therapeutic interaction* and the *patient's dynamics.* Part and parcel of the former is getting the student to talk about his own feelings and fantasies about the patient and helping him to identify countertransference when it occurs, but the supervisor stops short with the identification of it; it is up to the student and/or his therapist to analyze it. I agree with Tarachow (1963) that one addresses personality issues in the trainee only when it is apparent that they are interfering with the supervisory process and/or the patient's therapy. Then the supervisor does not at first address them directly, but rather modifies his approach in accord with what he knows about the student's style of interaction. With a trainee who is inordinately sensitive to criticism, for example, he might not address this directly but rather behave in such a way as to make things safer for him, softening his critical remarks and delivering them in conjunction with positive ones. Of course, if all else fails then the issues must be confronted directly, but the supervisor, again, stops with identifying them. If the issues need analysis he should suggest the student broach them with his therapist or enter therapy, if he has not done so already.

phone, as if they were chatting with a high-school sweetheart. Patients may act out oedipal issues by phoning you at hours when they believe they are taking you out of your marital bed. Others use phone calls, since they are often not charged for, to gain special favors. In all such cases, and when it is apparent there is no emergency, you should quickly but politely end the conversation, informing the patient that it sounds like the issue can wait until the next session. In the following hour you must then address both that which went into the phone call and the phone call itself. To do otherwise is to invite the patient to continue to act out rather than talk about his fantasies and feelings.

Apart from acting out, some patients use the telephone as a way of bypassing the resistance. They apprise you of important and sensitive issues over the phone which they cannot discuss face-to-face. To allow them to do so is to deny them the insight attendant upon coming to terms with the dangers surrounding these issues.

In short, the place for therapy is your office. The phone is reserved for emergencies.

## "HUMANNESS," FALLIBILITY, AND THE ANALYTIC WAY

There is currently much controversy in psychoanalysis, well summarized by Malcolm (1981), over the limits of the analytic attitude within the therapeutic hour. Strictly speaking, this dispute applies only to the practice of psychoanalysis. Nevertheless, because many students unfortunately interpret what they read about psychoanalysis to apply on a point-for-point basis to psychodynamic psychotherapy (and because some therapy supervisors fail to distinguish sufficiently between the two in their supervision of students), I feel it necessary to address briefly the issues here.

One contingent advocates that the analyst should do nothing more nor less than analyze, while the other contends that there are special situations, such as when the analyst himself commits major errors or when the patient has experienced a grave misfortune in external reality, when a more "real" or "human" response is in order.

The test cases most commonly cited are one's own tardiness and a death in the patient's family. The "hard-liners" argue that to apologize for the former or offer condolences for the latter might make it more difficult for the patient to talk about his various reactions to the events. In other words, to apologize or explain might defuse his feelings and fantasies about your lateness, while to proffer condolences might prevent the patient from expressing any sense of relief or triumph over the death. The "soft-liners" counter that failing to apologize or express condolences constitutes such a deviation from socially expectable behavior that this in itself becomes a major determinant of the patient's subsequent behavior.

I believe there is merit in both arguments. Indeed, you can behave in a way that impedes the patient's speaking his mind. However, you can also act in a manner that conveys callousness or indifference to the patient's plight. In some respects we are confronting a false dichotomy, for the psychoanalyst or psychodynamic therapist should always be concerned about, and empathic toward his patients. This should, as I have said, be the foundation for all his interventions.

Important technical errors, lapses, and misunderstanding should *always* be acknowledged to oneself and analyzed later. When indicated they should also be acknowledged, with a succinct apology and without prolonged explanations or self-analysis, to the patient. This would be indicated, for example, if one is tardy for a session, falls asleep in an hour, forgets an appointment, commits a major parapraxis, or egregiously misremembers or misquotes one of the patient's communications. After proffering your apology, you would then proceed to deal with the patient's feelings and fantasies about your behavior. Consider, for instance, the following vignette from my work with Mr. E:

> Because of a clinical emergency it was necessary for me to meet Mr. E. in the waiting room and explain that I would be a few minutes late. In fact, we ended up starting half an hour later than usual. I succinctly apologized and we began work. He said nothing more about my tardiness but, a few minutes into the session, began inveighing against a friend who was late meeting him for a prearranged visit to the exhibition of a well-known artist's work. After a few moments of this I asked him if this anger was also directed at me since I, too, had been late for a prearranged meeting with him. He stopped short and said, "But you had good reasons for it." I replied that, whatever my reasons, he was entitled to feelings and fantasies about my behavior. After we discussed his fear of offending me, he disclosed his anger and suspicion that my lateness meant he was less important to me.

It did appear that my apology had hindered his talking about his reaction to my lateness. Nevertheless, we dealt with his reaction to the apology just as we dealt with his feelings about my tardiness. I apologized because I felt that failure to do so would constitute a sufficiently radical departure from customary behavior that that in itself would determine his subsequent reactions more than would the apology itself. Had I said nothing I could not have treated his anger at me as merely an historically determined transference response because it would also have been a response to my acting as if I were somehow exempted from the universal requirement to apologetically acknowledge one's lateness.

Many of the same considerations hold true in the case of a patient's experience of grave external misfortune in the course of the treatment. In the case of a death, for example, there are ways of expressing concern without closing off discussion. An empathic and prolonged gaze and nodding of the head might do better than a hundred words. Your reaction is to some extent dictated by what you know about the patient's prior relationship with the deceased. In any event, you cannot appear indifferent to the matter. Greenson (1967) discussed the case of a therapist who omitted to empathically acknowledge the reality of a patient's concern about her severely ill child. Greenson rightly concluded that the woman's anger was a legitimate response to the analyst's behavior rather than merely an aseptic unfolding of her internal dynamics.

Nor is it catastrophic if a patient inadvertently stumbles upon a piece of your own neurosis or character style. Although we do not attempt to apprise him of them, he will, if he has any observational capacity at all, perceive some of our personal idiosyncrasies and sensitivities. Learning that we are not psychological saints but human beings like himself is harmful to neither his reality testing nor his self-esteem.

It is a fiction that if we can only be sufficiently neutral, impassive, and un-self-disclosing, we can then treat whatever emerges in the patient as simon-pure historically determined transference. Fromm-Reichmann (1950, p. 4) warns that, despite its usefulness, the "transference doctrine gave an opening to obviate the fact of the actual experiences between therapist and patient then and there. In practice, this at times has carried with it the danger of inducing therapists to neglect the significance of the vicissitudes of the actual doctor-patient relationship as opposed to its transference aspects." (Apropos this entire discussion, see Stone's [1961] *The Psychoanalytic Situation.)*

## DYNAMIC PSYCHOTHERAPY AND RELIGION, ETHICS, AND PHILOSOPHY

The relationship of dynamic psychotherapy to the patient's religious, philosophical, and ethical creeds is an important, though insufficiently addressed, topic. To begin with, a considerable percentage of patients profess, to some degree, religious convictions; many of them, whether religious or not, hold tenaciously to some philosophy of life; all espouse, practice, and (at times) violate personal ethical norms. In short, this is a topic that no therapist, whatever his particular persuasion, can afford to ignore. I have included this section in order to advocate humility, respect, and caution before the tenets and values that are among the most cherished possessions of many individuals.

I have previously provided several examples of psychopathological manifestations of religion. There is an unfortunate tendency, on the part of many therapists, to conclude from such cases that religious practices are psychopathological in and of themselves and that no healthy and mature individual would practice them, with the corollary that one test of a truly "complete" therapy is the renunciation of such beliefs. This is as illogical as deprecating the F.B.I. because some paranoids incorporate it into their delusional systems. To wit, any cultural institution can function as a socially furnished vehicle for symptom (compromise) formation or become built into idiosyncratic, maladaptive modes of being in the world. That this is the case no more devalues religion than any other institution.

Insofar as religious or philosophical convictions function, psychologically, as sublimations, you would tend to analyze them no more than you would occupation, hobbies, recreation, or any other form of sublimation. Sublimations in general are only dissected when they become somehow maladaptive or incorporated into psychopathological structures. To do otherwise might rob a precious adaptive behavior of its unconscious, psychodynamic fuel or give the patient the impression that it is somehow pathological.

When aspects of a person's religion become used symptomatically and maladaptively, then it is incumbent upon you to treat them analytically. But this must be done without conveying the impression that you view his religion as pathological through and through, that you view its maladaptive function as the only one, and that you intend to explain it away. One cannot, in any event, honestly do this last since psychodynamics can never exhaustively explain, without taking account of sociocultural and historical factors, institutionalized behaviors like religion. Nor can dynamic psychiatry contribute to the question of whether, after all the sociocultural and psychological factors are removed, there is a transcendent reality that corresponds to religious beliefs.[8]

If you must be careful not to engage in the psychodynamic reductionism of religious (and indeed philosophical) beliefs, you must also be on the alert for the defense of "transcendentalization." This is exemplified by patients who want to talk theology or draw you into, at times quite interesting, philosophical-ethical discussions and debates. (Your convictions on such matters should be open to discussion no more than any other area of your personal life; nor should you intrude them in any fashion upon the patient.) Often you will observe a relatively clear connection between the ethereal topic and its affective, interpersonal, earthly counterpart, but you must use even more caution in confronting it than you would with other defensive maneuvers. If you watch closely,

---

[8]If I see no basic incompatibility between adherence to religious convictions and the role of patient or therapist, I feel strongly that the consulting room is no place for a mixing of the roles of pastor and dynamic clinician. When the boundaries between the two are blurred, both psychiatry *and* religion suffer. Those interested in a more extensive treatment of the interface between religion and psychoanalysis are directed to my two essays, "Freud and Religion: A History and Reappraisal," *The Psychoanalytic Study of Society*, Volume X, 1983, and "Reflections on the Relationship Between Psychoanalysis and Christianity," *Pastoral Psychology*, in press, 1983.

the patient usually lets real persons and feelings into his conversation occasionally and you can use this as a vehicle to bring him back down to earth. If he persists, you must convey to him that you are learning more about philosophy than about his personal life. Or you might simply wait, saying nothing, for eventually he will feel irritated and hurt at your refusal to collaborate in his defensive maneuvers and to gratify his desires that you share yourself.

Commonly, this defense manifests itself in a desire to discuss "existential" issues, which are implicitly placed in opposition to "dynamic" ones. In fact, there is no hard-and-fast line between the two. Dynamic issues *are* existential issues. They are the existential issues of childhood and of the adult unconscious. Similarly, an existential issue like death, for example, cannot be considered without reference to one's personal experience with loss, separation, rejection, and the deaths of those around him. The question of the meaning and purpose of life cannot be considered apart from the meaning and purpose of one's own particular life. Nevertheless, if existential issues cannot be treated apart from the patient's psychodynamics, neither can the former be reduced totally to the latter. I concur with Frankl (1973) that there is a fundamental will to meaning in the human being which, if frustrated, can lead to suffering as surely as can the repression of historically determined conflictual strivings.

The dynamic therapist, like everyone else, has a more or less explicit code of ethics by which he lives his life and upon which he bases his moral valuations of the behavior of self and others. Although he makes every conscious effort to leave these categories at the door of his consulting room, as a human being he cannot help but find himself, almost reflexively, responding judgmentally at times to that which the patient has done or is doing. The therapist does not, however, act upon these sentiments and moralize against him; rather, he does nothing more than consistently attempt to *understand* and, when appropriate, convey his understandings to the patient. This does not mean that there are not occasions when, in the face of a patient's serious abuse or neglect of others, the therapist can profitably draw his attention to it by questioning him about his intentions toward, and understanding of his impact upon, them. Fortunately, however, most insight-oriented patients are nice people in the conventionally moral sense!

If you do not moralize against your patient, neither can you abet him in his attempts to evade the moral consequences of his own behavior. That is, occasional patients seem to feel, like Nietzsche's superman, that they can turn their own professed moral code upon its head when it suits their whim, and that you will somehow analyze their guilt away! One man, raised in a devout Catholic home, acted as if he ought to be able to have adulterous affairs without pangs of conscience. He saw as the problem not his repeated infidelity to his wife, but rather his guilty conscience in reaction thereto. He came to me, as his ancestors might have gone to a shrine, to exorcize it away. As it turned out, he did become less guilty as a result of the therapy, because some of his guilt was neurotic—related to the incestuous nature of his object choices and his identification with his hypocritical father. However, the guilt over his violation of moral norms that he still, both consciously and unconsciously, held sacred, remained and had to be dealt with. He finally decided, in part as a matter of taking the path of least resistance, that a life in accordance with his deeply rooted moral values was more pleasant and pain-free for all concerned than one which ran counter to it.

Nor is your attempt to instruct the patient on the role of history and the unconscious in his life an effort to absolve him from assuming personal responsibility for the consequences of his behavior and from morally evaluating his *actions*. To say that a person chooses for reasons of which he is partly unaware is not to deny that it is he, nonetheless, who does the choosing. Nor is your consistently nonevaluative stance, which is, in any event, part of the technical apparatus of dynamic psychotherapy and confined to the consulting room, meant to be taken up by the patient as a prescription for living. Analysis is a door to the freedom to choose a way of life; it is not that way of life itself.[9]

## DEATH

In your psychotherapeutic work you are confronted with death upon three levels: neurotic, symbolic, and real. As for the first, death anxiety or preoccupation with death can be a function of unconscious conflicts representing self-punitiveness for a variety of guilt-laden unconscious aggressive or sexual strivings, resulting from projected hostility, or being a function of castration or separation anxieties. As for the second, death (and rebirth) imagery can be prominent in nonpsychopathological states as well—during transitional periods in adult development, when

---

[9]The misapprehension of Freud as "instinctual" libertarian is by now so rampant, and its clinical and social implications so powerful, that it deserves address. Freud's thinking on the matter is nowhere better summarized than in that unblinkingly realistic work, *Civilization and Its Discontents*, where he asserts that the demands of one's impulses and those of society are irreconcilable beyond a barely tolerable degree. He keenly appreciated that there can be no civilization without self-restraint. His aim was to free up unconscious fantasies, not so they might be indiscriminantly acted upon, but in order that conscious deliberation and choice might replace automatic and pathogenic repression and compromise formation. This would lead to the prudent satisfaction of some inclinations, but the suppression and sublimation of others (Freud, 1909, p. 145; Freud, in Nunberg and Federn, 1967, p. 89).

contemplating major relocations or shifts in occupation or life-style, when confronted with overwhelming external catastrophe, upon ending important relationships, during religious transformations, and when, through psychotherapy, one is molting a neurotic identity for a healthy one. As for the third, dynamic psychiatry has inadequately acknowledged the most fundamental fact of human existence—that it ceases. Freud, with his emphasis on the neurotic and symbolic aspects of death and death anxiety and his idea that there is no notion of mortality in the unconscious, unwittingly set the tone for this. Be that as it may, we therapists collude, day in and day out and from our own anxieties, in our patients' denial of death.

I believe that there are at least two paradoxes in one's attitude toward death. The first, which Searles (1965) outlines, is that only a whole (intrapsychically and interpersonally integrated) person can come to terms with his mortality, and yet only by acknowledging death can one attain to such wholeness. The knowledge of one's finiteness, he says, should be the background for all life's experiences and decisions, including, of course, those of psychotherapist. Searles reinterprets certain forms of psychopathology (in particular schizophrenia) as, in part, attempts to deny the fact of death and to deal with the fear of death by numbing oneself to life. At times this is a function of the schizophrenic's omnipotently and guiltily owning responsibility for the very fact that people die.

The second paradox is that while there is no genuine wholeness and maturity without recognizing the finitude of one's biological existence, there is yet no possibility for peace and meaning in life unless one possesses some idea (or ideas) of immortality. This might be (to borrow Lifton's [1979] categories) a purely symbolic one (living on in one's work and in one's impact on others), a biological one (living on in one's children and in the flow of generations), a natural one (living on in the abundance of nature), a transcendental one (engaging in mystical and even athletic, aesthetic, and other peak experiences where one, however briefly, transcends the experience of self and its relationship to time and death), or the time-honored belief in spiritual immortality or resurrection.

Useful works for the student who would come to terms with death personally, clinically, and theoretically include: 1) Harold Searles' aforementioned (1965) essay, "Schizophrenia and the Inevitability of Death," 2) Robert Lifton's (1979) *The Broken Connection,* 3) Ernest Becker's (1973) *The Denial of Death,* 4) Philip Ariès' (1977) little book, *A History of Western Attitudes Toward Death,* 5) Carl Jung's (1934) essay, "The Soul and Death," 6) Jacques Choron's (1963) *Death in Western Thought* and 7) Paul Tillich's (1952) *The Courage to Be.* You could also profitably listen to Mahler's Ninth Symphony, written when its composer knew he stood at death's door.

## SUGGESTED READINGS FOR CHAPTERS 7 THROUGH 10

In general, I think it fair to say that reading plays a smaller role in the education of the dynamic psychotherapist than in that of almost any other medical specialist. I do not mean that the student should not read, that there is no clinical payoff from it, but only that the bulk of the learning occurs in supervised clinical work and case conferences. Most of the mileage from absorbing the literature comes only later, after one already has a basic grasp of the clinical method of dynamic psychiatry. However, if reading will take the novice only so far, he should at least let himself be taken this distance. Learning psychotherapy is anxiety-provoking and difficult enough without lacking the succor that is available in the good basic readings. These books will spare you some of the trial and error inherent in learning this craft. The following reading list is selective. I have included only what I feel are the best, and I encourage the student to read his choices more than once. Some, such as Fromm-Reichmann's text, should be all but memorized. It is far, far better to have drunk deeply at a few good wells than to have sipped superficially at many springs.

In reading, your constant aim should be to subordinate theory and technique to personal and clinical experience, and not the reverse. Each of you must produce the working concept of dynamic psychiatry that best meshes with your particular personality, thinking, and experience.

Altman, L.: *The Dream in Psychoanalysis*. New York, International Universities Press, 1962.

Frank, J.: *Persuasion and Healing*. New York, Schocken Books, 1974. Excellent for the "nonspecific" factors in psychotherapy.

Freud, S. (1899 [1900]): *The Interpretation of Dreams*. Standard Edition, Volume IV, Chapter 2. London, Hogarth Press, 1953. Unfortunately, Freud wrote relatively little on therapeutic technique such that it is necessary for you to treat the following papers as pure gold.

Freud, S. (1903): "Freud's Psycho-Analytic Procedure." Standard Edition, Volume VII. London, Hogarth Press, 1953, pp. 249-254.

Freud, S. (1910): "The Future Prospects of Psycho-Analytic Therapy." Standard Edition, Volume XI. London, Hogarth Press, 1957, pp. 141-151.

Freud, S. (1910): " 'Wild' Psycho-Analysis." Standard Edition, Volume XI. London, Hogarth Press, 1957, pp. 219-227.

Freud, S. (1911): "The Handling of Dream Interpretation in Psycho-Analysis." Standard Edition, Volume XII. London, Hogarth Press, 1958, pp. 91-96.

Freud, S. (1912): "The Dynamics of Transference." Standard Edition, Volume XII. London, Hogarth Press, 1958, pp. 99-108.

Freud, S. (1912): "Recommendations to Physicians Practicing Psycho-Analysis." Standard Edition, Volume XII. London, Hogarth Press, 1958, pp. 111-120.

Freud, S. (1913): "On Beginning the Treatment." Standard Edition, Volume XII. London, Hogarth Press, 1958, pp. 123-144.

Freud, S. (1913): "Fausse Reconnaissance (Déjà Raconté) in Psycho-Analytic Treatment." Standard Edition, Volume XIII. London, Hogarth Press, 1953, pp. 201-207.

Freud, S. (1914): "Remembering, Repeating, and Working Through." Standard Edition, Volume XII. London, Hogarth Press, 1958, pp. 147-156.

Freud, S. (1914): "Observations on Transference Love." Standard Edition, Volume XII. London, Hogarth Press, 1958, pp. 159-171.

Freud, S. (1916-1917): *Introductory Lectures on Psycho-Analysis*. Standard Edition, Volume XVI, Lectures XXVII and XXVIII. London, Hogarth Press, 1961, pp. 431-463.

Freud, S. (1918): "Lines of Advance in Psycho-Analytic Therapy." Standard Edition, Volume XVII. London, Hogarth Press, 1955, pp. 159-168.

Freud, S. (1920): *Beyond the Pleasure Principle*. Standard Edition, Volume XVIII, Chapter 2. London, Hogarth Press, 1955, pp. 7-64.

Freud, S. (1923): "Remarks on the Theory and Practice of Dream-Interpretation." Standard Edition, Volume XIX. London, Hogarth Press, 1961, pp. 109-121.

Freud, S. (1926): *The Question of Lay Analysis*. Standard Edition, Volume XX, Chapter 5. London, Hogarth Press, 1959, pp. 183-250.

Freud, S. (1932): *New Introductory Lectures on Psycho-Analysis*. Lecture XXXIV, Standard Edition, Volume XXII. London, Hogarth Press, 1964, pp. 136-157.

Freud, S. (1937): "Analysis Terminable and Interminable." Standard Edition, Volume XXIII, London, Hogarth Press, 1964, pp. 209-253.

Freud, S. (1937): "Constructions in Analysis." Standard Edition, Volume XXIII. London, Hogarth Press, 1964, pp. 257-269.

Freud, S. (1938): *An Outline of Psycho-Analysis*. Standard Edition, Volume XXIII, Chapter 6. London, Hogarth Press, 1964, pp. 144-207.

Fromm-Reichmann, F.: *Principles of Intensive Psychotherapy*, Chicago, University of Chicago Press, 1950. The single most successful introduction to dynamic psychotherapy. Her "humanness" and equally intense dedication to patient and craft come through on every page. For a patient-side view of this great therapist and human being, read Hannah Green's *I Never Promised You a Rose Garden*.

Greenson, R.: *The Technique and Practice of Psychoanalysis*. New York, International Universities Press, 1967. The best advanced text on dynamic psychotherapy.

Langs, R.: *The Technique of Psychoanalytic Psychotherapy*. New York, Jason Aronson, 1973. These two volumes are detailed expositions of many practical issues and questions the therapist faces.

Malcolm, J.: *Psychoanalysis: The Impossible Profession*. New York, Alfred A. Knopf, 1981. Entertaining and informative look at the psychoanalytic scene.

May, R., Angel, E., and Ellenberger, H.: *Existence*. New York, Basic Books, 1958. Existential thinking provides a useful complement to psychodynamics. This is an excellent introduction to phenomenological psychiatry and existential analysis.

Reik, L.: *Listening with the Third Ear*, New York, Farrar, Straus & Giroux, 1949. Falls in the category of inspirational literature for the dynamic therapist, of food for his soul.

Rieff, P.: *Freud: The Mind of the Moralist*. New York, Viking Press, 1959.

Rieff, P.: *The Triumph of the Therapeutic: Uses of Faith After Freud*. New York, Harper & Row, 1966. Both of Rieff's books constitute the foundation for the dynamic psychiatrist's humanistic and philosophical education.

Saul, L.: *Psychodynamically Based Psychotherapy*. New York, Science House, 1972. A good intermediate text with an excellent longitudinal account of an actual analytic treatment.

Searles, H.: *Collected Papers on Schizophrenia & Related Subjects*. New York, International Universities Press, 1965.

Searles, H.: *Countertransference & Related Subjects: Selected Papers.* New York, International Universities Press, 1979. Both Searles' books are beautiful treatments of countertransference and dynamically oriented therapy with disturbed individuals. They are written with the same soul as are the works of Sullivan and Fromm-Reichmann and fall, like Reik's book, in the category of inspirational literature for the psychotherapist.

Tarachow, I.: *An Introduction to Psychotherapy.* New York, International Universities Press, 1963. The best intermediate text on dynamic psychotherapy.

# 11

# Supportive Psychotherapy

The aim of supportive psychotherapy is to augment the patient's adaptive capacity and to reaffiliate him with his fellows. If this sounds familiar it should, because these are the goals of insight-oriented therapy as well. In other words, there is no difference between the ultimate objectives of insight-oriented and supportive approaches.

Where insight-oriented and supportive therapies differ is in their methodologies, in the routes which they take to this goal. In insight-oriented psychotherapy the ultimate objective is achieved through the intermediate one of personality restructuring. This fundamental realignment in the balance of mental forces is attained via an *interpretive* approach—that is, an approach that brings the patient to a cognitive-affective awareness of the historical dynamics of his behavior. Every departure from interpretation or from maneuvers (i.e., questions, confrontations, and clarifications) designed to prepare the patient for interpretation is a deviation from an insight-oriented approach and a move toward a supportive one. Such deviations are termed "parameters."

Nevertheless, even in the area of methodology there is much overlap between supportive and insight-oriented treatment. The most insight-oriented approach has supportive elements, and vice versa. To begin with, the nonspecific factors outlined in Chapter 7 are all supportive and operate in insight-oriented, as much as in supportive, psychotherapy. Furthermore, the most supportive factor in supportive therapy is also the most supportive in insight-oriented: to wit, *conveying to the patient (verbally or nonverbally) that his feelings and predicament are being accurately understood.* Finally, it is a rare, if nonexistent, patient who cannot profitably arrive at some insight into the motives and meaning of his behav-

**344**

ior. I am referring to attempts to bring the patient to insights that are accompanied by the therapist's empathy, that occur within the context of a strong therapeutic alliance, and that are keyed to the capacity of the patient's ego to make use of the insight (without excessive anxiety, undue regression, acting out, or other untoward consequences). Insights that decrease intrapsychic conflict and its attendant anxiety are by nature supportive. When the ego feels less endangered, it is supported and its functioning enhanced.

It is a common misconception that supportive treatment is easier than insight-oriented psychotherapy or psychoanalysis. This is emphatically not the case. Ideally, supportive therapy should be performed by one already adept at a dynamic interpretive approach. Supportive treatment is not simply showering the patient with warm feelings, saying whatever is on your mind, and trying to be a pseudo-friend or parent. Nor is it a welcome coffee break from the "more serious and demanding" work of insight-oriented psychotherapy, in which you can put your mind on "hold," lean back, relax, and just "be yourself" because, wonder of wonders, this felicitous state of mind is exactly what the patient needs.

In supportive treatment you take the same thorough history, compose the same rigorous formulation, spend just as much (or more) time on the treatment plan, and strive as strenuously to understand the patient dynamically as you do in insight-oriented treatment. Just as in insight-oriented therapy you are always asking yourself, "What does it mean that this particular person, with his particular history, current environment, and dynamics, is doing this with me right now?"

In contrast to insight-oriented psychotherapy, however, you must often decide more actively how to intervene on the basis of this comprehension. In other words, you must give more consideration to the *consequences* of your intervention, to its potential impact on the patient's ego strength, in supportive treatment than in insight-oriented. In addition, the situation is further complicated because the connections between psychodynamic theory and supportive psychotherapeutic technique are less clearly delineated than those between dynamic theory and insight-oriented technique. In other words, while the rules are not rigid in insight-oriented therapy, they are even more flexible in supportive therapy. Hence, the clinician's responses in supportive treatment are less predictable, chosen from a wider range of possibilities and in view of a wider range of considerations, and more a function of his idiosyncratic judgment than is the case in insight-oriented treatment.

In supportive therapy you cannot simply wait for the patient to make his connections. You must have ever at your fingertips a statement of his ego credits and debits, his superego assets and liabilities, and the overdue accounts in his id. You must decide now to speak to the ego, now to the superego or id; now to come down on the side of expressiveness, now of restraint; now to confront his intellectualization or reaction formation, now to support it; now to analyze the transference, now to utilize it as a suggestive or reinforcing lever; now to speak to a budding negative transference, now to try to defuse or circumvent it; now to be analytic, now to be "real"—now to ask him what goes into his question, now to answer it immediately and directly, now to gratify his request for coffee or advice, now to analyze it.

Apart from the active decision-making role that is required of us, there is another reason that supportive treatment is difficult. It calls upon us to have our own psychological houses in order even more than does insight-oriented work because of the more overt and intense expression of primitive affect (e.g., murderous rage, devouring infantile dependency, unbridled lust, frank exhibitionism, devastating fear, godlike idealization, bitter scorn, self-righteous reproach) that schizophrenics, manics, borderlines, and the other supportive clients can engage in. Essentially, many of these patients will be asking you to indulge and tolerate in a fully grown adult what you would barely countenance in a small child. This "irresponsible" behavior is guaranteed to rudely awaken the more or less slumbering infant that lives in all of us. To the degree that that infant feels frustrated and deprived, and therefore entitled to special dispensations, then to that degree will our patient's behavior evoke in us intense feelings such as anger, depression, envy, or anxiety. If we are unaware of these issues, then our feelings may be projected onto or otherwise acted out with the patient.

Patients who tend to profit from a more supportive approach include those with 1) insufficient verbal intelligence or psychological mindedness, 2) severely compromised ego function, 3) overwhelmingly powerful impulsions, 4) grossly impaired superego functioning, and 5) especially problematic and chaotic current environments. They include all diagnostic categories, though those with schizophrenic, major affective, organic, borderline, narcissistic, schizoid, schizotypal, and antisocial diagnoses are overrepresented among them. They fall into all age ranges, though the very young and very old seem to contribute more than their share. They come from all socioeconomic levels, though those from poverty stricken and culturally deprived environments are disproportionately present.[1]

## INDICATIONS FOR SUPPORTIVE TREATMENT

I shall elaborate on the five indicators for supportive treatment, beginning with *verbal intelligence and psychological* mindedness. It is obvious that, since the primary medium of communication in insight treatment is verbal, some facility with words is essential to insight formation.

---

[1]See page 347.

Related to, though to some extent independent of, this is the mysterious gift called "psychological mindedness." That is, the patient must have some capacity for access to the inner life and be willing to at least entertain the idea that autoplastic change is as, or more, valuable than alloplastic, that he should be able to identify and communicate his feelings, that he can spot themes and make connections, and that his defenses are sufficiently pliable that he can gain a controlled and modulated access to hitherto preconscious material. To the extent that a patient is lacking any of these qualities, then to that degree is he a more appropriate candidate for a supportive than an insight approach.

*Impaired ego functioning* is undoubtedly the most important and comprehensive of the criteria under consideration. (Indeed, psychological mindedness, broadly conceived, is itself an aspect of ego functioning.) This includes (and is evidenced by): inability to form stable and lasting relationships; difficulties with object constancy; identity diffusion and deficient boundaries between representations of self and objects; a paucity of stable sublimatory channels for the adaptive discharge of sexual and aggressive drives (e.g., little or no involvement in occupation, athletics, recreation, hobbies, religion); a preference for the more maladaptive and reality distorting defenses (e.g., projection, denial, splitting, projective identification); little tolerance for anxiety and dysphoric affect in general and a tendency to seek immediate relief through repression or through defensive or expressive acting out; little willingness or ability to endure frustration and postpone gratification, with a proneness to seek immediate release of tension through the acting out of drive derivatives; and consciousness of relatively primitive fantasies and feelings that would be unconscious in the neurotic.

For reasons of constitution and early environment, the underlying strength of affectionate, dependent, sensual, and aggressive strivings differs somewhat from individual to individual. The early experience of candidates for supportive therapy often includes degrees of stimulation, deprivation, and abuse that markedly strengthen their *impulsions*. When one couples this with an already compromised ego structure, the result

---

[1]De Wald (1971) has enumerated a number of reasons that he believes this is often the case, ranging from poor models of adaptation to deficient internalization of moral demand systems with a corresponding need for external controls. Be that as it may, the evidence for and against the suitability of insight therapy for lower socioeconomic patients is equivocal, with some studies suggesting they can profit from it quite as much as their more privileged counterparts. The needs and capabilities of each lower socioeconomic patient should of course be determined case by case, without preconceptions, just as with any patient. Some of them may expect you to behave in the prescriptive and hortatory manner of the general physician, but you then have the choice of conforming to their expectations or attempting to educate them to, and enlist their cooperation in, a different type of doctor-patient relationship.

can be great difficulty binding or appropriately channeling the derivative affect-laden fantasies. Depending upon a number of factors, this can lead to maladaptively rigid or reality distorting defenses, to acting out of the impulsions themselves, or to rapid and precipitous oscillations between defense and discharge. One cannot engage in anything remotely resembling insight-oriented work unless the patient is able to bind his feelings and fantasies sufficiently to talk about them rather than to act upon them.

*Superego disturbances* often reflect gross inconsistencies in the admonitions and behavior of the parental models, parents insufficiently present to identify with, parents sufficiently abusive and/or depriving so that the love and affection prerequisite to lasting identifications is absent, and the incorporation of extremely punitive parenting into the superego. The first three situations will lead to an inadequate internalization of society's normative values, while the last can lead to a vicious superego that may, in the interests of self-preservation, be projected onto the environment and rebelled against. Either of these outcomes poses special problems not usually encountered in the more adequately enculturated insight-oriented patients.

Finally, the patient's *current environment* may be such that, under the circumstances, his psychopathology is highly adaptive. For example, there may be family members whose vested interest is that the patient not change and perhaps place demands upon them they would be unwilling to meet. A woman whose husband is constantly battering her has good extrapsychic reasons to withdraw and deny her needs for sex and affection. A hostile and paranoid stance may not be so delusional in a setting where a patient's family or friends give him good reasons to mistrust them and where people abuse and exploit one another. Struggling to cope with these and other external stressors (e.g., finances, obtaining the physical necessities of life) may leave him with little or no energy to engage in a luxury like psychotherapy. It is difficult to talk with a woman about her Oedipus complex when her apartment is cold and her children are starving. Finally, financial and other secondary gains attendant to illness may make it maladaptive for the patient to recover. Returning to uninteresting work with low pay and little prestige may appear (largely unconsciously) less attractive than one's hysterical paralysis or back pain.

## THE NATURE OF SUPPORTIVE THERAPY

I shall elucidate the nature of supportive therapy by comparing and contrasting it to insight-oriented treatment along 12 parameters, among which there is much overlap.

*No more or even less than with insight-oriented psychotherapy can you mechanically apply the principles outlined herein and expect to obtain beneficial results.* Supportive patients differ one from another as much as insight-oriented ones. They defy pigeonholing and it is only in the school of supervised hard knocks that you will learn to apply these general principles in a way that does justice to their uniquely human individualities. Analytic priggishness or dogmatism have no place here.[2] *What* you do is less important than doing it within the context of a dynamic understanding of the patient and good supervision.

1. *A good history* of the present problem, past problems, and life course plays just as central a role in supportive treatment as in insight-oriented. As the only way of spotting patterns and significant concerns and arriving at a meaningful formulation, this history gathering must occur at the outset of treatment. I wish to reiterate that this activity is in itself therapeutic since it conveys your interest and competence and offers the patient what is often the first opportunity to obtain an overview of his life. Nevertheless, since many patients will be used to the briefer anamnesis and early advice-giving of the general physician, you should *warn* them that you will need far more information than the internist or surgeon and that they will play a correspondingly more active role in the treatment plan. If you do not so prepare them, then many will flee treatment, in disgust, after the first hour.

2. *A preliminary and tentative dynamic organization* of this history is next in order. *Your supportive interventions and treatment plan are guided by this formulation as much as are your insight-oriented ones.* This seems not to be understood since I have found that most trainees have considerably sparser history and a less rigorous formulation on those patients with whom they are doing "supportive" treatment than on those with whom they are doing insight-oriented. Indeed, I have seen charts of long-term clinic patients in so-called "supportive treatment" in which virtually no relevant information was available. This is an insult to such patients and is probably one of the reasons they receive so little real treatment and end up being considered as medication-maintenance cases.

Indeed, the supportive therapist must use his formulation *more* actively and creatively than the insight-oriented one. He must pay more attention to ordering the patient's defensive maneuvers on an adaptive

---

[2]Common to all supportive interventions is the aim to promote psychosocial adaptation. We are, after all, therapists first and simon-pure Freudians, philosophers, or scientists second. Consequently, we are, personal prejudices aside, *for* anything that seems hygienic for a particular patient, *against* anything that does not. This might even involve (as has actually occurred in transcultural psychiatry) calling in the witch doctor when his theory and therapy mesh better with the patient's belief-action system than our own. Nor shall we jealously begrudge kindly grandmothers, new romances, bartenders, job changes, hot-tub therapists, and winning lottery tickets their cures.

hierarchy, taking account of ego strengths and weaknesses, and discerning the health- and disorder-promoting factors in his environment.

*Unless you grasp the patient's dynamics, you will not know what any of your interventions will mean to him.* You will have no idea what, within the framework of his historically determined view of self and world, will constitute support, reassurance, and reward, nor what will be ego strengthening or the reverse. You will not know what it will mean if you give or deny him medication, if you gratify or analyze his request for a cup of coffee, if you lend or refuse him the bus fare, if you accede or not to the request for an extra session, and so forth. In some cases an ill-considered gratification of such requests has led to precipitous regressions, eroticized psychotic transferences, and homosexual panics, whereas in others a failure to do so has constituted an inappropriate deprivation and disturbed an incipient rapport or catapulted the patient out of treatment.

Understanding a patient's dynamics helps you in such practical matters as the attitude to adopt when instituting a medication. For example:

> I had suspected for some time that an antidepressant might be useful to Ms. R. However, since one of her strongest dynamics was a masochistic way of retaliating against others (which included foiling people's best intentions to help her), I held off until she herself raised the issue. I heard her out and unenthusiastically agreed that she might be right, that indeed such medications had helped many people with problems similar to hers, but that there was no guarantee this would be the case with her. In any event, I added, she should not expect too much improvement in the first few days since it usually took several weeks for these medications to take optimal effect. I behaved in this manner because I wanted her to feel in control of the pharmacological intervention and because I wanted to provide as little range of operation for her masochistic dynamic as possible.

Understanding his schizophrenic patient's dynamics and something about unconscious symbolism helped one of my residents to appreciate what otherwise appeared to be bizarre and inexplicable behavior and, consequently, to alter his own approach. The patient, a paranoid man, was receiving biweekly fluphenazine hydrochloride (Prolixin) injections from the male resident. After each injection, which was received in the arm, the patient would lower his trousers, ostensibly to tuck in his shirt. Each time he did so, his penis would fall out of his undershorts and the patient would shake it for a few seconds before pulling up his pants. After a few episodes the resident understood that this man, with a long history of gender identity and sexual orientation issues, was feeling sexually penetrated by his resident, and that pulling out his penis was a way of reasserting his masculinity to himself and to the physician. The resident henceforth arranged for a female resident to administer the injection.

3. The most important constellation of factors is, as I have said, one that supportive and insight treatment share in common: being consistently and visibly with the patient, listening attentively and empathizing, and conveying, verbally and nonverbally, that he is being *understood*. It is so important that you appreciate this last that I shall re-repeat it: *understanding is the most supportive thing you can do for a patient, whether he is in supportive or insight-oriented therapy*. If you grasp this, then you will hear him out and listen to his concerns rather than jumping in with the premature and facile reassurance or infantilizing and irritating advice that so many mistakenly feel is supportive, but is actually the reverse.[3]

For example, a patient is feeling guilty about something. Do not leap in right away, as would his neighbor, and say, "You shouldn't feel that way about such and such." Instead, listen to him, let him ventilate, be empathic, and *then* you can point out any extreme or unrealistic elements in his response or help him use his feelings constructively. The same is true if he expresses fears that he is going insane, that he might harm himself or others, and so forth. Encourage him to talk about what that is like and the foundation for his fears *before* you decide whether to *do* anything in particular.

Different patients require us to go to different lengths to convey our empathy. Some need it spelled out more plainly than others. Some must hear it repeatedly and in different contexts before it sinks in. This was the case with Ms. Y. It took considerable work to get her to appreciate that I understood something about her neediness, her sense of deprivation and frustration in our relationship, and her unresolved feelings about rejection by others that were resurrected each time I showed her the door. When she finally did, you will remember, she began to change. Her eventual appreciation of my empathy played as large a role in her transformation as my interpretive work.

4. Closely related to the previous parameter is helping the patient to *understand himself*. It is, as I have said, a rare patient who cannot form and profit from some insight about himself. Indeed, Mr. E. and Ms. Y., who often appear in my vignettes on insight-oriented treatment, would not be considered ideal candidates by many for an interpretive approach, the former because of the rigidity of his characterological defenses and the magnitude of his fears, the latter because of tendencies to acting out. Nevertheless, they thrived in what was predominantly an insight-oriented approach. We should make every effort to gauge our

---

[3]Most of the time it is accurate empathy alone that constitutes "reassurance." On other occasions it is empathy *plus* the explicit acknowledgment of the patient's past and present coping abilities.

patients' capacities for insight and give them as interpretive an approach as they can tolerate.

It is factors three and four, feeling understood and forming insight, that are often indicated when one is tempted to resort to advice, exhortations, commands, and instructions. These latter irritate, patronize, infantilize, and stir up erotic fears and fantasies in many patients. The following vignette illustrates my point.

> Mr. Z.'s central issues revolved around separation from his parents, by whom he was overprotected and yet still not nurtured in any meaningful emotional way. Much of his symptomatology was a means of simultaneously defending against, and yet obliquely expressing, powerful infantile dependency needs and overwhelmingly intense anger toward his parents, as well as an attempt to distance people out of his fears of closeness. Predictably, he began to experience the same conflicts vis-à-vis me, which he acted out in a variety of ways: making faces and bizarre noises in public and with friends and acquaintances, changing his tone of voice and gesturing bizarrely in therapy and at times outside it, periodically screaming from the balcony of his apartment, phoning and occasionally walking into various community and mental health agencies and frightening staff (to whom he was a total stranger) with suicide threats, acting foolish and idiotic at his job interviews, taking quizzes in his college courses without having opened a book, and persistently arriving late to therapy.

> I found myself, like his parents, becoming irritated with his behavior and, like them, I felt the impulse to tell him to "cut it out, shape up, and fly right." Indeed on the few occasions in which I did just this, he only escalated his "clowning," as he called it. It became plain that, if anything, he enjoyed my irritation as much as he did that of his parents. It was not until I calmed down enough to do with him what I would have done with any other patient—explore the meaning and purpose of this behavior— that we made progress and the acting out began to subside.

> Working together we discovered that his socially self-destructive behavior and acting out within the session served several functions. 1) They were a way of defending against his anger at his parents and me and at the same time indirectly, even pleasurably, expressing it (by embarrassing the former and by thwarting my good intentions to be a therapist) and punishing himself for it; 2) a way of insuring that he would remain dependent upon his parents and me, independence being associated with a fear of losing us; and 3) a way of dealing with his fears of rejection and of intimacy by distancing people in whom he was interested or who appeared interested in him. *In addition* to our dealing with these conflicts and the associated danger situations, it was necessary for me to point out, with concern but *not* oversolicitude (which would only have given him another self-destructive weapon against me), that he was gradually alienating people with whom he might at some point want to be friends, that his phoning up and visiting social service and mental health professionals was a way of keeping me from becoming too important to him and trying to distance me, that his lateness to therapy was serving the same function, and that if he continued to embarrass his parents that indeed he *was* going to bring them back into his life (which was what he professed to fear most).

As I succeeded in helping him to form insight *and* pointing out the consequences of his behaviors, his acting out began to subside and he began to verbally express his feelings and fantasies directly in the transference.[4]

5. *The transference* in supportive therapy is just as (or even more) powerful than the one in insight-oriented though, because you are more active, it is more "contaminated" than the one in the latter. Relative to insight-oriented psychotherapy, there is less resolution of this transference through analysis of its historical roots and more cultivation of the positive transference as a suggestive and reinforcing lever and as the medium in which constructive identification with you can occur. For both these reasons you strive to operate in the climate of a positive transference while not stimulating the negative one. In either case the transference would be interpreted only if it appears to be significantly impeding the therapy, if the patient is engaging in destructive acting out, or if it appears he may stop coming to the sessions.

Because of this positive transference and your status, the patient will value your time and comments more than those of friends and family members. Consequently, a perceptive remark or verbal reinforcement of an adaptive behavior will carry more weight when it comes from you than from his spouse or best friend. There is no better example of the supercharged nature of transference time than those schizophrenic patients who are maintained indefinitely, outside the hospital, with a mere 15 or 20 minutes of your time a month and who regress rapidly if and when you stop seeing them.

The positive transference is used *unobtrusively*. It is generally not, as I discussed earlier, capitalized upon directly but rather as a fringe benefit of one's reflective, confrontative, clarifying, interpretive, and other work. You accept graciously that it gives added clout to all your interventions (leading many of them to function, in effect, as *suggestions*), but you do not necessarily let this fact influence the nature of your interventions. It may come to your aid when you remind your patient, after you have heard him out and deemed his "catastrophizing" unfounded, that his past history shows he has more ability to contain his anxiety or rage than he seems to think. It often greatly strengthens the thought-provoking character of your query: what does it mean that, in the face of solid evidence that he functions best when he is working, he allows

---

[4]This is also an excellent example of failed empathy. I was so preoccupied with the maladaptiveness of the patient's defensive acting out (and so ensnared by my countertransference to it) that I lost sight of the incredible fearfulness that necessitated it. I was brought back to my senses by the patient himself who apprised me of my critical tone and reminded me that the most superficial social interaction was for him a mine field.

himself to remain unemployed with large quantities of unstructured, anxiety-laden, and "depressogenic" time upon his hands. It vastly empowers your reinforcement of his adaptive maneuvers, such as quietly nodding your approval of his decision to resume jogging and weight lifting as a means of discharging the aggression that he has previously internalized or displaced upon his spouse. It lends additional credence to your observation of the self-destructive effect of his continued alcohol abuse or the depressing effect on himself and the destructive impact on his family life of his continued inability to decide for his wife or his long-time girl friend. It adds salve to the healing effect on an inordinately strict and hostile superego of words like, "You seem to be pretty hard on yourself today."

In particular, the positive transference is a potent ally of your pharmacological interventions. With most patients you should administer the prescription with calm and confident, but not extravagant (lest you lose too much face if the medication fails), expectations of success. It will carry more transference clout if, as De Wald (1971) says, you spontaneously and willingly offer it than if you do so reluctantly or only after repeated demands and requests. For example, with a patient to whom I am giving an antidepressant medication I might say:

> These medications have helped millions of people with problems similar to yours. There are many from which to choose, but this one is generally the most effective for those whose depressive symptoms are similar to yours. It is important for you to understand that it takes several weeks for you to develop an optimum blood level of this medication. Consequently, we will not know exactly how much it will help you until you have been on it for about a month. Your sleeping, anxiety, and appetite should begin improving in the first few days though your mood will probably lag a bit behind. Although some people experience a lift in the first few days, most will not before two to four weeks. As to side-effects, you should expect to experience some dry mouth, but others, such as blurry vision, are much rarer and, if they occur, frequently subside after the first few days.

If the medication is effective it will play back positively upon the transference to augment its potency still further. Indeed, some patients, either because of a dependent and infantile character or because of their experience with general physicians, feel that you are not doing anything for them if you do not prescribe a medication and, consequently, do not return unless you at least explain your rationale for not doing so.

Because of the propensity of many supportive patients to develop exceptionally strong transferences in which they may forfeit all observing ego (i.e., the "transference psychosis"), it is often necessary to do some reality testing for them and to minimize the exotic fantasies that would flourish in the face of a too-strenuous neutrality and blankness. For example, you literally might have to remind a raging paranoid that you are not his father. Whereas to the neurotic patient of the opposite sex who queries, "Doctor, have you ever had an affair with any of your patients?" you reply with a question about his or her fantasies, to the borderline or schizophrenic you unhesitatingly respond with a "no." In addition to interpreting the historical roots of certain expectations of, and attitudes toward you, you might have to point out their lack of justification in reality. This would be the case, for example, with a patient whose sense of entitlement leads him to miss scheduled appointments and then become enraged when you cannot drop everything and see him when he arrives unexpectedly. The following is an example of the clarification of reality within the transference:

> Mr. Q. was virtually ignored by his parents in childhood. He was allowed to go his own maladaptive way with little or no direction or encouragement from them. He interpreted my refusal to tell him what to do, to manage his life between the sessions, and to be available whenever he wanted to see me as meaning that I was as little interested in him as his parents were. Indeed, he even accused me of reveling in depriving him. I had to point out to him, repeatedly, that because of his unfortunate experiences in childhood, he interpreted my adherence to the therapist role as meaning I did not care about him. I reminded him that if I told him what to do I would be fostering the illusion that he could receive from me what his parents had failed to give him.

6. *Gratification* is the most problematic parameter of all. It is true that there is more gratification of the transferential strivings in supportive than in insight-oriented therapy. Indeed, appropriate and timely gratification is one of your most powerful tools. However, if engaged in indiscriminately, without reference to the patient's particular history and dynamics, it can prove disastrous. Before discussing the actual mechanics of such maneuvers, I wish to emphasize that, by and large, people in supportive treatment are probably capable of tolerating, in the interest of insight formation, more deprivation than most of us are aware.

The rule of thumb is that your gratification, when indicated, should be as *unobtrusive* as possible. Much of it is carried by the vehicles that also operate in any insight-oriented therapy: being interested, attentive, empathic, and visibly present. This can be augmented by nonverbal maneuvers as gentle as a smile, leaning forward at the right moment, concerned and knowing nods, and so forth. Simply talking a bit more than you might otherwise constitutes gratification for some. Much of the gratification accrues to that which you do *not* do, rather than to anything that you do in particular. Every time you do not analyze the transference you are permitting it to be real, hence to some degree gratifying.

You express this last by returning, rather than analyzing or keeping silent in the face of, the patient's comment upon the weather; laughing at his joke; tolerating a certain amount of his idealization of you; allowing yourself to be drawn at times into a brief chat about sports or current events; or occasionally answering a direct question about yourself or making a judicious self-disclosure.

As much (or more) forethought must go into whether to gratify a patient's explicit or implied request in supportive treatment as in insight-oriented. This is exemplified in the following vignette:

> One hospitalized young man, with dynamics similar to Mr. E.'s, was late to the point that it appeared that he would not come at all to three sessions in the first few weeks of therapy. I pondered, as I sat in the office each time, whether to phone the nurses's station and remind him of our hour. Because one of his central dynamics was withdrawal from others out of the fear that he was unimportant to them, I elected to give him the behavioral message that I valued our time together. Consequently, I phoned the ward each time. When some weeks later this occurred the fourth time, however, I was in more of a quandary about what to do. Because, at this point, I felt our rapport was sufficiently established and his awareness of his dynamics sufficiently preconscious, I elected *not* to phone the ward. He came in the following Monday in a silent boil. With but a little encouragement he was able to express his fury at me for "allowing" him to sleep through the session. To help him modulate his rage and sense of rejection, I apprised him that I had given some thought to the matter and decided that by calling him I was doing him no favor, but rather allowing him to bypass issues that should be aired in the hours. He responded by opening up the hitherto avoided constellation around rejection and self-esteem. It emerged that he felt he was taking less risk when others "made the first move" than when he himself initiated the contact. My phone calls functioned as invitations which diminished his fears that I would see how important I was becoming to him and use or reject him.

When you do gratify a transference derivative, it is important to know that it is always possible to go back later and analyze it, but that it should not be done simultaneously. For example, on one occasion I briefly hospitalized Mr. Q. for a suicidal gesture. Feeling that he was probably capable of containing himself, I yet opted for admission in order to convey the message that I, unlike his parents, took him seriously and cared about him. Much later we were able to go back and analyze this episode, but had we done so at the time, it would have robbed my intervention of its supportive effect.

However, it is paramount that you appreciate that any gratification must be dispensed within the context of a thorough history and sound dynamic understanding of the patient. You must possess this in order to know *what* constitutes an appropriate gratification and *how* it will be perceived by him. The cup of coffee that is supportive for the infantile character or regressed schizophrenic may be perceived as a seduction by the hysteric and a homosexual assault or power play by the paranoid. The bus fare loaned to one psychotic depressive is taken as emotional nourishment and augments your rapport while it induces guilt in another. Being a "real person" might bolster the self-esteem of a depressed and rejected patient and frighten off or incite violence in the paranoid. Direct expression of concern and caring is therapeutic for some, undermines the ego of others (e.g., making them feel they must be fairly disturbed for you to talk like this), and is used by still others as a club with which to beat you over the head. Complying with the request for an extra session enhances the ego of one and leads the other to feel you view him as incapable. Filling out a disability form is sustenance for one, an insult to another.

I shall illustrate how a harmless compliment (around obtaining and keeping a job, let us say) is not at all the same compliment when transmitted to six different individuals by the same male therapist:

a. To one ambulatory schizophrenic, with a virtually nonexistent self-esteem and few social contacts, it is taken as a real reward and incentive to work still harder.
b. To a male latent homosexual it represents the desired and feared penetration and a panic is precipitated.
c. The moral masochist feels guilty at his "greediness" and out of his sense of unworthiness, and self-punitively regresses at work.
d. The borderline, out to defeat the therapist, interprets it as an invitation to sabotage his employment.
e. The dependent individual, heavily laden with issues of separation and loss, fears he is recovering too rapidly and in imminent danger of being terminated or of being burdened too quickly by adult responsibility; he regresses.
f. The female hysteric sees it as a seduction and begins to act out her erotic transference at work, to call the clinician between the hours, and to harbor the illusion that at last she has found the "right man."

In short, gratifications have their place, but are not to be doled out indiscriminately. When in doubt about a gratification, as with any other intervention, the best policy is to refrain from it. When in doubt about how to respond to a patient's request, the best tack is to ask him to clarify it.

7. Closely related to the sixth factor is that of *"being a real person."* Discriminating and well-titrated doses of this are a powerful tool. Paradoxically, much of the power of your real person for the patient resides in largely transference factors. In other words, it is the patient's perception of you as a powerful parent imago that gives the reality of your person more clout than the reality of the others with whom he is in contact.

Being there, honestly and directly, without lying or subterfuge, is the most important part of being real. You must be there, as a whole person, with a whole person, continually. Your empathy as well is quite real; there is nothing contrived about that. Because I have touched upon most of the aspects of being real in the discussion of transference and gratification, I shall cover only two touchy topics: moralizing and expressing anger.

As for the first, I have inveighed against it in earlier chapters. Nevertheless, modulated and against a ground of caring and acceptance, moralizing has its place with certain patients—to wit, the psychopath or antisocial personality. Both on the ward and in outpatient treatment, there are times when you must explicitly represent the normative values of civilized society and your own moral code to such a patient. Generally, these are justified to him by invoking pragmatics rather than moral absolutes, i.e., the maladaptive and destructive consequences for himself, as much as for others, of his playing outside the rules. At times this course involves ensuring that the patient does face the consequences of his behavior. I was once in the position of pressing charges against one borderline male who calmly broke out several plate-glass windows as a means of embarrassing his parents, who had visited the clinic for an appointment with a social worker. Involved in this was pointing out to him 1) his implicit conviction that, because he had suffered certain deprivations in the past, he was entitled to receive special dispensations and to break the rules with impunity, 2) his use of his psychiatric diagnosis to relinquish responsibility for his actions, and 3) the possibility that he could have seriously injured some passerby.

Anger, I have argued, is generally used silently to further one's knowledge about the patient's intentions toward you and/or to give you clues to countertransference *mishegoss*. Like other information it is factored into the equation that leads eventually to your intervention. Actually expressing anger to a patient, on the other hand, is like dynamite. It is seldom indicated, is used only *after* other maneuvers have failed, and is utilized carefully and in controlled amounts. As a trainee, you should use it only after consultation with your supervisor.

To begin with, if you have conveyed your anger, unintentionally, to a patient and he perceives it and queries you about it, you should not lie lest you disturb an already compromised reality testing. I confessed to one severely borderline young woman that indeed I was irritated with her but that *I* was responsible for it, that it had to do with *my* impatience with her difficulty recognizing the role of her parents in her problems, with *my* failure to appreciate just how disturbing this issue was for her.

Situations in which the communication of irritation may be appropriate (and again this must be decided *in the light of each individual's dynamics*) include: a patient's persistence in occupationally and socially self-destructive behavior despite considerable awareness of the motives and maladaptive consequences of such behavior; a perennial circumvention of the treatment through tardiness, absences, acting out, and other means; and a failure to take the initiative in activities that he clearly understands are in his best interests (e.g., joining AA, keeping his appointments with his cardiologist, looking for a job when he is down to his last funds). A little irritation may convey, in such situations, 1) that you feel him *capable* of more constructive behavior and that you view him as *responsible* for the conduct of his life and 2) that you care enough to become a little "discombobulated" in his own best interests.

Anger is at times indicated with patients who persistently cross the line of limits you have set. Some borderlines can be famous for their cruelty in the transference and for evoking murderous feelings in their therapists.

One young borderline woman repeatedly abused me in a variety of ways: by calling late at night from phone booths simultaneously threatening suicide and pointing out my impotence to do anything about it, by dropping out of treatment every other day, by persistently refusing to pay her bill, by going to other physicians for medication, and so forth.

I knew that much of her behavior was a way of dehumanizing me as she had been dehumanized, of simultaneously paying me back for refusing to meet her needs and trying to cajole me into it, of rejecting me before I could reject her, of keeping me at a distance out of fears of closeness, and of turbulently defending against her softer, warm, and sad feelings vis-à-vis me. All this was gradually and repeatedly interpreted to her and she developed some insight into her behavior. However, she used this very insight to taunt me still further, saying, literally, "Yes, I know what I'm doing, you bastard, but you know what, I don't give a damn and there's nothing you can do about it." Her behavior did not change until I dropped my aspirations to beatification and let her hold a little of my anger. I pointed out to her that it was extraordinarily disconcerting to see someone who was capable of doing good therapeutic work continue to behave so cavalierly. I communicated to her that, although I understood just how much distress she felt and what she had been exposed to and although I wanted to stick with her and help her reach the other shore, that I, like every other human being, had limits beyond which another could not trespass. Finally, I pointed out that it was indeed possible for her, like any other human being, to behave in such a way as to push another away, that she, like all of us, possessed the power to do this. This, coupled with a clear delineation of the conditions under which I would continue to treat her and the consequences should she depart from them, turned matters around swiftly and some real work began.

Some time later she was able to reflect on this period. My angry limit-setting was reassuring and supportive to her in several ways. It conveyed to her 1) that she was sufficiently present in my life to get me angry, 2) that I was interested enough in her welfare to become incensed at her self-destructiveness, 3) that I dispelled her fear that she must be unspeakably and basically terrible if I could not react in a human way to her abusiveness, 4) that I viewed her as capable of more adaptive behavior and of tolerating a little direct feedback, 5) that I helped her diminish the guilt she was feeling about her abusiveness to me, and 6) that I restored her respect in my competence.

Excessively angry or rageful responses, on the other hand, should not be shared with patients but should be allowed to abate and be treated self-analytically after the session. Such feelings usually stem from 1) the therapist's psychodynamics and the manner in which the patient's behavior impinges upon them, 2) a failure to set limits sufficiently early in the treatment and, related to this, 3) inappropriate gratification of the patient's acting out and demands which lead him to escalate them until you can no longer abide them. An inability to say "stop" or "no" when it is therapeutically indicated makes a therapist all but useless to many dependent, borderline, and narcissistic personalities.

8. *The lending of ego and, at times, superego* are among the most important maneuvers in supportive treatment. The patient acquires new and more adaptive ego, superego, and ego ideal functions through identification with you and through internalization of the therapeutic, problem-solving interaction with you. This is furthered in a number of ways.

Once you have assessed a patient's ego strength and determined that he is capable of talking about certain feelings and fantasies without acting on them, then one of the most important things you can do is simply allow or encourage him to talk about these emotionally charged issues which he may have viewed as particularly dangerous. By so doing you implicitly communicate (and in supportive psychotherapy a good many of your communications are *implicit* or *behavioral*[5]): "I think you are capable of modulating this feeling sufficiently to discuss it. Talking about something is one thing, acting on it quite another. I am not afraid, nor need you be, that merely by telling me about it you will thereby act upon it." The patient, through identification with you, may come to view his fantasies as less threatening such that he can begin to talk them through. This was the case with Mr. Z., who could only begin dealing with his anger directly and non-self-destructively after he found he could verbally express his angry fantasies about me without my immediate disintegration.

-----

[5]For example, by refusing to see a narcissistic patient who missed, without prior notice, two sessions, and who then showed up unannounced for a make-up session, I behaviorally communicated to him: 1) "You are not the only person in my life. You cannot disown your responsibility for coming to the sessions and then show up at your whim and expect to be gratified. There are other people in the world besides you, and you must take account of their particular needs and constraints." 2) "I feel that you are capable of containing yourself until the next session. You are not so disabled that I need to absolve you from the requirements for responsible adult behavior. You are not so disturbed that you need to be treated with kid gloves or given special dispensation." When we did meet again he confessed that although he was at first irritated by my not seeing him, he was reassured that I was treating him like a man, not a child, that I thought him capable of more.

"Decatastrophizing," related to encouraging ventilation, is another important part of lending ego and is useful in times of apparent crisis. Many patients' intolerance for dysphoria and stress is such that their turbulent *reactions* to depression or anxiety become worse than the *underlying feeling* itself. The classic example is the anxiety attack, where the patient's "awfulizing" around his initial mild tension pushes him into a spiral of ever intensifying anxiety. Merely sitting calmly and letting the patient ventilate his feelings and concerns, without becoming caught up in his urgency, and pointing out to him he has weathered such storms in the past, usually helps him to regain his composure because you undercut the fantasy that something terrible will happen. Unnecessary and precipitous hospitalizations and pharmacological interventions can seriously weaken the patient's ego and foster dependency and a sense of helplessness. Similarly, refusing to respond to an "hysterical" phone call with the immediate offer of an extra session can, in the long run, be more ego strengthening than gratifying this request. If there is any indication that the patient can contain himself without patronizing and infantilizing "special favors," he is better off without them. Some patients even resent you for acceding too readily to them. What we are talking about essentially is 1) *always speaking to such conscious control over his behavior as the patient possesses,* of addressing, in more technical terms, the healthy part of his ego, and 2) recognizing the tremendous influence of your explicitly and implicitly communicated expectations on the patient's behavior (e.g., what we usually mean when we speak of "suggestion").

Of course, when past history and current behavior lead you to concur with the patient's catastrophic assessment, then providing the requested external structure *is* the supportive maneuver. Some patients who could not otherwise contain their destructive or self-destructive urges will be able to do so if you remind them that you are willing, not to assume total responsibility for them, but to serve as a sort of auxiliary ego—to be available by phone and, if they feel it indicated, to briefly hospitalize them. With some this is sufficiently reassuring that you will never hear from them between the sessions.

At times it is necessary to choke off, rather than encourage, ventilation and to otherwise set limits. Many have understood the repression theory of psychopathology to mean that the aim is to get the patient to "let it all hang out," to "get it off his chest" in any way, shape, or form that he chooses. The current social climate seems to favor this misconception as well. Sheer affective discharge, while essential, by itself accomplishes nothing lasting. It must be performed in a manner that does not impugn the human dignity of either the patient or you and that allows him to form some insight into its nature and origins.

You are doing neither yourself nor your patient a favor by allowing him to put you in physical danger, destroy your property, make a scene in your waiting room, open your windows and scream out of them, undress or masturbate in your office, or grovel on your rug in the fetal position. Some patients derive so much gratification from these and other primitive discharges that such behavior becomes an end in itself and an impediment to the therapeutic enterprise. You learn from your patients' histories and your experiences with them which ones are likely to escalate the expression of certain feelings into a full-blown affective storm. Because it is easier for anyone to contain such feelings at the outset rather than in full bloom, you need to nip them in the bud. This entails reminding the patient that there are appropriate and verbal ways to express anger, sensuality, and so forth, but that you refuse to tolerate his *acting them out* within the sessions. *Limit setting* is communicating to the potentially obstreperous patient that your aim is to understand and be of assistance to him, but that there are lines beyond which he cannot cross and be permitted to remain in your office. Moreover, allowing a patient to abuse you or continue to place unreasonable demands upon you ensures that you will eventually, consciously or unconsciously, become resentful of him, which is helpful for neither of you. Even if you were able to tolerate the perennial abuse and cater to his unreasonable demands, however, such saintliness (or masochism) would be bad for his reality testing for it would foster the illusion that he had finally acquired the omnipotent, omnibenevolent parent.

Helping patients set limits can also involve pointing out that it is possible to entertain fantasies without acting on them and to experience an impulse and yet refrain from indulging it. This might simply entail encouraging the patient to stop and think before acting in certain situations or to remind himself of what you and he have discussed on the matter (including the functions and consequences of the behavior). It was fascinating, over the months, to watch Mr. Z. building our interactions into his ego. He went from instantly enacting his desire to clown, to hesitating a few seconds before doing so, to painfully deliberating for minutes before making a halfhearted face, to finally giving it up altogether and proceeding immediately to talk about the feelings involved.

Limit setting is only effective within the context of a strong transference valence to you. Limit setting before the transference is established may carry no more clout than if the patient's bus driver or next-door neighbor delivered it.

Occasionally it is necessary to set limits to sexual, as much as to aggressive, expressiveness. One patient was becoming so obviously titillated by her minute accounts of her numerous sexual encounters and her erotic fantasies about me that she was ignoring virtually everything else. It was necessary for me to point out that this was both becoming an end in itself and allowing her to avoid problematic feelings and aspects of reality. In other words, the erotic transference had come to operate, in effect, as a resistance to the therapeutic work.

When a patient engages in behaviors that are destructive to the treatment (e.g., erratic attendance, refusals to take medications that are essential to his treatment, refusals to cooperate in a withdrawal from drugs or alcohol that not only jeopardize his life but make psychotherapy unworkable) and refuses to respond to confrontations and attempts to explore his purposes, then one is obligated to apprise him that therapy cannot be carried out with only one participant. It is hypocritical to pretend otherwise (that you can treat a patient who will not allow you); you are not that powerful. It becomes necessary for you to inform him of the conditions under which you can treat him and of the consequences should he not want to meet them. At times it is helpful to draw up a written contract of these conditions and consequences and sign it with the patient. You then have a concrete document to which you can refer him should he become tempted to resume acting out. Regrettably, there will be some people who will simply not let you help them and whom you will have to discharge from treatment. Such terminations may even have a therapeutic effect over the longer term in that they may make it possible for such a patient to work more realistically and effectively with another therapist in the future.

An important aspect of lending ego is modeling problem-solving behavior. This is usually what is indicated instead of direct advice or engaging in the delusion that you are intelligent enough to tell the patient what to do or powerful enough to see that he does it once you tell him.[6] You tell a patient what to do only in life-threatening circumstances and when you are prepared to implement what you say (i.e., civil commitment for extreme suicidal or homicidal tendencies).

For example, if a patient asks you whether he should take a particular job or get an apartment with a certain person, it is far better to first ask him what it means that he is asking you. Second, you should encourage him to explore his feelings on the matter and weigh the pros and cons. For example, with Mr. Q. it was necessary for me to point out that he was trying to make me give him the advice that he had never received

---

[6]The more active and intrusive maneuvers such as giving advice and encouragement should always be viewed in terms of a costs-benefits ratio. In other words, do the advantages accruing to possibly constructively influencing the patient on a particular issue outweigh the disadvantages of infantilizing him? Furthermore, there is a large class of patients (the so-called "help-rejecting complainers") who will beg you for advice and instructions only to enjoy the pleasures of rejecting them out of hand or of halfheartedly implementing them and proving you wrong.

from his father and that he took my refusal to do so as a sign that I was as uninterested in his welfare as the father had seemed to be. From there we went on to explore his options together. Eventually he was able to internalize the problem-solving interaction between us. He had acquired a movable skill rather than the dependency that advice would have fostered. Furthermore, I believe his self-esteem was improved by my implicitly communicating to him that he was capable of making his own decisions, whereas telling him what to do would have been precisely the *un*supportive course to follow.

The only situations in which advice and instructions are indicated are those treatments where you are satisfied that the patient will need pharmacological and psychotherapeutic maintenance for the duration of his existence; where it seems to be virtually the only way of building an initial rapport (as is the case with some especially dependent and infantile characters who will feel too deprived and will leave treatment if you do not); or where it appears the patient is about to make a precipitous decision with potentially major consequences for his family life, career, and general well-being. In the case of this last you still stop short of telling him *what* to do, only advising him of the possible negative repercussions and recommending that he postpone his decision until the two of you have talked about it further.

When one is tempted to proffer advice or instruction, questioning the patient about the meaning of his behavior, then pointing out, if necessary, the maladaptive consequences of it, and asking him if there are not other options at his disposal are among the best routes to take. This transmits your concern at the same time that you do not engage in the pretense that *you* can *do* anything about it.

Helping the patient form a new self-image and more positive self-esteem are also important parts of lending ego. This, here again, is accomplished unobtrusively. You need not say anything in particular. Simply being there, empathically, day after day and treating him like an autonomous and responsible human being will have wondrous effects. Gradually, he will begin to view and esteem himself as you view and esteem him.

With a frankly psychotic patient, lending ego may involve reality testing around hallucinations, delusions, and so forth. This should not occur before rapport has been established and before medication has rendered him amenable to a verbal approach. Oftentimes this results in his spontaneous awareness of the fantastic nature of his hallucinations and delusions, or they simply move from his center of consciousness. When this does not occur, you must first hear him out and attempt to understand his psychotic world before apprising him of alternate interpretations of reality. To do so prematurely would produce arguments that lead nowhere. Once you learn his psychotic vocabulary you will appreciate that his bizarre communications are metaphorical messages about himself. There are even delusional systems with elements of which you will never tamper. The only barrier between one chronically depressed paranoid schizophrenic and suicide was his conviction that he was suffering, in some mysterious way, for the benefit of all mankind.

Part of supporting the patient's reality testing includes consensually validating his perceptions and interpretations of others' (and your own) behaviors that appear well founded. This might entail, for example, agreeing with his concerns about whether a person is exploiting him or whether his mother is accurate when she repeatedly denies her attempts to control him and curb his independence.

Under "lending ego ideal" (and also, to some extent, self-esteem) I shall consider encouragement and exhortation. Pep talks do have a place in supportive psychotherapy, albeit a more limited one than is usually imagined. Because these maneuvers have infantilizing and patronizing potential, they should be used sparingly and only after a more insight-oriented approach has failed. One 30-year-old woman, for example, had gone far toward realizing the historical sources of her dependent attitudes, low self-esteem, and work inhibitions. She did not, however, make any changes in the outside world until I 1) pointed out the secondary gain for her in the patient role and her dependency on me, 2) told her I thought her fully capable of getting and keeping a job, and 3) encouraged her to begin taking social risks.

Finally, as for lending superego, you do this when you accept, rather than punish, the patient for his fantasies and feelings, when you point out the difference between a wish and a deed, when you alert him to unrealistic elements in his guilt, when you show him he is assuming responsibility for that over which he has no control, and when you help him to use his realistic guilt in a constructive way. You lend ego ideal when you help him reward himself for mundane accomplishments and small, but tangible, signs of progress and when you keep your expectations of him realistic. Burdening him with your own agenda and aspirations for him is countertherapeutic. Developing more realistic expectations of life and of himself is one of the most constructive outcomes of supportive, as well as insight-oriented, treatment. In short, by "lending" ego ideal and superego, you allow the patient, in his identification with you, to adopt your constructive attitudes toward himself.

9. Another factor in supportive therapy is *dealing with the patient's defenses*. Already touched upon in the discussion of limit setting and implied in that on lending ego in general, it nevertheless deserves a separate section unto itself. There is, as I mentioned, greater onus on the supportive therapist to decide which of his patient's defenses are more adaptive, and which more psychopathological. He must then facilitate

the atrophy of the former, the hypertrophy of the latter. This means that he will be concerned with analyzing some defenses more than others.

For example, with an alcoholic you might, in addition to trying to understand the sources of his addiction, help him to exchange denial (e.g., drinking) for reaction formation (e.g., Alcoholics Anonymous). With a depressed, obsessional personality you might foster a return to his workaholic isolation of affect in exchange for turning anger against the self. Or you might, as I did in the following case, promote catharsis and the substitution of intellectualization for projection.

> Mr. J. entered treatment in the midst of his first, acute paranoid episode. Almost before sitting down he looked at me and said, "Doctor, there's one thing I want to get straight right now. And that's that I am not a homosexual. I have never had gay feelings or participated in such acts. Do you understand me?" After assuring him that I did, he then shared a delusional system involving the spreading of snide rumors about his masculinity, sexual potency, and penis size. He almost got into several fights with his persecutors—all men.

> Upon taking a history I discovered that there were many oedipal issues related to a smothering mother and coldly distant but harshly domineering father. The latent homosexual elements were easily inferred from the history as well as from his initial negation and paranoid complaints. It also became apparent to me from this history, and his behavior in my office, that his best premorbid level of functioning was an obsessive-compulsive one with a good deal of intellectualization.

> In addition to hearing him out about his present complaints and encouraging him to ventilate his feelings about his father, I opted to give him what Glover (1955) terms "inexact" or "incomplete" interpretations which he could then use as intellectualized defenses against his homosexual impulses. For example, I focused on the elements of aggression and dominance-submission vis-à-vis males and their genetic origins in his relationship with his father rather than on the more important, but more unconscious, more ego dystonic, incestuous hetero- and homosexual fantasies. In other words, I gave him a partial truth which he could then use as an intellectualization in exchange for his more maladaptive projection. Since my interpretations also symbolically represented gifts, they functioned as ego-syntonic gratifications of his otherwise unacceptable and unconscious dependent desires.

Not only is it incumbent upon you to rank order your patient's defenses on a scale of adaptiveness and shore up some and dissect others, it is necessary to decide whether his preferred defense or that which is defended against is more maladaptive.

> For example, one young business executive came in on the brink of psychosis, experiencing incipient somatic delusions (regarding his inner ear) and preoccupied with ruminations about two groups of individuals, the "number ones" and "number twos," which latter he felt himself a member of. His life was characterized by a paralyzing array of inhibitions

so that he could not parcel out responsibilities to subordinates, write his reports, support his own interests in company meetings, and complete his application for promotion. His diffidence was such that he could barely go to the grocery store and be assertive enough to take a place in line at the cash register. After several weeks it became apparent that he had profound conflicts over aggression. The resident's task was to decide whether his aggression was so overwhelming that his severe inhibitions and reaction formations were the lesser of two evils. Whenever the subject of anger was broached, the patient indeed behaved as if he were sitting atop a volcano and would go off on some bizarre philosophical discussion about number ones and twos or experience the hurting in his inner ear. The resident finally concluded, from his history and ongoing mental status, that the depth of this man's fears about his anger was unjustified. His inhibitions, not his anger, were draining his energy, crippling him, and moving him toward psychosis. Consequently, the resident began a gingerly dissection of these defenses and an exploration of the danger associated with them. As this man became less frightened of his anger, began to decompress it, and escaped the grip of his omnipotence of thoughts, the inhibitions and somatic delusions began to subside and he dropped his bizarre, intellectualized "number one, number two" metaphors in exchange for a direct discussion of the aggressive and self-esteem issues which they both concealed and expressed.

Akin to this issue is the identification of formerly constructive factors in a patient's life which have, for some reason, been given up. You should question him about this. If, after so doing, it seems there is still some hygienic element there, then you may want to promote it.

If athletics once provided a ready and pleasurable discharge of anger and anxiety and a prop for self-esteem, then by all means encourage it. If a hobby once served as an enjoyable sublimation, then why not promote it? With a socially isolated and guilt-ridden depressive you might encourage a return to the church or temple which once functioned as a source of meaning, affiliation, catharsis, and absolution or to the civic work that was formerly a source of self-worth and self-transcendence.

10. Related to points eight and nine is *dealing with the greater propensity of many supportive patients for regression* to infantile, hitherto unconscious, primary process modes of cognition and handling of drives. Whereas the neurotic needs to loosen up enough to have access to such material, the borderline or psychotic may be in danger of being overwhelmed by it. Whereas the obsessive-compulsive needs to let go sufficiently to free-associate, the schizophrenic needs to tighten up and organize his thinking.

With such patients, you want to minimize regression-promoting factors such as analytic neutrality, long silences, deep interpretations of dreams and other material, and unstructured interactions between the two of you. With some, shorter sessions are less regressive than longer ones. You want to keep the schizophrenic focused on the major issues lest he become lost in his defensive-expressive ramblings. You encourage him, as De Wald (1971) says, to "think first and speak later," as opposed to the neurotic whom you want to "speak first and think later." You should not allow him to talk about his rich and bizarre fantasy life to the exclusion of issues in current reality. You are interested primarily in his conscious concerns. In an effort to help him regroup, you might point out when only five or ten minutes are left in the session and you might, in an effort to organize his thinking and help him maintain the continuity between the sessions, recapitulate and summarize the salient themes of the hour.

There is more emphasis on the "here and now," with many of your interpretations being designed to make him aware of the connection between current situations and his fantasies, feelings, and behaviors: i.e., that the voices he heard over the weekend seemed related to some set of feelings about his brother's visit, that he began seeing devils right after you announced your impending vacation, that his confusion began right after the two of you started taking about his employer, that the hallucinations telling him he is worthless seem to intensify as he leaves your office, and so forth. Indeed, premature or excessive focusing on historical factors will detract from your message about the more pressing current and transference factors. Excessive genetic interpretations may also provoke unmanageable regression and the patient's confusion of you with a variety of historical objects.

11. *Explicit education* plays a greater role in supportive than in insight-oriented psychotherapy. You might have to correct misconceptions about bodily functions and myths and misinformation about sexual practices and their supposed noxious effects. Chronic manic-depressives and schizophrenics need to understand the nature of their disorders and how best to cope with them. Patients on medication need to know the rationale for the drug and the dosage schedule and to be apprised, in a matter of fact fashion, about any troublesome side-effects that are likely to occur. Insomniacs often profit from a little knowledge about normal sleep and processes that impede it (i.e., caffeine, late-night cigarettes or exercise, mid-day naps) or facilitate it (i.e., regular daily exercise, the consumption of substances containing tryptophan, paradoxical intention). Patients with chronic anxiety might profitably learn the Jacobson and other relaxation-inducing maneuvers.

12. Finally, *alloplastic* or environmental manipulations play a greater role in supportive therapy than in insight-oriented. The current environments of many severely disturbed patients are quite as pathogenic as their historical ones. Consequently, any real change may be impossible unless one can extricate them from their vital niche in a pathological ecosystem. With a regressed ambulatory schizophrenic or otherwise infantile individual, you might have to intervene, directly or through a social worker, with his family, friends, and employer or take steps to

implement his admission to a hospital, boarding home, supervised apartment, or halfway house. You should encourage and, if necessary, guide him to the appropriate social clubs and community activities in an effort to reconnect him with people and get him involved in activities outside himself—what Frankl (1973) calls "decentering" or "dereflection."

You resort to such direct advice and implementation only if less directive interventions have failed and if it is clear that the patient is incapable of realistically assessing his situation. Otherwise, you limit your activity to encouraging the patient to express his thoughts and feelings about his situation, what he sees as its advantages and disadvantages, and what options he has.

Table 11-1 summarizes my discussion of the similarities and differences between supportive and insight-oriented therapies.

**TABLE 11-1. Comparison and Contrast of Supportive and Insight Therapy**

| Supportive | Insight |
|---|---|
| 1. Thorough history and rigorous formulation prerequisite to treatment. | The same. |
| 2. All interventions are based upon this dynamic understanding. | The same. |
| 3. Necessity to rank order patient's defenses on an adaptive hierarchy and decide which to dissect, which to support. | Less so. |
| 4. Conveying your empathy and understanding is the prepotent therapeutic factor. | The same. |
| 5. As much insight formation as the patient can tolerate and is capable of. | The same. |
| 6. Proportionately greater emphasis on nonverbal and behavioral communication; interpretations more likely to be incomplete and may simultaneously serve a variety of functions such as (a) facilitating insight and the diminution of one defense and the shoring up of another and (b) gratification of transference strivings. | Proportionately greater emphasis on verbal interventions; interpretations generally designed to diminish defenses and pave the way for complete interpretations. |
| 7. Important aspects of the transference are left unanalyzed or utilized as subtle suggestive levers. | More complete interpretive resolution of the transference. |
| 8. Less analytic neutrality, hence more gratification of transference strivings (e.g., medications, "real" person comments). | More deprivation in the transference. |

## TABLE 11-1. (Continued)

| Supportive | Insight |
|---|---|
| 9. More "real." | More analytic. |
| 10. More lending of ego and superego occurs both (a) implicitly by allowing him to talk about his feelings and fantasies and serving as an object of identification, and (b) explicitly and actively by "decatastrophizing," conveying of positive expectations, appropriate limit setting, reality testing. | Lending of ego and superego occur, but are more implicit (a) simply by allowing the patient to talk about whatever he pleases with a calm and nonjudgmental acceptance, and (b) by being available as an object of identification. |
| 11. Little place for advice and none for telling a patient what to do, except when he is acutely suicidal or homicidal and commitment is required. | No place for advice and telling him what to do. |
| 12. Regression-promoting factors generally minimized; includes more structuring and focusing of session. | A regression in the presence of an observing ego is the vehicle of treatment. |
| 13. Alloplastic interventions may occur. | Hardly ever. |
| 14. Explicit education often important. | Much less so. |
| 15. Aims more at symptomatic relief or overt behavioral change than personality restructuring. | Aims at understanding and personality restructuring, from which symptomatic relief and behavioral change will follow. |
| 16. Interpretations are keyed more to the transference and the "here-and-now." Excessive genetic interpretation may provoke unmanageable regression and an inability to distinguish the therapist from historical figures. | Aims at complete interpretation and genetic reconstruction. |
| 17. Because of the patient's propensity to forfeit observing ego or develop transference psychoses, the reality aspects of the therapist-client relationship must often be clarified. | Seldom any need for this. |

## BRIEF TREATMENT

One species of supportive therapy, brief treatment, is sufficiently important (and neglected) to deserve special mention. Having been both treated and trained in a long-term insight-oriented mode, I, like most of my colleagues, initially looked askance at brief therapy. Not until I began work in a public mental health clinic did I awaken to the popular demand for, and therapeutic possibilities in, this modality.

Year after year, in our public clinics, approximately 50% of all patients referred to individual psychotherapy terminate treatment by the sixth session (see Garfield and Bergin, 1978, pp. 195-210). Looking at the other end of the spectrum, only a small percentage of patients stay for the 40 to 50 or more sessions that most would consider to constitute a longer-term therapy. A questionnaire, administered by Anthony La Bruzza to 100 consecutive "walk-ins" at the Connecticut Mental Health Center, found that 50% desired one-to-one treatment of eight sessions or fewer.

Patients appropriate for a brief approach range from ego-abundant creatures suitable for psychoanalysis but who, for various reasons, do not want it, to marginally functioning individuals with a past history of noncompliance beyond a handful of sessions. Indeed, I was continually amazed by those relatively disturbed and chaotic outpatients who were effectively treated in our brief treatment unit at the Connecticut Mental Health Center. Mann (1973), Sifneos (1972), Malan (1976), and Davanloo (1977) propose useful models for working with many of the patients a brief therapist is apt to encounter. The therapist is careful, from collaboration with the patient, to set a clearly delineated focus around which most of the work occurs, to keep the goals realistic, and (usually) to set a prearranged termination date.

Popular demand requires that each therapist familiarize himself with the briefer approaches, which can be learned only *after* he has obtained some grounding in the practice of long-term insight-oriented psychotherapy.

## SUGGESTED READINGS FOR CHAPTER 11

De Wald, P.: *Psychotherapy: A Dynamic Approach.* New York, Basic Books, 1971. Section III contains a good comparison and contrast between supportive and insight-oriented psychotherapy.
Easson, W.: *The Severely Disturbed Adolescent.* New York, International Universities Press, 1969.
Giovacchini, P.: *The Psychoanalysis of Character Disorders.* New York, Jason Aronson, 1975.
Kernberg, O.: *Borderline Conditions and Pathological Narcissism.* New York, Jason Aronson, 1975. Contains a discussion of treatment.
Langs, R.: *The Technique of Psychoanalytic Psychotherapy.* Volume I. New York, Jason Aronson, 1973. See Chapter 16 for an excellent discussion of supportive psychotherapy.
Masterson, J.: *Psychotherapy of the Borderline Adult: A Developmental Approach.* New York, Brunner-Mazel, 1976.
Miller, D.: *Adolescence: Psychology, Psychopathology, and Psychotherapy.* New York, Jason Aronson, 1974.
Searles, H.: *Collected Papers on Schizophrenia and Related Subjects.* New York, International Universities Press, 1965.
Searles, H.: *Countertransference and Related Issues.* New York, International Universities Press, 1979. Both his books are excellent on psychotherapeutic work with schizophrenics and borderlines.

# 12

# The Dynamic Model on the
# Inpatient Unit

## REASONS FOR HOSPITALIZATION

The first point to be emphasized about psychiatric hospitalization is *"whenever possible, avoid it."* This is so for a number of reasons. First of all, hospitalization is the most active and controlling intervention that you can make and, as such, cannot help but foster a bit of dependency and a sense of helplessness. Second, it is a communication to the patient that he has somehow failed to succeed on his own. Third, it fosters the identity of "chronic mental patient" which, coupled with the first two factors, lowers self-esteem and makes it easier to resort to hospitalization in future times of stress. Fourth, there is evidence that it fosters guilt feelings in many patients which increase progressively with the number of hospitalizations (see Ermutlu, 1977).

For these and any number of other reasons hospitalization should be used, not to augment the psychiatrist's income, but when the patient is unable or unwilling to retain vital responsibilities for his life and well-being. It has been my experience that there is more tendency to err on the side of overutilization than underutilization of this resource.

Before hospitalizing any patient you should consider the list of alternatives. There are ways of injecting increased structure into his life and lending ego other than this highly restrictive and infantilizing procedure. You might temporarily increase the number of sessions, remind the patient of your accessibility by phone, explore the possibility of his staying with a concerned friend or relative, intervene pharmacologically, or involve him in a day hospital or other form of organized activity.

Of course, when hospitalization is indicated, it is ego weakening to do otherwise. The most important indications for admission are grossly destructive or self-destructive urges. I refer you back to Chapter 5 for the assessment of these tendencies. When past history and current mental status indicate that the patient or someone else is in imminent danger at his hands, then it is incumbent upon you to advise him to admit himself. If he refuses, you must then apprise him that the only alternative is commitment. However enraged at you such patients might be at the moment, most will eventually feel relieved and supported by your taking control of the situation.

Socially and occupationally destructive or self-destructive behavior, incapacitating symptomatology or impaired judgment and reality testing, the need to extricate the patient from a noxious environment, and failure to comply with crucial aspects of outpatient treatment all constitute a second, less compelling set of criteria for admission. Any decision must be based upon the severity of disturbance and the patient's inclinations in the matter. If the patient does not raise the issue himself, then you should broach it in a manner befitting his dynamics and the severity of the problem, ranging from a query about his thoughts on hospitalization to an unambivalent statement that he would profit from it and how. The rule of thumb is that the patient should feel in as much control of this process as possible. Indeed, unless he is quite severely disordered, he is in control, for he is otherwise not committable.

Next, is that large group of patients who, in times of mild to moderate crisis, will request hospitalization. It is never wise, for the reasons in the first paragraph, to precipitously acquiesce. Considerable time should be spent in evaluating the nature of their distress, its past history, and any alternatives before resorting to admission. Such patients, like many people, may be requesting something they really do not want, and will thank you and see it as a vote of confidence in the end if you do not admit them.

## THE HOSPITALIZATION

Having made the most important point in this chapter, I shall now discuss the actual hospitalization itself.

To begin with, you should admit your patient yourself or, if the ward has its own admitting clinicians, you should at least accompany the patient to the floor. Your therapy sessions should continue as usual, with the focus being the problems that precipitated the hospitalization and discharge planning.

There are all sorts of hospital units, from the briefest to the longest term. If the aim of hospitalization is to contain a relatively well functioning patient around a temporary crisis, then that should be the message at the outset. You then want to minimize the development of any particular attachment to, and dependency upon, the ward and its staff and activities. You want to keep your interactions with the patient at the vital center of treatment, making certain that, if you are not in formal administrative charge, you are at least maintaining a tight liaison with the patient's administrator.

The intermediate to long-term hospitalization is another matter, and most of this chapter is related to this subject. Such a facility affords you a high-powered view of processes that are barely visible, if at all, on shorter-term units. I shall be referring primarily to the role of the psychiatrist as hospital physician, as *clinical administrator*, rather than as ongoing therapist of a patient who happens to be hospitalized.

Long-term inpatient units are organized in various fashions. In most a psychiatrist is administratively in charge, though in others he functions as co-administrator with the head nurse, and in some as an administrative back-up or consultant to the nurse. Some units are further divided into ward groups, each with its own treatment team and administrator, ultimately responsible to the chief of the ward. In some the same individual may be both therapist and clinical administrator for the patient, whereas in others different clinicians occupy these respective roles. This latter, known as the "T-A," or "therapist-administrator," split is utilized in some of the established private mental hospitals such as Chestnut Lodge and the Yale Psychiatric Institute. It has the advantage that the transference is less contaminated by the therapist's intrusion into the day-to-day issues and decisions of the patient's life and that it often allows the patient to feel freer in what he can say to his therapist. Its disadvantages are 1) if the team is mismanaged, power struggles and schisms can develop within it with the resultant transmission of mixed and confusing messages to the patient; 2) the therapist may sometimes find himself in the dilemma of whether to represent to the patient administrative policies about which he is lukewarm or disagrees; and 3) the therapist is tempted to resort to the hypocritical conceit that he plays no administrative role vis-à-vis the patient, when this is simply not the case.[1]

Whatever the organization of the intermediate to long-term unit, the *treatment team* is its common denominator. This is a group of mental

---

[1] In such splits your therapy patient may try to play you off against the hospital, inducing you to keep matters secret that would greatly affect his ward management, for example. Although you should not make a routine of disclosing to the treatment team any more than the broad strokes of your sessions with him, it is foolhardy to promise your patient, *in advance* of a particular communication, that you can withhold it from the rest of the staff. Tell him you will do your best to honor his request but you cannot make any guarantees before hearing him out. If he then refuses, treat it like any other resistance, exploring his fears.

health professionals brought together in an integrated and differentiated way to plan and implement the treatment goals of the patient. The typical team consists of a clinical administrator, nurse, social worker-family therapist, psychiatric aide, activities therapist, and the patient himself. The patient should participate in a real and active way, to the extent of his capacities, in the decisions of the team lest he be infantilized and patronized. It is essential that he is always present through his primary representative, whether that is his aide, social worker, or therapist, and that he be physically present at least some of the time, and certainly whenever he requests it.

The psychiatric hospital team is unlike that of any other clinical team. It does not, like the medical or surgical one, have a scalpel- or chart-wielding attending physician at its head. Its model is more egalitarian and its clinical administrator must, to some extent, earn his authority by proving his usefulness to the team and the patient. This is the case because psychiatry is a less technical specialty than internal medicine or surgery and because it is possible for mental health professionals and workers to become, with supervised experience and inservice education, adept in roles for which they were not originally trained. This is not to say that you engage in the democratic delusion that the team is a Hydra in which one head can function much like another. Obviously only the administrative psychiatrist can perform physical examinations and prescribe medication, the nurse dispense them, the psychologist perform testing, and the social worker do case work. However, apart from a few specialized skills, I suggest that you respond to people on the basis of their knowledge, experience, and demonstrated competencies as much as on that of their particular training or discipline.

As an inpatient psychiatrist you must know a good deal about all of your patients and make rounds on them regularly. It is important that you make your rounds individually, or with no more than one or two additional staff persons (perhaps the head nurse) and that no other patients be in his room (which is usually preferable to your office). The quality of your time with him, the degree that you are really present, is more important than the quantity itself. It is possible to seat yourself and convey, though you have only a few minutes, an air of timelessness such that the patient will feel that he has received a good deal from you. However, it is also possible to enter the room, lab coat flying, with one eye on the clock and one foot out the door, spend the same number of minutes, and leave him with the feeling that you have not been there at all.

In addition, I encourage every administrative psychiatrist to spend a little time staying on the floor, participating in both informal and structured interactions. This is anxiety-provoking at first and your inclination will be to avoid it, but if you relinquish the security of your office, you will not only learn things about ward sociology you would otherwise never know, but you will experience the pleasures and pains of interacting with patients in a way that the psychotherapist must deny himself.

Nevertheless, you are deluded if you think you can be directly responsible for your patients' treatment. The bulk of your impact will be *indirect*, through your ward staff. If you, like so many clinicians, view one-to-one work with patients as "real" psychiatry, and anything else as menial drudgery, then you will never make a good hospital psychiatrist. Those who know the most about the patient and who do most of the treatment are those who spend the most time with him: the nurses, or rather, the psychiatric aides. *Your unit is only as strong as your weakest aide.* Since it is he who will make or break the back of the treatment plan, you are well advised to value, as did Harry Stack Sullivan, your interaction with him.

You are called upon, at various times, to be an administrator, consultant, educator, and even therapist to your staff. These multifarious tasks make this sort of work both more draining and more rewarding than purely outpatient psychotherapy. As an *administrator* you exercise your authority quietly, permitting your individual staff members to play as large a role as their competence and experience allow. You should be neither diffident nor ostentatious with your knowledge that, in the event of deadlock, the final decision-making authority lies with you. (You carry, after all, the overwhelming majority of the medicolegal responsibility.) As Jay Haley (1978) advises, there should be no doubt to any about where the power lies, but it should not be made explicit any more than absolutely necessary.

Once a treatment plan is arrived at, you cannot assume that merely because you murmur or scribble an order it will be carried out. You should keep close touch with what transpires on the ward to know whether your staff are following through. If you do not, some of them will doubt that you take the proposals seriously. Personnel need periodic energizing around particular plans, especially those for the more withdrawn and chronic patients who are apt to become lost in the woodwork.

## EDUCATION OF THE STAFF

The *consultative* and *educative* functions blend into one another. They constitute a two-way process with the staff member giving you information that would otherwise be inaccessible and with you helping him to organize, formulate, and apply it. If you both graciously accept what he has to offer and spell out the rationale for your suggestions and decisions, he will feel like a respected colleague and value both you and his own work the more for it. Furthermore, people who understand the thinking that goes into a particular plan are more likely to help you implement it.

Your educative efforts entail teaching the staff what constitutes relevant information, what to ask and look for, and how to understand and act upon it. This last does not entail lecturing about dynamic theory—though a certain amount of this, in inservice seminars, can profitably occur—so much as it does *transmitting your dynamic comprehension into plain English, and demonstrating its relevance to day-to-day interaction with the patient.* I shall give two examples to emphasize this point:

> In one hospital where I worked the staff were allowing J., a schizophrenic adolescent, to withdraw, to isolate herself. This was partly because of her abusiveness whenever they tried to draw her out. Consequently, their efforts to involve her became only token ones. After asking once or twice if she wanted to join the group, they would accept her "no" and walk away. I explained to them that they were repeating the way her family had treated her, that they, like her parents, were inadvertently conspiring with her illness. It was pointed out that the patient had experienced her parents' acquiescence in her withdrawal as lack of caring. In other words, there was a part of her, even if only a small one, that knew that regression was unhealthy and that wanted to be pulled out. Her negativistic behavior functioned as a defense against rejection and as a test to see how much the staff really wanted to get through to her. When they understood this, they made a first-rate effort to get her out of that room and they succeeded. This, rather than anything that happened in individual psychotherapy, proved to be the turning point in her treatment. The patient had learned that the staff really wanted her with them and that they saw her as capable of more mature behavior.

> Mr. U., a young adult male schizoid personality, was doing all that he could to avoid and distance his primary aide, a woman. He treated her with the utmost arrogance and contempt, when he was not outright verbally abusive, skillfully homing in on her most sensitive points. She became hurt and angry, as would any human being, and repayed him in similar coin. Only after I apprised her that his behavior was actually *intended* to produce her disgust and withdrawal, as his way of avoiding a variety of fears associated with intimacy (chief among which was that he was such a nonentity that she would reject any of his attempts to draw closer to her), was she able to contain her feelings and keep at it. Somewhat later it became apparent, from his continuous erotic-dependent preoccupations with her and his attempts to act out some of these, that she had gone overboard in the other direction. It was then necessary to apprise her of this so that she could more appropriately modulate the closeness.

Part of this function is helping the staff appreciate the "dynamic," in the strictest sense of the word, nature of the therapeutic process. The following example illustrates how a particular stance toward a patient may be appropriate at one phase, but not at another.

> Mr. M., a young schizotypal adult, had gone through a period in his early hospitalization when he was acutely suicidal and when immediate attention and special precautions were the correct response to his self-destructive threats. As he became more direct in his expressions of anger and

sadness the suicidal tendencies subsided. However, in his last months of treatment, the threats returned and the staff reinstituted its solicitude and precautions. They had to be informed that this was not the same suicidalness that they had previously witnessed. The earlier episodes were genuinely life-threatening internalizations of anger, to which the solicitous and restrictive response *was* the ego-supportive one. The recent episodes were manifestations of his fears of discharge and independence and attempts to convince us to change our minds, to which the old response was *ego weakening*. When they understood this, they were able to calmly, but empathically, encourage him to focus on his feelings about leaving, implicitly communicating to him that talking of suicide was a defensive maneuver and that he was fully capable of controlling such impulses.

In your educational-consultative work with staff, you must help them distinguish between psychotherapy on the one hand and the sociotherapeutic function of the milieu on the other. Although there are some similarities between the functions of the therapist (particularly the supportive one) and those of the floor personnel, there are absolutely essential differences which must be appreciated lest the patient become confused.

In educating the staff to a patient's dynamics, your aim is not to clone an army of mini-therapists, but to facilitate their performance of the *sociotherapeutic* tasks.

Therapy is the place where the patient is as expressive (within the accepted limits) as he dares be and where he learns something about the meanings and motives of his most persistent and troublesome behaviors. It is, in many respects, like nothing else that he will encounter anywhere. The milieu, by contrast, is meant to be a little more like outside reality, with some of the attendant responsibilities and opportunities that accompany it. The ward personnel should be enough like people on the outside that the skills the patient learns from interacting with them will be transferable to the "real" world, and yet sufficiently unlike those outside that they will not be offended by his transference behavior.

The milieu is an improved, microcosmic version of the world from which the patient comes, where he can experiment with the new options that psychotherapy is giving him, where he can garner success experiences with people in a less threatening environment, where he can incorporate some of the rules of civilized interaction, where he can identify with and learn from mature and adapted role models, where he can receive constructive feedback about his presentation to others, where he has the opportunity to internalize some of the structure and predictability of the milieu into a hitherto chaotic ego, where he can gain (particularly from the activities therapies) a sense of mastery, creativity, and leisure skills, and where, from participating in patient government and other hospital community projects, he can learn how to interact with others around both task and playful orientations.

The following vignette illustrates the importance of not confusing the psychotherapeutic and sociotherapeutic roles.

> B. was a schizoid adolescent male, with a low self-esteem and many conflicts over intimacy deriving from his experience with cold and distant upper-class parents. He consistently took issues from his therapy to various staff members, broached concerns with them he never raised with his therapist, and baited them, with flattering comments about how they were more understanding than his therapist, into making inappropriate and "deep" interpretations. With this behavior B. was acting out his fears of intimacy with his therapist. Furthermore, what appeared to be close interactions with staff were really structured and intellectualized ways of avoiding more emotional and spontaneous interactions with them. When the staff appreciated this, they were able to direct him to his therapist on certain issues and to function as no more nor less than a laboratory for him to experiment on being with people in a less fearful way.

As in supportive therapy, *expectations* play a prepotent role in the sociotherapeutic work. The old adage "you get what you expect" is truer of human behavior than of anything else. If you expect adaptive reality-oriented behavior from a patient, and consistently convey this to him, you are more likely to get it than if you permit him to engage in prolonged regression, allow his fellow patients and staff members to laugh at and otherwise reward his crazy antics, let him loose-associate and speak bizarrely without encouraging him to organize his thoughts and check the flow, allow him to shirk the responsibilities attendant upon adulthood and to engage in socially destructive and self-destructive behavior or destroy property without facing the consequences. There is no place for an analytic neutrality about what constitutes expected and acceptable behavior in the ward culture.

I have seen the most out-of-touch schizophrenics turn round and astound one with the level of maturity of which they are capable if the staff (and their less regressed fellow patients) consistently convey a raised, but realistic, set of expectations to them.[2]

Every administrative psychiatrist should know, and communicate to his staff, the most basic principles of learning theory and their role in behavior modification. The concepts of modeling, classical and operant conditioning, positive and negative reinforcement, and punishment are useful, and not incompatible with thinking dynamically. Modeling concerns identification, in dynamic terms, and is one of the reasons you want to hire staff members who seem to be experiencing some success at the business of living.

---

[2]Of course, if your expectations are extravagant relative to the patient's capabilities or are raised too precipitously, then they can backfire and you will encounter less, rather than more, adaptive behavior.

Positive reinforcers are responses (rewards) that, when they occur in conjunction with or subsequent to the performance of certain behaviors, increase the frequency of those behaviors. You must know some information about the patient's history and dynamics to appreciate what constitutes a reward for him.

When the reinforcement occurs simultaneously with the behavior, this is known as classical conditioning. An example would be managing the milieu in such a way that the patient associates pleasurable experiences with his contact with people. This might include having tasty snacks and drinks, interesting games and activities, a pleasantly decorated ward, music, and the like. When, by contrast, the patient must perform a certain behavior for the desired response to occur, this is known as operant conditioning. With rather regressed patients this might involve well-systematized schedules of responding to appropriate and reality-oriented behaviors with reinforcers as tangible as candy, cigarettes, or coffee. With more reality-oriented patients, the reinforcers should be less tangible and less obtrusive lest they be patronizing: for example, rewarding adaptive behavior with increased attention or non-verbal communications of approval.

*Negative reinforcement* is the application of an unpleasant stimulus, the removal of which is contingent upon the performance of the desirable behavior (or the cessation of the undesirable one). This might entail the patients and staff in a group meeting ignoring a patient or forcing him to leave the room while he is being bizarre or verbally abusive and paying attention to him or allowing him to return only when he begins behaving more appropriately. This is also an example of how much negative reinforcement amounts to the withholding of positive reinforcement until the undesirable behavior ceases or the desirable behavior occurs, ignoring him being both a noxious stimulus and the withholding of gratification.

*Punishment* is something we dislike admitting we ever mete out to patients. Indeed, the intellectual gymnastics I saw one administrative psychiatrist perform, to convince a patient that his afternoon in the seclusion room was not punishment, were wondrous to behold. The floor staff uses punishment all the time: telling a patient he is being "inappropriate" (the most widely used of the psychiatric "moralisms"), withdrawing his privileges for a violation of the rules, or withholding cherished positive reinforcers (such as cigarettes).

Educating the staff to the general concept of countertransference and dealing with individual and group instances of it are functions on the boundary between your role as staff educator and staff "therapist." It is essential that they understand that patients can evoke in us, out of realistically provocative behavior and *through* our own particular histories, countertherapeutic responses. It is necessary that they comprehend that they may approach all, or only certain types of, patients with a preconceived set of attitudes and expectations that may interfere with treatment.

When this is a particular individual's problem, it should be dealt with on a one-to-one basis, lest he lose face before his peers. Oftentimes this is best accomplished through the head nurse (who often has more rapport with the nurses and aides than do you and who plays a larger, if more subterranean, role in determining the ward culture than do you). However it is done, it is tactful to keep the focus on the *patient* and the particular ease with which he can elicit counterproductive responses in staff members. The employee must understand how his inadvertent response feeds back in a negative way on the patient's dynamics, how the patient is attempting to get him to act like his father, mother, sister, brother, and so forth. Only as a last resort, and when it appears all else has failed, is it indicated to remove an employee from a particular patient's treatment team and induce him to enter therapy himself.

When our responses to patients are sufficiently countertransference-ridden and inappropriate, then it is difficult to determine how much of what we see is historically, and how much situationally, determined. Attributing everything to transference can be a way of avoiding the common-sense fact that the patient's dynamics do not merely impinge upon us, but *we* upon them. Whole ward policies can amount to an institutionalization of somebody's (usually the administrator's or head nurse's) countertransference *mishegoss*.

For example, I have witnessed ward rounds conducted in an utterly dehumanizing way. A score of staff members and trainees would parade behind a white-coated general who then proceeded to ask each patient, as the patient stood at attention before his bed and in the presence of his roommates, meaningless stock and canned, or else insensitively personal, questions and then give each about 30 seconds to answer them. In such circumstances, when most patients are tight-lipped or utter polite banalities, you can hardly attribute their reaction solely to historical factors within them. Irving Goffman (1961) and others have demonstrated brilliantly that much so-called "psychotic" behavior (social withdrawal, passivity, helplessness, and ego regression in general) is an adaptation to the hospital environment and staff needs and expectations as much as a manifestation of psychopathology.

One of the most important, anxiety-provoking, infuriating, and rewarding roles of the clinical administrator is that of "therapist" to his staff. Hospital psychiatry is hard, draining work for all concerned and you must accept that your personnel have feelings and the vulnerabilities to which flesh is heir as much as your patient and you. If you are insensitive to their needs and tensions, then not merely they, but your patients and, ultimately, you will suffer. Frozen resentment toward an administrative or attending psychiatrist or disgruntlement with the institution in general are particularly likely to be displaced upon patients. I have seen beautifully conceived treatment plans sabotaged and certain patients declared *persona non grata* not because of anything they did, but because of something their attending physician did or did not do to, or for, the staff.

Taking care of the staff is as much a part of your clinical work as your direct rounds on patients and your leadership of treatment teams. The preventive part of this task is making sure they know just how important their work is and how much you value it. Periodic demoralization is an occupational hazard of the worker on an intermediate or long-term ward and you must do as much as possible to circumvent it or nip it in the bud. Occasional pep talks are indispensable, as are informal cups of coffee, which are not only as much a part of your job as prescribing medications, but also more enjoyable. Creative inservice education, stimulating case conferences (in which the staff play key roles in the presentation and discussion), and outside speakers accomplish much toward fostering a sense of professional and personal growth and development and counteracting one of stagnation and despair.

This task entails being as aware as possible of particularly troublesome personal issues on the part of any of the personnel and being empathically present if called upon, or at least taking this information into account in your interactions with them and looking for any untoward ramifications on their work with patients. Just as importantly it involves being aware of the "systems" issues in and around the hospital that impinge upon your unit and affect its efficacy. Stanton and Schwartz (1954) wrote a fine description of how vibrations beginning in the most exalted institutional administrative offices or committee rooms can be transmitted through the ward chief, head nurse, and floor personnel right on down to influence the behavior of the most withdrawn and regressed schizophrenic. This can be the case, or indeed is *more* likely to be the case, even when these issues are not overtly discussed. It was striking, in one hospital where I worked, to see the remarkable increase in psychotic, violent, and agitated behavior in the weeks before the imminent arrival of the new psychiatrist-in-chief.[3]

---

[3]By contrast, staff navel-gazing is the cancerous proliferation of healthy introspection. I have been in "treatment teams" where the personnel were so busily engaged in the "shrinkage" of each other or the administration that there was no time left for the patients. It is always necessary to remember that such "therapeutic" work as you engage in with your staff is not an end in itself, but rather a *means* to an end: the optimal treatment of the patients.

## SUICIDAL TENDENCIES ON THE WARD

Although we have already examined the topic of suicidal tendencies in general and particular, the ward management of the self-destructive individual is special enough to deserve separate treatment. When you treat an episodically suicidal person as an outpatient, you do not foster in him the fiction that you can protect him from himself between the sessions. You can do no more than be available by telephone. When, however, you deem his suicidal tendencies sufficiently severe to hospitalize him, you are explicitly communicating to him that you *will* assume the auxiliary ego function of inhibiting these impulses.

It is not sufficient that he, alone, receive this message. His *staff* must receive it *clearly* and *unambivalently* as well. They must know that 24-hour observation means being with him 86,400 seconds a day. Since hurt and internalized rage attendant upon rejection constitute the major dynamic in suicide, the patient must feel that the attendant *wants him alive.* Turning one's back on him for but an instant, to get a cigarette or cup of coffee, can represent a rebuff that sets off unresolved feelings about countless previous rebuffs and eventuates in a belt around the neck or a piece of glass to the throat. I know of several instances in which death occurred in just this way.

Professionally unpreventable suicides occur only outside hospitals, not within them. If they occur within, they do so because the attending psychiatrist was not perceptive enough to recognize the patient's subtle cues, because he recognized them but did not spell out his concerns clearly enough to the staff, or because he spelled them out and somebody did not believe him.

## RESTRAINTS

In 1856 an Englishman named John Conolly wrote a book proposing the then newfangled notion that it is possible to manage severely disturbed mental patients without mechanical restraints. From the attitudes occasionally encountered on hospital wards today, one wonders if that idea has lost its novelty. *If the staff really understand their patients' dynamics and what constitutes provocation or ego weakening of them, then there is little indication for the use of physical restraints.*

Laughing at or patronizing patients, setting limits in such a way that they lose face with their fellows, using confrontative, "macho" behavior toward them, failing to give them sufficient space when they need it, indiscriminant physical touching, and communicating excessive fearfulness can all precipitate violence in those who could otherwise contain it.

Since the advent of the psychotropic drugs, which not only provide symptomatic relief but function for some as chemical restraints, there has been less need for the older, mechanical restraints. Nevertheless, the latter are indicated at certain times. You never do a patient or his staff a favor when you allow him to be physically abusive. It dehumanizes both him and his fellows and leaves him with a residue of guilt. When it is clear that the individual is asking you to assume control over his impulses, then restraining or secluding him *is* the ego-supportive intervention. Indeed, after his initial frustration and rage subside, he is likely to respond to you with relief, if not gratitude. In any event, he must not be allowed to see you as a bogeyman, but must clearly understand the role that *he* is playing in getting you to respond to him in this manner.

When, however, restraints are *not* indicated, they are the opposite of ego-supportive. They cause the patient to feel needlessly controlled and hemmed in, increase his agitation, and perhaps make it even more likely, by conveying negative expectations of him, that he will relinquish control in the future. I can speak of the anxiety-provoking role of mechanical restraints, when they are not indicated, from personal experience. On my last day as a senior resident on a particular ward, the staff, in good fun, placed me in arm and leg restraints and in a wheelchair! Even though I was aware it was to be a time-limited experience and was, in some ways, an expression of their affection for me, I still found it a bit disconcerting and was relieved when I was freed.

## PSYCHIATRIC CONSULTATION ON THE MEDICAL-SURGICAL WARD

This is a highly specialized area of psychiatric practice and will receive no more than a brief footnote in this volume. Strain (1979), Strain and Grossman (1975), and Hackett and Cassem (1978) have written works on the subject which are part of the general education of any psychiatrist.

My primary point is that your history-taking ability and dynamic understanding will be of equal service in the surgeon's and internist's ward as in your office and on the psychiatric ward. In practice, this might involve helping a physician understand 1) that his patient's medication noncompliance is a self-destructive way of getting back at his spouse; 2) that what he interpreted as hypochondriasis is really depression; 3) that the patient's hostile and rebellious attitude hides an abject fear of the authority that the doctor represents; 4) that his coronary patient's too early and strenuous exertion is a way of covering up his underlying sense of weakened masculinity, and 5) that his orthopedic patient's rejection is a way of dealing with underlying conflicts around dependency.

These and other dynamic understandings are communicated to the consultee, not in complicated psychoanalytic jargon, but in plain English. You should show him that this is not merely esoteric knowledge, but that it can eventuate in concrete, practical interventions with the patient. For example, consider each of the five instances just cited: in the first case you might get the patient to begin to ventilate a bit to you and his doctor about his marriage; in the second, you might recommend the institution of an antidepressant; in the third you might counsel his physician to assume as egalitarian and collaborative a role with him as possible; in the fourth you might encourage his physician to speak to his strength and fortitude in dealing with this difficult hospitalization, to empathize with the problems encountered by a previously active man in adapting to enforced passivity, and to give him some harmless finger or other exercises; and in the fifth you might encourage him to give the patient as active a role as possible in the treatment, such as determining when the nurses will come or when certain medications will be dispensed.

Because many of these patients will be psychiatrically untouched, working with them is often refreshing. At times you can make seemingly obvious observations and connections which help the patient see himself and the world in a different light. Or, you can make simple pharmacological interventions that make a great difference. Although the need to form a relatively rapid assessment and put yourself on the line with your medical colleagues makes this work a bit more stressful, your absolution from the responsibility for making a full and ongoing descent into the patient's pain and misery makes it less so.

Finally, your attitude toward your fellow physician is more important than anything else in determining whether the patient profits from your recommendations. You must educate the doctor without his knowing that he is being educated, lest he feel patronized. You must recognize plainly that your consultation constitutes information and recommendations, not commands, and that he is under no moral or professional obligation to utilize or follow them. This education begins with teaching him how to consult you and how to frame his questions and concerns as specifically as possible. If you do not tactfully shape his behavior in this area, you will continue to receive vague and meaningless consultation requests such as, "Please do a psychiatric evaluation on this patient."

## SUGGESTED READINGS FOR CHAPTER 12

Cumming, J., and Cumming, E.: *Ego and Milieu.* New York, Atherton, 1962. Good theoretical and practical exposition of milieu therapy.

Edelson, M.: *Ego Psychology, Group Dynamics, and the Therapeutic Community.* New York, Grune and Stratton, 1964.

Edelson, M.: *The Practice of Sociotherapy: A Case Study.* New Haven, Yale University Press, 1976.

Hackett, L., and Cassem, N.: (Eds.): *Massachusetts General Hospital Handbook of General Hospital Psychiatry.* St. Louis, C.V. Mosby Co., 1978.

Kubler-Ross, E.: *On Death and Dying.* New York, Macmillan Publishing Co., 1969. Propounds her famous five stages in the dying process: denial, anger, bargaining, depression, and acceptance. Useful not only for your work with the terminally ill patient, but for your consultations upon the medical-surgical inpatient in general, since each of them, to some degree and at some level, fears he will not leave the hospital alive.

Stanton, A., and Schwartz, M.: *The Mental Hospital.* New York, Basic Books, 1954. The preeminent classic in the field. A *must* for every psychiatrist.

Strain, J., and Grossman, S.: *The Psychological Care of the Medically Ill: A Primer in Liaison Psychiatry.* New York, Appleton-Century-Crofts, 1975. An excellent introduction to the practical application of dynamics on the medical-surgical ward.

Strain, J.: *Psychological Interventions in Medical Practice.* New York, Appleton-Century-Crofts, 1979. More of the above. Keyed to the special problems posed by chronic cardiac, renal, and other patients.

Wolpe, J.: *The Practice of Behavior Therapy.* New York, Pergamon Press, 1973.

# EPILOGUE

"Just as a golden apple overlaid with a network of silver, when seen at a distance, or looked at superficially, is mistaken for a silver apple, but when a keen-sighted person looks at the object well, he will find what is within, and see that the apple is gold."

Moses ben Maimon (Maimonides), 12th Century A.D., on interpreting the biblical text, from *The Guide for the Perplexed*.

Every human being is a universe in himself, a rich and complicated psychic organism with his own more or less idiosyncratic and absolutely irreproducible style of wishing, feeling, fearing, avoiding, perceiving, thinking, and being-in-the-world. The most prosaic person recalcitrantly refuses to be snared by the most complete of "complete" formulations. And yet we strive, in the face of each individual's ambiguity, to understand him as well as we can.

In the pursuit of our craft we are constantly confronted by this dialectic between intelligibility and obscurity in human behavior. Although my book has perforce been concerned with emphasizing the former, it would be disastrous to both the soul of the patient and to your own empathy and modesty if you were to lose sight of the latter. *Homo sapiens* might be defined as that animal who is always capable of surprising us, who reserves the right to act "out of character," to cussedly break out of any theoretical corral into which we have herded him.

We never see, for the silver lattice, all of the apple of gold.

## BIBLIOGRAPHY

Aichorn, A. (1925): *Wayward Youth.* New York, Viking Press, 1975.

Altman, L.: *The Dream in Psychoanalysis.* New York, International Universities Press, 1962.

American Psychiatric Association: Diagnostic and Statistical Manual III. Washington, D.C., 1980.

Ariès, P.: *A History of Western Attitudes Toward Death.* Baltimore, John Hopkins University Press, 1977.

Bateson, G., Jackson, D., Haley, J., and Weakland, J.: "Toward a Theory of Schizophrenia." *Behavioral Science,* 1:251-264, 1956.

Becker, E.: *The Denial of Death.* New York, Free Press, 1973.

Bleuler, E. (1911): *Dementia Praecox or the Group of Schizophrenias.* New York, International Universities Press, 1950.

Blos, P.: *On Adolescence: A Psychoanalytic Interpretation.* New York, Free Press, 1962.

Boisen, A.: *The Exploration of the Inner World.* New York, Harper & Row Publishers, 1939.

Brenner, C.: *An Elementary Textbook of Psychoanalysis.* Revised Edition. New York, International Universities Press, 1973.

Brenner, C.: *Psychoanalytic Technique and Psychic Conflict.* New York, International Universities Press, 1976.

Bruch, H.: *Learning Psychotherapy.* Cambridge, Harvard University Press, 1974.

Choron, J.: *Death and Western Thought.* New York, Macmillan Publishing Co., 1963.

Conolly, J.: *Treatment of the Insane Without Mechanical Restraints.* First published in 1856; reprinted by Dawsons of Pall Mall, Kent, England, 1973.

Cumming, J., and Cumming, E.: *Ego and Milieu.* New York, Atherton, 1962.

Davanloo, H.: *Basic Principles and Techniques in Short-Term Dynamic Psychotherapy.* New York, Spectrum Books, 1977.

DeWald, P.: *Psychotherapy: A Dynamic Approach.* New York, Basic Books, 1971.

Dodds, E. (1951): *The Greeks and the Irrational.* Berkeley, University of California Press, 1973.

Dollard, J., and Miller, N.: *Personality and Psychotherapy.* New York, McGraw-Hill Book Co., 1950.

Easson, W.: *The Severely Disturbed Adolescent.* New York, International Universities Press, 1962.

Edelson, M.: *Ego Psychology, Group Dynamics, and the Therapeutic Community.* New York, Grune & Stratton, 1964.

Edelson, M.: *The Practice of Sociotherapy: A Case Study.* New Haven, Yale University Press, 1976.

Ellenberger, H.: *The Discovery of the Unconscious: The History and Evolution of Dynamic Psychiatry.* New York, Basic Books, 1970.

Erikson, E.: *Childhood and Society,* Revised Edition. New York, Norton, 1963.

Erikson, E.: *Identity, Youth, and Crisis.* New York, W. W. Norton & Co., 1968.

Ermutlu, I.: "The Effect of Hospitalization on Guilt and Shame Feelings." *Psychiatric Forum* 6, 18-22, 1977.

Fenichel, O.: *The Psychoanalytic Theory of Neurosis.* New York, W. W. Norton & Co., 1945.

Foudraine, J.: *Not Made of Wood: A Psychiatrist Discovers His Profession.* New York, Macmillian Publishing Co., 1974.

Fraiberg, S.: *The Magic Years.* New York, Charles Scribner's Sons, 1959.

Frank, J.: *Persuasion and Healing.* New York, Schocken Books, 1974.

Frankl, V.: *The Doctor and the Soul.* New York, Alfred A. Knopf, 1973.

Freedman, D., Kaplan, H., and Sadock, B., (eds.): *Comprehensive Textbook of Psychiatry* (3 volumes). Baltimore, Williams & Wilkins, 1981.

Freud, A. (1936): *The Ego and the Mechanisms of Defense.* The Writings of Anna Freud, Volume II. New York, International Universities Press, 1967.

Freud, A.: *Normality and Pathology in Childhood.* New York, International Universities Press, 1965.

Freud, S., and Breuer, J. (1895): *Studies on Hysteria.* Standard Edition of the Complete Psychological Works of Sigmund Freud,* Volume II. London, Hogarth Press, 1955.

Freud, S. (1900 [1899]): *The Interpretation of Dreams.* Standard Edition, Volumes IV and V. London, Hogarth Press, 1953.

Freud, S. (1901): *On Dreams.* Standard Edition, Volume V. London, Hogarth Press, 1953, pp. 633-686.

Freud, S. (1901): *The Psychopathology of Everyday Life.* Standard Edition, Volume VI. London, Hogarth Press, 1960.

Freud, S. (1903): "Freud's Psycho-Analytic Procedure." Standard Edition, Volume VII. London, Hogarth Press, 1953, pp. 249-254.

Freud, S. (1905): *Fragment of an Analysis of a Case of Hysteria.* Standard Edition, Volume VII. London, Hogarth Press, 1953, pp. 7-122.

Freud, S. (1905): *Three Essays on the Theory of Sexuality.* Standard Edition, Volume VII. London, Hogarth Press, 1953, pp. 130-243.

Freud, S. (1905): *Jokes and Their Relation to the Unconscious.* Standard Edition, Volume VIII. London, Hogarth Press, 1960.

Freud, S. (1909): *Analysis of a Phobia in a Five-Year-Old Boy.* Standard Edition, Volume X. London, Hogarth Press, 1955, pp. 5-149.

Freud, S. (1909): *Notes Upon A Case of Obsessional Neurosis.* Standard Edition, Volume X. London, Hogarth Press, 1955, pp. 155-249.

Freud, S. (1910): "The Future Prospects of Psycho-Analytic Therapy." Standard Edition, Volume XI. London, Hogarth Press, 1957, pp. 141-151.

Freud, S. (1910): "'Wild' Psycho-Analysis." Standard Edition, Volume XI. London, Hogarth Press, 1957, pp. 219-227.

Freud, S. (1911): *Psycho-Analytic Notes On An Autobiographical Account of a Case of Paranoia.* Standard Edition, Volume XII. London, Hogarth Press, 1958, pp. 9-82.

Freud, S. (1911): "The Handling of Dream Interpretation in Psycho-Analysis." Standard Edition, Volume XII. London, Hogarth Press, 1958, pp. 91-96.

Freud, S. (1912): "The Dynamics of Transference." Standard Edition, Volume XII. London, Hogarth Press, 1958, pp. 99-108.

Freud, S. (1912): "Recommendations to Physicians Practicing Psycho-Analysis." Standard Edition, Volume XII. London, Hogarth Press, 1958, pp. 111-120.

Freud, S. (1912): "On the Universal Tendency to Debasement in the Sphere of Love." Standard Edition, Volume XI. London, Hogarth Press, 1957, pp. 179-190.

Freud, S. (1913): "On Beginning the Treatment." Standard Edition, Volume XII. London, Hogarth Press, 1958, pp. 123-144.

Freud, S. (1913): "Fausse Reconnaissance (Déjà Raconté) in Psycho-Analytic Treatment." Standard Edition, Volume XIII. London, Hogarth Press, 1953, pp. 201-207.

Freud, S. (1914): "Remembering, Repeating, and Working Through." Standard Edition, Volume XII. London, Hogarth Press, 1958, pp. 147-156.

*Hereafter referred to as "Standard Edition."

Freud, S. (1914): "Observations on Transference Love." Standard Edition, Volume XII. London, Hogarth Press, 1958, pp. 159-171.

Freud, S. (1914): "On Narcissism: An Introduction." Standard Edition, Volume XIV. London, Hogarth Press, 1957, pp. 73-102.

Freud, S. (1916-1917): *Introductory Lectures on Psycho-Analysis.* Standard Edition, Volumes XV and XVI. London, Hogarth Press, 1961.

Freud, S. (1917): "Mourning and Melancholia." Standard Edition, Volume XIV. London, Hogarth Press, 1957, pp. 243-258.

Freud, S. (1918): *From the History of an Infantile Neurosis.* Standard Edition, Volume XVII. London, Hogarth Press, 1955, pp. 7-122.

Freud, S. (1918): "Lines of Advance in Psycho-Analytic Therapy." Standard Edition, Volume XVII. London, Hogarth Press, 1955, pp. 159-168.

Freud, S. (1920): *Beyond the Pleasure Principle.* Standard Edition, Volume XVIII. London, Hogarth Press, 1955, pp. 7-64.

Freud, S. (1921): *Group Psychology and the Analysis of the Ego.* Standard Edition, Voume XVIII. London, Hogarth Press, 1955, pp. 69-143.

Freud, S. (1923): *The Ego and the Id.* Standard Edition, Volume XIX. London, Hogarth Press, 1961, pp. 12-66.

Freud, S. (1923): "Remarks on the Theory and Practice of Dream-Interpretation." Standard Edition, Volume XIX. London, Hogarth Press, 1961, pp. 109-121.

Freud, S. (1924): "The Loss of Reality in Neurosis and Psychosis." Standard Edition, Volume XIX. London, Hogarth Press, 1961, pp. 183-187.

Freud, S. (1926): *Inhibitions, Symptoms and Anxiety.* Standard Edition, Volume XX. London, Hogarth Press, 1959, pp. 87-174.

Freud, S. (1926): *The Question of Lay Analysis.* Standard Edition, Volume XX. London, Hogarth Press, 1959, pp. 183-250.

Freud, S. (1932): *New Introductory Lectures on Psycho-Analysis.* Standard Edition, Volume XXII. London, Hogarth Press, 1964.

Freud, S. (1937): "Analysis Terminable and Interminable." Standard Edition, Volume XXIII. London, Hogarth Press, 1964, pp. 216-253.

Freud, S. (1937): "Constructions in Analysis." Standard Edition, Volume XXIII. London, Hogarth Press, 1964, pp. 257-269.

Freud, S. (1938): *An Outline of Psycho-Analysis.* Standard Edition, Volume XXIII. London, Hogarth Press, 1964, pp. 144-207.

Fromm-Reichmann, F.: *Principles of Intensive Psychotherapy.* Chicago, University of Chicago Press, 1950.

Garfield, S., and Bergin, A. (eds.): *Handbook of Psychotherapy and Behavior Change: An Empirical Analysis,* 2nd edition. New York, John Wiley & Sons, 1978.

Giovacchini, P.: *The Psychoanalysis of Character Disorders.* New York, Jason Aronson, 1975.

Glover, E.: *The Technique of Psycho-Analysis.* New York, International Universities Press, 1955.

Goffman, E.: *Asylums.* Chicago, Aldine Publishing Co., 1961.

Green, H.: *I Never Promised You a Rose Garden.* New York, Holt, Rinehart & Winston, 1964.

Greenson, R.: *The Technique and Practice of Psychoanalysis.* New York, International Universities Press, 1967.

Hackett, L., and Cassem, N. (eds.): *Massachusetts General Hospital Handbook of General Hospital Psychiatry.* St. Louis, C.V. Mosby Co., 1978.

Haley, J.: *Problem Solving Therapy.* New York, Harper Colophon Books, 1978.

Herbart, J.: *Psychologie als Wissenschaft (Psychology as Science).* Koenigsburg, 1824.

Hill, L.: *Psychotherapeutic Intervention in Schizophrenia.* Chicago, University of Chicago Press, 1955.

Jung, C. (1934): "The Soul and Death." in *Psychology and the Occult*. Princeton, Princeton University Press, 1977, pp. 126-137.

Kardiner, A. (1939): *The Individual and His Society*. New York, Columbia University Press, 1961.

Kernberg, O.: *Borderline Conditions and Pathological Narcissism*. New York, Jason Aronson, 1975.

Kernberg, O.: *Object Relations Theory and Clinical Psychoanalysis*. New York, Jason Aronson, 1976.

Kohut, H.: *The Analysis of the Self*. New York, International Universities Press, 1971.

Kris, E.: *Psychoanalytic Explorations in Art*. New York, International Universities Press, 1952.

Kubie, L.: "The Retreat from Patients." *International Journal of Psychiatry*, 9:693-711, 1970.

Kupers, T.: *Public Therapy: The Practice of Psychotherapy in the Public Mental Health Clinic*. New York, Free Press, 1981.

Langs, R.: *The Technique of Psychoanalytic Psychotherapy*, Two Volumes. New York, Jason Aronson, 1973.

Levinson, D.: *Seasons of a Man's Life*. New York, Alfred A. Knopf, 1978.

Lidz, T., Fleck, S., and Cornelison, A.: *Schizophrenia and the Family*. New York, International Universities Press, 1965.

Lidz, T.: *The Person: His and Her Development Throughout the Life Cycle*. New York, Basic Books, 1976.

Lidz, T., Blatt, S., and Cook, B.: "Critique of Danish-American Studies of Adopted-Away Offspring of Schizophrenic Parents." *American Journal of Psychiatry*, 138:1063-1068, 1981.

Lifton, R.: *The Broken Connection*. New York, Simon and Schuster, 1979.

Lindemann, E., "Symptomatology and Management of Acute Grief." *American Journal of Psychiatry*, 101:141-149, 1944.

Lindner, R.: "The Jet Propelled Couch." In *The Fifty Minute Hour*. New York, Holt, Rinehart and Winston, 1954, pp. 221-293.

Mackinnon, R., and Michels, R.: *The Psychiatric Interview in Clinical Practice*. Philadelphia, W.B. Saunders Co., 1971.

Mahl, G.: *Psychological Conflict and Defense*. New York, Harcourt, Brace, Jovanovich, 1969.

Mahler, M., Pine, F., and Bergman, A.: *The Psychological Birth of the Human Infant*. New York, Basic Books, 1975.

Maimonides, M.: *The Guide for the Perplexed*. New York, Dover Books, 1956.

Malan, D.: *The Frontier of Brief Psychotherapy*. New York, Plenum Publishing Corp., 1976.

Malcolm, J.: *Psychoanalysis: The Impossible Profession*. New York, Alfred A. Knopf, 1981.

Mann, J.: *Time Limited Psychotherapy*. Cambridge, Harvard University Press, 1973.

Masterson, J.: *Psychotherapy of the Borderline Adult: A Developmental Approach*. New York, Brunner/Mazel, 1976.

May, R., Angel, E., and Ellenberger, H. (eds.): *Existence: A New Dimension in Psychiatry and Psychology*. New York, Basic Books, 1958.

Miller, D.: *Adolescence: Psychology, Psychopathology, and Psychotherapy*. New York, Jason Aronson, 1974.

Moore, B., and Fine B. (eds.): *A Glossary of Psychoanalytic Terms and Concepts*. New York, American Psychoanalytic Association, 1968.

Niederland, W.: *The Schreber Case*. New York, Quadrangle Books, 1974.

Nunberg, H. and Federn, E. (eds.): *Minutes of the Vienna Psychoanalytic Society*, Volume 2. New York, International Universities Press, 1967.

Reich, W.: *Character Analysis*. New York, Farrar, Straus and Giroux, 1945.

Reik, T.: *Listening with the Third Ear*. New York, Farrar, Straus and Giroux, 1949.

Rieff, P.: *Freud: The Mind of the Moralist*. New York, Viking Press, 1959.

Rieff, P.: *The Triumph of the Therapeutic*. New York, Harper and Row Publishers, 1966.

Saul, L: *Psychodynamically Based Psychotherapy*. New York, Science House, 1972.

Schafer, R.: *A New Language for Psychoanalysis*. New Haven, Yale University Press, 1976.

Schafer, R.: *Language and Insight*. New Haven, Yale University Press, 1978.

Schur, M.: *The Id and the Regulatory Principles of Mental Functioning*. New York, International Universities Press, 1969.

Searles, H.: *Collected Essays on Schizophrenia and Related Subjects*. New York, International Universities Press, 1965.

Searles, H.: *Countertransference*. New York, International Universities Press, 1979.

Shapiro, D.: *Neurotic Styles*. New York, Basic Books, 1965.

Sifneos, P.: *Short Term Psychotherapy and Emotional Crisis*. Cambridge, Harvard University Press, 1972.

Stanton, A., and Schwartz, M.: *The Mental Hospital*. New York, Basic Books 1954.

Stoller, R.: *Sex and Gender*. Volume II. New York, Jason Aronson, 1975.

Stone, L.: *The Psychoanalytic Situation*. New York, International Universities Press, 1961.

Strain, J., and Grossman, S.: *The Psychological Care of the Medically Ill*. New York, Appleton-Century-Crofts, 1975.

Strain, J.: *Psychological Interventions in Medical Practice*. New York, Appleton-Century-Crofts, 1979.

Sullivan, H.: *The Interpersonal Theory of Psychiatry*. New York, W.W. Norton & Co., 1953.

Sullivan, H.: *The Psychiatric Interview*. New York, W.W. Norton & Co., 1954.

Tarachow, S.: *An Introduction to Psychotherapy*. New York, International Universities Press, 1963.

Tillich, P.: *The Courage to Be*. New Haven, Yale University Press, 1952.

Torrey, E.F.: *The Mind Game: Witch Doctors and Psychiatrists*. New York, Jason Aronson, 1977.

Vonnegut, M.: *The Eden Express*. New York, Praeger Publishers, 1975.

Wachtel, P.: *Psychoanalysis and Behavior Therapy: Toward an Integration*. New York, Basic Books, 1977.

Wallace, E.: "Freud's Mysticism and Its Psychodynamic Determinants." *Bulletin of the Menninger Clinic*, 42:203-222, 1978.

Wallace, E.: *Freud and Anthropology: A History and Reappraisal*. Psychological Issues Monograph #55. New York, International Universities Press, 1982.

Wallace, E.: "Freud and Religion: A History and Reappraisal." In *The Psychoanalytic Study of Society*, Volume 10. Edited by L. Boyer, W. Muensterberger, and S. Grolnick. New Jersey, Lawrence Ehrlbaum. In press, 1983.

Wallace, E.: "Reflections on the Relationship Between Psychoanalysis and Christianity." *Pastoral Psychology*. In press, 1983.

Wallace, E.: "Historiography in History and Psychoanalysis." *Bulletin of the History of Medicine*, 57(2). In press, 1983.

Whyte, L.: *The Unconscious Before Freud*. New York, Basic Books, 1960.

Wolpe, J.: *The Practice of Behavior Therapy*. New York, Pergamon Press, 1973.

# INDEX

Page numbers followed by 't' indicate tables; page numbers followed by 'n' indicate footnotes.

**393**